W9-CSN-683

Mental Health, Cultural Values, and Social Development

PRIORITY ISSUES IN MENTAL HEALTH

A book series published under the auspices of The World Federation for Mental Health

VOLUME 4

Mental Health, Cultural Values, and Social Development

A Look into the 80's

Edited by

RICHARD C. NANN, D.S.W.
The University of British Columbia

DORCAS SUSAN BUTT, Ph.D.
The University of British Columbia

and

LOURDES LADRIDO-IGNACIO, M.D.
University of the Philippines

Contributing Staff, WFHM

ROBERTA L. BEISER, M.Ed., *Executive Director*
MICHELLE BOURRÉE, *Administrative secretary*

D. REIDEL PUBLISHING COMPANY

A MEMBER OF THE KLUWER 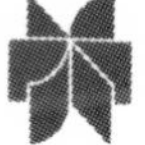 ACADEMIC PUBLISHERS GROUP

DORDRECHT / BOSTON / LANCASTER

Library of Congress Cataloging in Publication Data

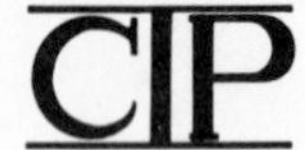

Main entry under title:

Mental health, cultural values, and social development.

(Priority issues in mental health ; v. 4)
Proceedings of the 1981 World Congress on Mental Health held in Manila, the Philippines, sponsored by the World Federation for Mental Health.
Includes index.
1. Mental health—Developing countries—Congresses. I. Nann, Richard C. II. Butt, Dorcas Susan. III. Ladrido-Ignacio, Lourdes. IV. World Congress on Mental Health (1981 : Manila, Philippines) V. World Federation for Mental Health. VI. Series. [DNLM: Mental health—Congresses. 2. Culture—Congresses. 3. Socioeconomic factors—Congresses. W1 PR524R v. 4 / WM 31 M549 1981]
RA790.7.D44M46 1983 362.2 83–13779
ISBN 90–277–1622–6

Published by D. Reidel Publishing Company,
P.O. Box 17, 3300 AA Dordrecht, Holland

Sold and distributed in the U.S.A. and Canada
by Kluwer Academic Publishers
190 Old Derby Street, Hingham, MA 02043, U.S.A.

In all other countries, sold and distributed
by Kluwer Academic Publishers Group,
P.O. Box 322, 3300 AH Dordrecht, Holland

Printed in The Netherlands

FOREWORD

It is not easy for a layman to attract attention to a book like this. Most who open the cover will be professionals in one of the many aspects of mental health. A moment's thought tells us, however, that if there is a distinction between laymen and professionals it makes no difference to a book like this. Both laymen and professionals care about what will be. That is why this book, the Congress it reports and the World Federation for Mental Health itself can be meaningful to both laymen and professional people. A look into the 80's from the point of view of mental health, cultural values and social development is for all who care about the future.

The 1981 Manila Congress of the World Federation for Mental Health was a unique and special gathering. It was the first time the Federation assembled for a Congress in a developing country. In the Philippines we enjoyed the overwhelming hospitality and charm of the people and a place where past and future seem as important as the present. All who attended from outside those magic islands will always remember the occasion as a special life experience. For those of you who did attend, this book can revive the stimulation and satisfaction of the Congress. For those of you who did not share the Manila experience, this book can inform and interest you about matters which are important.

To Chief Justice Roberto Concepcion, Judge Eduardo Tutaan, Mrs. Edita Martillano, Professor Charlotte Floro, Judge Oscar Inocentes, Judge Regina Ordonez-Benitez, Mrs. Flor Castelo, Professor Virginia Agbayani, Mrs. Juliet Luat, Dr. Romualdo Anselmo, Dr. Concordia Pascual, Justice Corazon Agrava, Attorney Rosalinda Sebastian-Lohla, Dr. Erlinda Lolarga, Director Gregorio Cendana, Commissioner Godofredo Asuncion, Dr. Artemio Cabrera, Attorney Salutario Fernandez, Mr. Leonides Valdez and all the others in charge of local arrangements, the World Federation for Mental Health will always be indebted. I know it is the sincere hope of all of us who came to you from abroad that somewhere, somehow we will be able to repay at least in part the kindness you showed to us.

To our own Organizing Committee members and particularly my predecessor in office Dr. Tsung-yi Lin, the Executive Director during my term Mrs. Roberta Beiser, Dr. Lourdes Ladrido-Ignacio and Dr. Morton Beiser, the Chairpersons of our Program Committee and to Drs. Nann, Butt and Ignacio as Co-Editors of these Proceedings, I owe a special debt of gratitude. I want to express the appreciation of all who benefitted from the Congress they planned, produced and epilogued.

I cannot conclude without thanking the President of the Philippines and Mrs. Marcos for their sponsorship of our Congress. The First Lady entertained us with

Richard C. Nann, Dorcas Susan Butt, and Lourdes Ladrido-Ignacio (eds.), Mental Health, Cultural Values and Social Development, v–vi.

warmth. The President in his keynote address reminded us that mental health is often a product of social, cultural and economic conditions. To both of them I express my personal appreciation.

When you read this book and consider the ideas in it, whether for the first time or as a reminder of your thoughts in Manila, remember there is much evidence today to confirm the feeling many of us had in Manila that we are living in a time when the world is changing faster and the future is less clear than at any time since our Federation was founded in 1949.

When the future is unclear it is a time of unusual opportunity. It is more relevant at such a time to build than tear down. It is more important to create than to regret or resent. I hope you will feel when you read these proceedings that the future was indeed the focus of the Manila meeting. I hope you will be inspired to join with others in the World Federation for Mental Health to make the future a priority for mental health as they look into the eighties.

Vancouver, B.C.

GOWAN T. GUEST
President, 1979–1981
World Federation for Mental Health

TABLE OF CONTENTS

SECTION TWO

WORKSHOPS REPORTS

PREFACE

This volume presents the proceedings of the 1981 World Congress on Mental Health which met in Manila, The Philippines, during the latter part of July and early August. The general theme of this conference was a call for world cooperation to seek ways of resolving social and personal conflicts which endanger the mental health of the peoples of the world. From the gathered representatives of both developed and developing countries alike, the call was for a respect of moral, ethical and cultural values in the common struggle for physical, psychological and economic security.

Concerns for the health and stability of the individual and his or her society in today's world were heightened by such observations as the following, heard in a workshop addressing the problems of children in stress:

> The coping strategies that are required if a child is to survive in today's world would seem to veer toward adults who are self-centred, socially isolated, detached and individualistic . . . although competent and efficient.

If human survival is to mean something other than a self-centred, isolated and detached existence, then new enlightened policies and action are obviously required. Such was the challenge confronting this conference.

The 1981 World Congress involved participants from 31 nations. They comprised lay contributors, government leaders, mental health workers and professionals, academics and social scientists of various disciplines and professions. The conference had welcome input and direction from the mental health workers of the host country, The Philippines, a nation which is experiencing rapid social and economic change with all of its concomitant pressures and conflicts. As noted by both President and Mrs. Marcos in their welcome remarks, the dilemmas encountered by many developing nations are experienced today in the Philippines. A central problem is how to modernize without succumbing to the insular materialism of the West. The traditional values of family and community are deeply ingrained in the psychology of the people and yet they must increasingly respond to economic necessities through technological development.

During the course of this conference, a variety of issues were examined in plenary sessions, lectures, workshops, and symposia relating to problems and dilemmas which threaten mental health. These are described in the pages which follow. We think the underlying themes generated by the conference participants cannot be overly emphasized. The major one is clear. It stands out in all of the papers in this volume. *Can the people of this planet move through the 1980's without losing their spirituality, their humanity, and their feelings of community*

Richard C. Nann, Dorcas Susan Butt, and Lourdes Ladrido-Ignacio (eds.), Mental Health, Cultural Values and Social Development, xi–xiii.

with other human beings? The world is in a state of flux. There is much need for intelligent and passionate advocacy and action if we care about the outcome.

Not all of the facts and evidence presented, sifted, and analyzed during the 1981 World Congress are of a negative nature. Indeed, a number of significantly positive elements in the world scene are cited. The conference heard accounts of effective social planning and cooperative effort. Particularly impressive are some developments in the country of Japan. Although not without significant psychological and social problems amongst its population, the Japanese are planning far into the future for events that other nations have not as yet prepared for. Two such examples are the Japanese representatives at this conference providing leadership in the areas of leisure planning, and life planning for the aged.

A conference, if successful, should generate direction and guidelines for future courses of action. Problems have been identified, and solutions offered, or at least possible avenues to travel in seeking solutions. We consider it of great importance that others hear these themes.

In 1962, Gerald Sykes wrote a book called *The Hidden Remnant*. This title referred to a small minority of scholars who concerned themselves with seeking knowledge of the human psyche. The author cited scholars with humanistic concerns as those few pioneers keeping alive interest in the subjective side of human nature which provides, in his view, the potential for infinite development. In a sense, we have an "expanding remnant" at this conference in people willing and able to explore social, cultural and psychological processes. It is our sincere concern that the results of their deliberations do not remain hidden.

With the great diversity of persons, nations and interests represented at the 1981 World Congress and in the pages of these proceedings, and with the strong forces that back this type of examination throughout the world today, we think we can be confident in the strength and commitment to mental health and to what has now become the *social health movement*. A woman formerly associated with out Federation, the late Barbara Ward Jackson, stated in 1972:

> To act without rapacity, to use knowledge and wisdom, to respect independence, to operate without hubris and greed are not simply moral imperatives. *They are an accurate scientific description of the means of survival.*

With its focus on the theme of *cultural values, social development and social health*, the 1981 World Congress is a step toward the goal of survival with the greatest amount of health and happiness.

The editors have found it a privilege to organize this volume of proceedings. Except for minor deletions and editing, few changes have been made to the original papers and presentations. These changes are for the purpose of obtaining consistency and smoothness of text. The volume is separated into three sections. The first section presents papers and commentaries given in plenary sessions. The second comprises summaries of workshops and small group discussions. Section Three presents the proceedings from a special Pre-Congress International Seminar on the topic, "The Disabled and Mental Health". This pre-congress feature was scheduled in observance of the International Year of Disabled Persons, and was sponsored by the following four organizations: The Philippine Foundation of Disabled, Inc., Rehabilitation International, The Philippine Mental Health Association, and the World Federation for Mental Health.

This volume is the result of the work and contributions of many people throughout the world, including those who organized the 1981 World Congress, as well as those who coordinated, facilitated, attended, and presented papers. A number of formal papers were presented in the Workshops, but limitations of space do not permit their inclusion in this volume. Copies of these papers, however, may be available through the World Federation for Mental Health Secretariat Office at #107 – 2352 Health Sciences Mall, University of British Columbia, Vancouver, British Columbia, Canada V6T 1W5.

We wish to acknowledge our appreciation to Mrs. Edita Martillano, and all of her staff and volunteers who so ably assisted in compiling the original workshop reports for these proceedings. We wish to express special acknowledgement and thanks to Susan Johnston for her editorial assistance, and to Roberta Beiser, Executive Director of the World Federation for Mental Health, and to Michelle Bourrée in the Secretariat Office, for their great assistance in helping us to compile these proceedings.

RICHARD C. NANN
School of Social Work
D. SUSAN BUTT
Department of Psychology,
University of British Columbia,
Vancouver, Canada

LOURDES LADRIDO-IGNACIO
Department of Psychiatry,
University of the Philippines,
Manila, The Philippines

FERDINAND E. MARCOS, President of the Philippines

WELCOME REMARKS

On behalf of the people and government of the Philippines, I welcome you all to Manila and tender you our very best wishes for a most fruitful Congress.

You have travelled great distances to come for this 1981 World Congress on Mental Health, and we are fully conscious of the honour that you bestow upon our country in holding this Congress here in Manila. To the World Federation for Mental Health, which has joined the Philippine Mental Health Association (PMHA) in the sponsorship of this Congress, I wish to express our heartfelt appreciation. To the PMHA, its officers and its members, I extend my sincere congratulations for ensuring adequate preparations for this conference. Your conference, ladies and gentlemen, addresses an issue that has long been a deep and abiding concern of all our societies, but it is also paradoxically an issue that has not always invited wide public attention, or enough global concern. This is partly because mental health as a social concern embodies also its opposite – the miseries and the plight of those who do not enjoy it, and indeed if the truth be told, it is in the effort to reach out to these benighted souls in human society that we customarily measure the worth and the compassion and the effectiveness of our programs for mental health.

The century in which we live has blessed the greater part of mankind with much fuller and longer lives. It has produced unparalleled comfort for many, especially those living in our more advanced societies. Yet this century of unparalleled progress has not provided fulfillment for all. We shall not remark here upon the searing issues of mass poverty and inequalities in the world today, but shall merely observe that this spectacle of contemporary deprivation is nowhere more clearly underlined than in the field of mental health. And I can think of no other social issue that touches so deeply the conscience of mankind than the states of care for the mentally ill. The awakening of conscience, and the effort to deal in a more practical and humane way with the problem of mental health, are to my mind one of the more salutary developments in recent decades of human history. When in 1946, the World Health Organization was formed, and it was stated in its constitution that "health is a state of complete physical, mental and social well-being, and not merely the absence of disease or infirmity", the family of man articulated for the first time its collective desire to move more decisively into the realm of mental health care. Hitherto, efforts were isolated and random, largely inspired and led by a few individuals of great compassion and vision, and by a few societies that were advanced in their humanitarian concern for the mentally ill.

From this landmark event, there emerged a fairly worldwide effort to pay greater attention to mental health care. In 1948, the World Federation for

Richard C. Nann, Dorcas Susan Butt, and Lourdes Ladrido-Ignacio (eds.), Mental Health, Cultural Values and Social Development, xv–xx.

Mental Health was formed. Under the impact of these developments, the pioneering activities of earlier years – at civic, national and international levels – began to be focused more on the linkage of researches and action programs. And what we know today of the problems of mental health and the ways of coping with them in a more decisive way are largely the produce of developments during the last three and a half decades of the 20th century. One cannot say enough about the work of the World Federation for Mental Health, and of the efforts of the various national organizations that constitute its membership. And it is all the more remarkable because this work has had to be undertaken in the face of very real public fear of and revulsion to the issue, which since time immemorial has characterized the instinctive response of human beings to mental disturbance among their brethren.

At this time the world is more aware than ever of the wider compass of mental health concerns: of how they touch a society's aspiration to development and progress, of how they relate to population pressures and social unrest, of how modern civilization impinges upon the mental well-being of people, and of how problems can be better managed for the rehabilitation and care of the mentally ill and the prevention of mental disorder in social life. Yours then is a task of advancing yet further what has been so impressively pushed forward by pioneers. Yours is the task of creating new initiatives for more beneficial change in the realm of mental health care. In our diverse and multiple world, there is wide disparity in the problems we face in this area, and consequently variations in the kind of responses that will avail. In our respective societies, there are variations of causes that underlie mental disorders, owing to different social pressures and experiences. But while we acknowledge this, and must be conscious of it, our solutions nonetheless spring from a common fount of knowledge and from the spirit of exchange among nations and medical communities. This is the value of a Congress of this nature: that in our great diversity as nations and societies, our common humanity links our experiences, our problems and our aspirations together. Speaking for the Philippines, we need all the help we can get. This is the reason why we are deeply gratified by your decision to hold this conference in our country. Our delegates have been encouraged to learn as much as possible from the discussions on mental health during this meeting. From their observations and the counsels of the world experts on this matter, as well as from the findings of our government's own researches we hope to be able to adopt a far more effective program on mental health.

Instinctually, we feel that the incidence of mental instability in our country is linked to and is partly a consequence of the process of modernization. Even as it affords a broader range of opportunities for material advancement, modernization also demands readjustment, sometimes radical, of previously established norms, attitudes and customs, Social relationships that thrived in more traditional milieu have been breaking down. We have found, for instance, that even the most fundamental unit of society, the family – which once was held in nearly reverent regard in our society, as in most Asian cultures – has lately been undergoing significant decline. In turn, values that once were not important or even alien to the sensibilities of our people have become, by material necessity, ascendant. Competitiveness, for example, was not a value that could be equated with traditional Filipino culture. But with the advent of new methods of work and the widening sprawl of urbanization, competitiveness has not only become acceptable but also desirable as a means to attaining yet another ideal, a prosperous lifestyle premised on the amenities and comforts that generally are perceived to accompany modernity.

Modernization has brought along with it glimpses of a culture that the foreign and local mass media have conditioned our people to aspire for and covet. Against a backdrop of underdevelopment it is practically impossible to create much less make accessible to every citizen all these desirable objects, which in the first place may not entirely be suitable to our requirements. The fact is that our people's expectations have been raised to such an extent and such a level that many of them tend to believe that they too have a right to the amenities of advanced societies. When they are finally made to realize that this is just not possible, mass frustration results. In more concrete terms, this frustration is manifested in a number of aberrant behavioural modes including crime, cultural and political rebellion, and dementia.

I must stress that these are mere theories that have yet to pass the test of empirical verification. However, I feel it would not be wrong to say that a nation's state of mental health is a product of existing social, cultural and economic conditions. In the individual this can be extended to mean that his capacity to remain sane and productively functional depends on the basic material security that he enjoys; that a society which cannot fulfill very basic needs and which does not instill a sense of purpose to their individual lives within the social and national framework could never expect any lasting relief from mental disorders.

In a setting like ours therefore, the mental health issue is inextricably linked to the so-called more fundamental issues. In a developing country, mental aberration can be and is a debilitating factor for further growth. We are at a critical point in our nation's development where every citizen must do his/her share and perform to the fullest his/her role in the collective task of fashioning a better quality of life for our people. We cannot afford the luxuries of other more advanced societies; we cannot allow to persist for long those factors that prevent us from harnessing the full potential of our human resources. The attainment of a reasonable level of mental health must not be viewed from a purely medical or psychological viewpoint. Mental health is a national concern that calls for nationally supported undertakings.

Lest I be misunderstood I must make clear that our quest for development is not a myopic obsession with mere material progress. Our concept of social growth envelops both material and spiritual advancement. We look around the world today and we see many advanced nations entrapped in a battle to recover their spiritual heritage. We see nations that have developed the technology to feed, clothe and shelter their citizens, nations that have begun exploring outer space, apparently caught in cyclical waves of crime, senseless violence, and other forms of anti-social behaviour. Our lateness in the ascent to modernization ought at least to spare us from these problems. We have been going to great lengths to ensure that progress for us does not result in the same problems that currently bedevil the advanced societies. With the benefit of hindsight we should perhaps be better able to plot out the course that we must take.

If I draw here a parallel between the struggle of mankind to cope with the problems of mental health and the struggle of developing societies like ours to achieve development, I do not mean merely that the two are intimately related. That is fact. I mean also to commend, and with this I will conclude, the principle which your Federation has always espoused, that we must do our very best in our efforts to promote mental health insofar as circumstances are alterable. That can also be said of the struggle for development. It is never easy to pursue ideals and visions in the development of human beings and human societies, but we must ever apply ourselves to the effort of making change.

Thank you and good day.

IMELDA ROMUALDEZ MARCOS, First Lady; Governor, Metro Manila; Minister, Ministry of Human Settlements; Chairperson, Executive Committee, 1981 World Congress on Mental Health

THE NEED FOR SANITY

It is with pride and joy that we welcome you, the delegates to the 1981 World Congress on Mental Health, to the Capital City of our new republic, Metro Manila, our City of Man. In the past few decades, mental health has become a great problem in a rapidly changing world, most particularly in the developed societies. We in the third world of developing countries are also beset with many complex problems which have far-reaching consequences for mental health. Poverty often breeds ignorance and disease, malnutrition and deterioration. But for our spirituality, we would have had in Asia, Africa and Latin America much mental illness.

Problems of mental health are different among the first, second and third worlds. But there is common ground of anxiety over the prospects of the human race in an environment torn by enmity and strife. There appears to be a neurosis among nations which cry for peace and arm themselves for war. While there is a general recognition of the necessity for a changed international economic order, there is a persistent effort to retain the old relationship of exploiter and exploited. Philosophers have pointed out that mankind because of his horrifying weapons of destruction, is under sentence of death. The sensitive mind and the delicate heart which perceive these conflicts must necessarily be disturbed.

Where do we begin? With the symptoms of disease or with its roots? In the Philippines, we begin with the family, the first and fundamental environment of the child. It is said that the Filipino parent loves the child not wisely but too well. This could well be our strength and our weakness, but we see around us that the world is not suffering from too much love, rather from too little. Love has become the victim of modernization without soul, or development for its own sake. Materialism has made impersonal relationships a norm. Development has been an iron-and-steel process ignoring, as it were, the promptings of the human heart. It is the attitude of progress, the soul-less technical pursuit of material improvement, which brings about an unhealthy mental atmosphere for mankind. The only way out, it seems is to place the human being at the centre of development, and to restrain him/her from gaining the whole world at the cost of his/her own soul or feelings.

You have set before you difficult tasks, as your 35 workshops covering different sectors, fields or studies, priorities and strategies, attest. We all hope that programs can be agreed upon and vigorously implemented. Perhaps we may consider the human being as the centre of our concern. Be it in development or progress, the development of the human being entails three levels: body, mind and spirit or feelings. As we have done here in the Philippines, in the Ministry of Human Settlements of which I am privileged to be Minister, we approach the problem from the perspective of human settlements, the bigger family, by providing the person in his/her family and community, the eleven basic needs – water, power, food, shelter, clothing, health, education, livelihood or economic base, sports and recreation, ecological balance and mobility. This leads to the new republic's national program of livelihood for every Filipino based on self-reliance nationally known as "Kilusang Pang Kabuhayan".

Beyond this, what is our program for the elite – for the few men and women in the social hierarchy of the world? These are the makers of far-reaching political decisions, the makers of histories, the manufacturers of engines and weapons of destruction, the manipulators of markets. These are the few, whether in democratic or non-democratic societies, who daily make the decisions which can save or destroy our planet. In sum, what about their mental health?

It is perhaps too idealistic to expect a world leadership which concerns itself not with power, but with service; not with competitive goals but with co-operative goals; not with conquest, but with love and compassion. But surely, they can perceive the peril of humankind. We can expect them to dispel the peril with action suitable to the perception. If there ever was a need for sanity in the world, it is now. That realization can lead to a global change of heart.

The poet W. H. Auden reminded us: "We must love one another or die." He did not mean mere physical death, but the death of our consciousness, our capacity to love and the abysmal end of all that is noble, beautiful and human in us. This is the most dismal of all tragedies.

The human race has not been created to live on this earth in mere material comfort; rich but not enrich, existing but not alive. The human mind is a gift of creation. No one has the right to debase it. Our commitment therefore is to the right of the mind, to be what God has intended it to be. On this note, let us all begin our task.

Again, welcome, good-day and mabuhay!

Dr. HIROSHI NAKAJIMA, WHO Regional Director, Western Pacific Region

GREETINGS FROM WHO

It gives me great pleasure to address this World Congress on Mental Health, organized by the World Federation for Mental Health and the Philippine Mental Health Association.

Allow me, first of all to extend the greetings of the World Health Organization to all participants attending this Congress in Manila.

The World Federation for Mental Health has a distinguished record and, under the able guidance of its Executive Board, has made a significant contribution to the progress of mental health in the world.

The Philippine Mental Health Association, as one of the most influential agencies in this field has done much to promote mental health activities in the Philippines under the kind patronage of the Government of the Philippines.

Mental health care is a subject of great concern to WHO and activities in this area have gained momentum in the past few years in the Western Pacific Region.

In 1977, the World Health Assembly decided that the main health target of governments and of WHO should be the attainment by all the peoples of the world by the year 2000 of a level of health that would permit them to lead a socially and economically productive life. This is popularly referred to as "Health for all by the year 2000".

In 1978, an International Conference on Primary Health Care, held in Alma-Ata, declared primary health care to be the key to attaining this goal.

The strategy for attaining health for all relies heavily on the development of the health system infrastructure, starting with primary health care for the delivery of countrywide programs that will reach the entire population.

These programs include measures for health promotion, disease prevention, diagnosis, therapy and rehabilitation. The strategy for mental health must also be formulated in the light of health for all by the year 2000.

At the present time, some 40 million people in the world are said to be suffering from severe mental illness and at least twice as many again are seriously disabled by drug dependence, alcohol-related problems, mental retardation and organic disorders of the nervous system leading to psychiatric and neurological conditions.

The estimated number of less serious but nonetheless incapacitating mental disorders varies but no less than 2000 million people are believed to be involved.

In many countries mental disorder is the main cause of disablement in two out of five disabled persons. In economically developed countries, every third hospital bed is occupied by a psychiatric patient and there is every reason to believe that the already high prevalence of mental disorders will grow over the next few decades.

Richard C. Nann, Dorcas Susan Butt, and Lourdes Ladrido-Ignacio (eds.), Mental Health, Cultural Values and Social Development, xxi–xxii.

For all these reasons, mental health care has become a subject of great concern to the World Health Organization, which has elaborated a mental health program.

The objectives of the mental health program are, first, to prevent or alleviate psychiatric neurological and psychosocial problems, including those related to alcohol and drug dependences; second, to increase the effectiveness of the general health services through appropriate utilization of mental health skills and knowledge; and third, to develop strategies for intervention based on an increased awareness of the mental health aspects of social action and change.

Particularly in many of the developing countries of the Western Pacific Region, mental health services have so far been insufficient and too sparsely developed.

Even in developed countries, the public mental health services which are in operation tend to be institutionalized. In many countries in this Region, mental hospitals are overcrowded, and understaffed, and rely predominantly or exclusively on custodial care and basic pharmacotherapy, while staff intensive and budget demanding activities such as activation and rehabilitation are insufficient or lacking.

There is now an urgent need to promote mental health, including the prevention of mental diseases, alcoholism and drug abuse, through psychosocial research, dissemination of information and development of low-cost strategies within the community and in the general health services.

I believe that an international congress such as this provides the opportunity for an invaluable exchange of information and ideas, as well as promoting discussions on future activities.

I would like to express to all members of the Executive Board my sincere appreciation of their initiative in organizing this very important Congress and to extend to all participants my best wishes for a highly stimulating and rewarding meeting.

SECTION ONE

PLENARY PAPERS

INTRODUCTION

Examinations of, and reflections on, social and cultural values provide the building blocks for the contents of this volume. Throughout the papers which follow, there is the theme that the mental health of the individual cannot be separated from the social health of the system in which a person is destined to live and to die. Thus, the issues examined by the speakers and discussants involve conflicts at both the societal and individual levels that are generated by economic and physical privation, uprooting and migration, family breakup, industrialization, urbanization and rapid social change. As so many of the papers in this volume profess, the rapid development in the world today is not serving the world population well. Are we correct in the assumption that people now face more human generated stress than in past decades? There has always been mental illness, but it seems this is increasingly a social problem and not confined to the traditional (medically defined) 3% of the population. Some of the figures and projections are alarming. For example, there is the WHO study cited in the opening plenary paper which reports that some 25–30% of the population in impoverished urban areas suffer from psychological disorders.

Understandably, there are compelling reasons to devote attention and help to those who display such disarray. But, effective intervention requires that attention must also be given to the social systems that generate such disarray. In light of the magnitude of the problems, we may well ask – what is the price of the accumulated conflicts; and do such difficult events in the lives of significant numbers of people produce any motivation for world leaders to find better alternatives?

And, what is the role of the mental health field? Social development implies social actions. Are mental health workers able to have any significant impact on major national or world events? In his opening paper, Dr. Stein, a senior policy advisor to UNICEF, proposes several potential points of intervention. In the same positive vein, Dr. Miller, the Discussant, expresses the need for the passionate advocacy of the mental health worker on behalf of people who need and deserve care in a competent health care system.

MENTAL HEALTH AND SOCIAL DEVELOPMENT – POSITIVE CONCEPTS

The general theme of the 1981 World Congress connotes a set of affirmative and positive paradigms. In identifying various levels of environments which affect the human condition, Dr. Pierce views mental health, social development and cultural values as terms relating to the same issue; that is, positive mental health

Richard C. Nann, Dorcas Susan Butt, and Lourdes Ladrido-Ignacio (eds.), Mental Health, Cultural Values and Social Development, 3–5.

is shown by those who attend to the social development of their society while at the same time providing an example of their culture's mentally healthy person. Social development, then, is the practice of positive mental health. A similar message is found in the paper by Dr. Abdel-Al, who reminds us that we do not live in an environment but rather, are part of an environment, and that this fundamental fact must be taken into account in considering both the goals and the processes of social development. Speaking to the ideas presented by these two speakers, Dr. Beiser suggests that an essential need is the development of a vocabulary dealing with health rather than illness. Many persons survive major change without psychological distress and we should, therefore, be giving more study to their strengths and adaptation patterns if we are to learn how mental illness can be prevented and positive mental health promoted.

CULTURAL VALUES AND VALUE CONFLICTS

One of the main messages coming out of the 1981 World Congress is a need for merging the social and cultural needs of people with developmental interests. This view is heard from the representatives of various regions of the world. It comes, for example, from Dr. Binitie of Nigeria who speaks of the African's need to reconcile conflicts between indigenous cultural values and a super-imposed alien culture brought by colonial powers; it comes from the representative of youth at the conference, Ms. Amor of the Philippines, who speaks emphatically for the preservation of family and traditional morality in the face of industrial development; and it comes as well from Dr. James of New Zealand, who speaks of the need for social planning and the making of legislation and policies which are informed by, and reflective of, sound mental health principles.

MENTAL HEALTH AND DEVELOPED COUNTRIES

The developed world has much to learn from the developing. In many ways, the privileged, who are often the isolated, may rediscover the potentials of humanity and community from those in developing countries. A cross-cultural examination of the healing arts provides an example wherein the impoverishment and the limitations of certain modern treatment technologies stand in contrast to healing practices and orientations of the traditional world which feature a much broader underlying model of the human. This message is highlighted in the plenary paper on mental health and culture by Dr. León and in the accompanying commentary by Dr. Spiegel.

Thus, it is not only the developing countries of the world that are pressed for change and development. Those living in highly industrialized societies are also under pressure, and the mental health concerns of the economically successful comprised important items on the conference agenda. These included: the paper by Dr. Cooper which analyzes the economics of health and mental health care in relation to such variables as life expectancy in countries of the western world;

the paper by Dr. Watanabe, which posits some rather unconventional views of the rights (or non-rights) of the mentally ill as an example of the problem of social and legal priorities in modern society; and the response to these two papers by Mr. Okura.

MENTAL HEALTH AND THE DEVELOPING COUNTRIES

This issues of conflict and change are experienced by both the affluent as well as the poor. But the latter, understandably, will press more and more significantly for a fairer distribution and use of resources, for a just political and economic leadership, and for commitment to community, identification and self assertion. Their task, however, will not be an easy one. In the memorial lecture in honour of the late Dr. Margaret Mead, Dr. Tsung-Yi Lin gives stark evidence of the problems and difficulties of Third World nations where developmental efforts based on western models have not significantly turned around mass poverty and inequality. An earlier sense of optimism and faith in the universality of Western technology and methods has given way to the recognition that a developing country must formulate approaches that are more consonant with its own wants, needs and resources – in short, its own culture. Dr. Lin's assessment suggests that the future of the delivery of mental health services in the Third World depends largely on how well mental health care can be integrated into primary health care delivery.

RELIGION AND MENTAL HEALTH

Religion is both an important source and expression of cultural values. In the Mary Hemingway Rees Memorial Lecture, Dr. Mansell Pattison observes that the relevance of religion to mental health has been generally neglected in western culture because of a separation of the two areas that reflects a process of western secularization. There is, however, a renewed interest today in religious cosmology, and this paper sets forth an analysis of the influence of religion on human behaviour in terms of general culture, social network, family and individual. Dr. Pattison discusses the relationship of religious philosophy and psychiatric thought, and produces a set of fundamental questions about religious assumptions and their effects upon mental health delivery systems in a specific culture.

HERMAN D. STEIN D.S.W. (U.S.A.)

THE WORLD IN CRISIS: MENTAL HEALTH IMPLICATIONS

ELEMENTS OF CRISIS

Is the world in crisis? An educator recently said: "Living in the late twentieth century is a hazardous adventure. Ours is not the only generation ever to have sensed that we live on the edge of doom, but we surely have more hard evidence than ever before to prove it" (Posvar, 1980).

That is so, and the evidence continues to mount, and it is as if a doomsday clock keeps ticking. It is not difficult to identify with those of old who conjured up dread apocalyptic visions – wars, famine, persecution, earthquakes – of cosmic proportions, some timed to go off in explosions with terrifying impact, and some – like the long-lasting pills glorified on American television – erupting quietly and steadily with cumulative and eventually devastating effect. Moreover, to contribute to the sense of crisis, the processes and institutions of our separate societies, let alone our world society, appear too weak and too irresolute to prevent, control or repair disasters created by man or natural disasters, some to which man is directly contributing.

What is the evidence that we may be living on the edge of doom? I will not recite the entire litany. Just a few reminders in case anyone's defenses have succeeded in blocking them out. Let us take war. From 1945 to 1976 there have been 120 armed conflicts involving governments, 5 in Europe and 115 in the Third World (Galtung, 1981). The rate is not declining, and the unspeakable nightmare of nuclear devastation – beyond even the horrors dreamt of in the Books of the Apocalypse – grows closer to reality. It is even becoming speakable, in the quaint technocratic jargon of national "tolerance levels", for millions to be killed.

At the beginning of 1981, some 12.5 million people were refugees from their homelands, or displaced from their homes within their own countries. In Africa, amid political turmoil and drought, the number of refugees and displaced persons jumped from 4 to 6.3 million.

Africa has in a sense replaced the Indian subcontinent as the focus of world famine. So far this year, the whole of Africa has secured about half of what it needs to import for food. Food-stocks worldwide have fallen critically and the nations of the world failed to implement decisions made at the 1974 World Food Conference to set up a system of grain reserves to act as a buffer against famine.

Writing in *The Lancet* early this year, one writer states: "It is estimated that in the present East African crisis hundreds of thousands died; over 90 million suffered abnormal hunger; 14 million contracted serious diseases; at least 40

Richard C. Nann, Dorcas Susan Butt, and Lourdes Ladrido-Ignacio (eds.), Mental Health, Cultural Values and Social Development, 7–16.

villages were wiped out; and the area is ripe for another famine". Elsewhere he comments: "Until we can somehow transcend the data and penetrate the human anguish, we can never understand the global insanity that will soon become impossible to ignore" (Meegan, 1981).

In the report of UNICEF's Executive Director on the Situation of the World's Children in 1980/81, the first sentence notes that of the 122 million children born during the International Year of the Child, 1979, one in ten is now dead and almost all of those 12 million children died in conditions of hunger, disease and poverty. Out of a total of 4.4 billion in the world population, 780 million are estimated to be in absolute poverty in the developing countries of the world, with their children dying by the millions, filling up scores of tables in hundreds of reference books, but each unit a child dying one at a time. No sudden explosion, no blaring headlines for world attention.

Two social scientists have established what they call "Hiroshima equivalents" (Galtung, 1981). They refer to "the difference between the actual number of deaths and the hypothetical number"; that is, the excess deaths in given countries equivalent to the total of those who died when the atom bomb was dropped on Hiroshima and Nagasaki, to what might have been expected had the same death rate existed that now exists in the United States. "Excess mortality" of children one to five years old alone in 1978 would correspond to 236 Hiroshima equivalents. These are among the children of the Third World who would have lived, had they been born in the richer countries.

In the past five or six years, since the mid-1970s, the world economy has suffered. In the industrialized countries, the rate of economic growth was 4% from 1950 to 1975. By the end of the 1970s, an annual growth rate of 2% was common. In developing countries the per capita gross domestic product, which had been increasing at a 3% yearly rate during 1950 to 1975, was generally sharply reduced in the late 1970s. The world as a whole is experiencing an economic downturn that shows no signs of abating. The consequences in unemployment, grave hardship, and social unrest, need no detailing.

I doubt that I need go on to recite the evidence of crisis, and the world in mounting danger – the population projections, the menacing disease rates, environmental destruction, the threat of nuclear cataclysm, the East-West and North-South conflicts and the growing disparity between rich and poor within countries and among countries.

IMPLICATIONS FOR MENTAL HEALTH

What then are the mental health implications of a world situation – even if one chooses not to call it crisis – composed of malignant elements of this order of magnitude? I will reflect on these, not to presume to give final answers, but to help launch the Congress theme.

Let me begin by venturing the premise that the mental health professions by themselves are not going to have any vital impact on issues of war and peace, on the direction of world trade and economy, on military expenditure, on nuclear proliferation, or directly on any of the overpowering global factors contributing to crisis.

This is not to say that individual movers and shakers in the world would not benefit from some professional therapeutic attention, and so possibly benefit the rest of us, or that mental health practitioners in their citizen roles might not join movements or political parties that could have a bearing on the shape of world events. But it is difficult to see the mental health professionals, or the mental health movement, if you will, having a direct bearing on the macro systems of the world, or indeed on power conflicts within individual nations.

Does this mean that the mental health professions have little to contribute? Not at all. There are direct and important contributions to be made – far more, I believe, than have been made to date – to the mitigation of distress related to these elements of crisis and to constructive social development. These contributions are not at the level of international politics and power relationships, nor at the level of direct treatment services, at least in the developing countries, but at middle levels, affecting policies, institutions and social processes involving masses of people.

First, let us clear away some underbrush by identifying a number of propositions amply discussed and documented in several publications, notably the issue of the *International Journal of Mental Health* devoted to the International Year of the Child, and the essays published from the Vancouver Mental Health Congress. These propositions are the following:

(1) The incidence of severe mental and emotional problems is variously estimated as 2.3% for those with severe disorders and over 10% for less severe disorders throughout the world. (However, a WHO study in developing countries of children attending general health centres showed 13 to 18% in rural areas, and 25 to 30% in urban slum areas suffering from psychological disorders.) WHO estimated that a total of 40 million people have a functional psychiatric disturbance and another 40 million are mentally retarded.

(2) There is a severe shortage of mental health professionals in the Third World. There is also an almost complete absence of epidemiological and prevalence data; on disability prevention surrounding birth, and on normative data on child psycho-social development (WHO, 1980).

(3) Mental health programs are given very low priority, particularly in the developing countries. This is not surprising when the health budgets of developing nations amount to 1% per head of what is spent in the industrialized world and rarely exceeds $5 per capita per year in Africa and Asia, including private spending (Grant, 1981).

(4) In the developing world, 80% of the people who receive medical attention do not receive it from a doctor, but more likely a nurse or paraprofessional. Doctors, including psychiatrists, have not generally been engaged in selecting auxiliary health workers and training them, and doctors will not likely be administering general health care (Sondhi, 1978).

My thesis for the essential contribution of mental health to help stave off the forces of darkness and death is not primarily to produce more professional therapeutic personnel, important as they are, but to penetrate relevant social systems and develop social policies and practical methods mainly for preventive, but also for diagnostic and treatment purposes.

In the developing world, the principal system to be affected, but not the only one, is that of primary health care, as promulgated by the WHO/UNICEF Conference in Alma Ata. Mr. Sartorius, who is present, and WHO/UNICEF publications, can best interpret how mental health concepts can be incorporated. For now, suffice it to say that the primary health care approach relies on villages and communities developing their own paraprofessional health competencies, backed by a framework of government resources for referral, training and supplies. In this approach, prevention is foremost through health education and sanitation, and there is no choice but to be as economical as possible, and as unprovincial and cross-sectoral as possible in the perspective on what contributes to well-being generally as well as health services specifically; with attention to food production and nutrition, availability of potable water, environmental sanitation, and at least basic education.

A comment may be in order about China, in this connection, since I have been asked about my recent visits, but I hesitate to speak with any authority. The rural barefoot doctor system in China, backed by resources at commune and county level, and the analogous array of health centres in industrial enterprises and neighbourhoods in the urban areas, has yielded very impressive results, which have been widely heralded. Maternal, neonatal, infant and child mortality have been sharply reduced, with health services seen as part of a broader array of social provisions. I must confess, however, that I am still not well enough informed on mental health conditions among the children because, in the rural areas I visited, mental health disorders affecting children were not seen as problems affecting more than the rare child, with the exception of occasional mental retardation. With adequate nutrition, clean water and general environmental sanitation, regular health examinations, and quick treatment of mother and child, and every child assumed to be a "wanted child" – particularly in the light of the campaign for the one-child-family – a great deal of pathology arising from gross malnutrition of expectant mother and child, and of fetal abnormalities, has without doubt simply been prevented. In certain of the large urban areas, facilities exist for psychiatric diagnosis and treatment of children and adults, and barefoot doctors in surrounding rural areas, and their equivalents in urban areas, are given training in recognizing possible pathology in order to make referrals and to provide care after return of patients to the community. Mental health problems, however, apparently remain at the periphery of China's mass health concerns; diagnostic prevalence studies exist only sporadically, and one can hardly say that China's mental health problems have been broadly assessed, let alone solved.

Elsewhere in the developing world, the prevalence of mental health problems has occasionally been quantified, almost always with the observation that they are related to conditions of abject poverty, hunger and disease. I am not sure, however, what good it does to categorize apathy, reduced responsiveness, and irritability of children suffering from marasmus and kwashiorkor, as mental health problems, any more than to refer to the somatic pathologies these poverty-stricken, starving children are prone to as disease problems, or to their malnutrition as problems of food production and storage, or of nutritional ignorance. All of these conditions are related. Most of the problems are preventable only through multi-sectoral approaches at local community level, what UNICEF refers to as a Basic Services Approach.

The availability of health workers in each community, even with only an initial modicum of training, can bring untold dividends. Since this is the International Year of Disabled Persons, permit me to quote one statistic. In the field of blindness, 250,000 children a year lost their eyesight for lack of Vitamin A. The cost of providing Vitamin A to those who need it is five cents (U.S.) a year – provided there is a health worker in the community (Grant, 1981). Similar levels of cost effectiveness should be aimed for in the mental health field, and a number of such efforts are in progress, for example in Colombia. With respect to mental health services as part of primary health care, Zaki Hasan makes the point that the very fact that such services have only started to emerge in the developing countries makes it easier to orient and adapt them to a primary health care approach. He noted that a major impact can be made on many forms of mental disorders – mental retardation, sensory impairment, epilepsy, psychosomatic illnesses – not through separating them under mental health labels but through joining with efforts to mobilize community resources to improve nutrition, promote immunization and better sanitary conditions, and expand maternal and child care services (Hasan, 1947/48).

This is, I believe, the fundamental approach to take, for in the developing world the priority is not more mental health specialists, needed as they are, but the incorporation of essential and elementary concepts of prevention, diagnosis, care and rehabilitation within primary health care programs, as part of overall essential services that are community-based. Unless the total environment is one that provides at least minimal conditions for physical growth and development, under conditions of some dignity, mental health specialists can do little but despairingly identify and count the wreckage.

There are other systems that the mental health field can and, to a very limited extent, has penetrated, both in developing and industrialized countries. One is primary education. Examples of problems and the efforts to resolve them, in developing countries, were brought up at a special meeting called by the World Federation for Mental Health, after the regular Congress in Salzburg in 1979, with the co-operation of WHO and UNICEF. Two programs covering primary and secondary education were among those described (Chintu and Hayworth, 1979; Kapur and Cariappa, 1978), in India and Zambia. The first identified and dealt with misconceptions about behavioural problems of the students and the consequent aggravation of those problems; the second analyzed the psychological trauma caused by a school system built on extreme competition. These are hardly the only instances of study and recognition of emotional and educational problems caused by the schooling itself – "pedagogenic", if you will permit coinage of a term – but they represent for the poorer countries of the world the kind of insight and impact that professionals could bring to bear on hundreds of thousands of children, even without professional treatment services.

A second illustration of potential system impact is the current campaign to promote breastfeeding generally and reduce aggressive marketing of infant food substitutes, especially in the developing countries. Dr. Martin Gittelman (1978) is among those psychiatrists who referred to this. He noted the formula feeding of infants in poor and developing countries as "perhaps a source of serious mental health problems" as well as a cause of malnutrition, disease and developmental deficits. Here is a movement that mental health can join, drawing on its own expertise and trying to influence not only government positions but hospital practices themselves, which often makes it impossible for a women even to have the choice of breastfeeding. I know how difficult it is for one branch of medicine to influence another, or for any branch to modify hospital practices, but practices have undergone change, sometimes kicking and screaming, as a result of study and research in which mental health disciplines have formed a prominent part.

I also know it is not easy. Some 22 years ago one of my own children, then four years old, was hospitalized for acute appendicitis. Her mother was not permitted in the room to soothe and interpret. A nurse uttered the magical phrase "hospital policy" and the surgical resident brusquely and naively told the child a series of falsehoods about what was going to happen to her. I was aghast, for this was one of the most prestigious hospitals in the United States, with a strong department of psychiatry and scores of psychologists and professionally qualified social workers. I knew this because I was myself then offering them a seminar. I communicated with the Department of Psychiatry, not only with respect to the treatment of my own child, but on behalf of all children undergoing pediatric surgery, and received a sympathetic but lame reply, testifying to the impotence at the time of psychiatry vis-a-vis surgery in the hospital. I know all of this has changed in that hospital and most modern hospitals, but I also know that vested interests and set patterns take a lot of undoing – even in the medical profession.

The breastfeeding issue is important not only in developing countries – although bottlefeeding in such countries is a wide source of disease and death. The issue of availability of choice for breastfeeding is also important for the health and well-being of mothers and children everywhere for reasons of mental health, physical health and economy. The mental health professions have an opportunity to strengthen the coalition of interests concerned with this issue, and to affect the well-being of multitudes of future generations.

A third illustration is in the care of children uprooted as a result of wars or other disasters. Mental health resources are available, to some extent, in the care of resettled refugees, especially in the more well-to-do countries, but rarely figure in affecting the emergency operations that have such bearing on exacerbating or mitigating the emotional trauma of being forcibly uprooted, especially when the children are separated from their kinfolk. Again, I am not primarily referring to treatment, or separating out mental health as a service sector, but to measures affecting administration, physical planning, orientation of staff, and, indeed, to psychological support to staff themselves.

Recently, a number of mental health professionals concerned with such issues met with us in informal discussions. Widely differing as these disaster situations are, some general principles could be identified. Among them, for example, are the importance of building routine into the daily lives of children, especially, for older ones, in some form of education or training; of assuring them of physical protection; of seeing that any direct relationship in care-taking, individually or in groups, is performed by those from the same culture, not by strangers, no matter how expert; by supporting, and not interfering, with traditional medicine to cope with psychic problems and co-operating with traditional healers in general health care, wherever feasible; by supporting religious and cultural norms generally, and not confusing or interfering with them; by not demanding too much trust from children too early after disaster, especially those torn from their kin; of encouraging older children to be part of groups; of ensuring a reliable means of communication in the camp; of enhancing relevant and culturally congruent participation of residents in camp matters; of orienting camp staff to recognize psychological as well as physical problems, and of helping staff cope with their own, often severe stress reactions.*

Those professionally competent in mental health can have considerable influence in working with those who are running the camps and others in the system, co-operating with UNHCR, ICRC and the League of Red Cross Societies, voluntary agencies and others with long experience in disaster work.

One of the problems is that mental health specialists are not generally drawn to collaborative efforts affecting social systems, any more than medical clinicians and researchers are generally attracted to public health or even community medicine. Research results are hard to come by, the subject matter is "soft", prestige and income are not increased as much as by more conventional avenues. But for exercising a social development function, having impact at low per capita cost on multitudes – cost-benefit impact, if you will – there is, to my mind, none more effective than to contribute positively to the workings of indigenous institutions, provided there is a genuine understanding of the larger and institutional culture within which one is operating – particularly where they are not one's own – sufficient to navigate with confidence.

One might add to such systems those concerned with management of the workplace. In industrialized countries, mental health professionals specializing in work with executives and in management policies is hardly rare, although such work is not always oriented to safeguarding the mental health of the workforce as much as in enhancing productivity. The proposition is hardly new that the impact of management systems, and of executives, on the mental health of people is considerable, and there is a significant body of professional concern with the mental health of executives themselves. In developing countries, however, the incorporation of mental health concepts into management, along with efficiency and productivity considerations, is rare.

POSITIVE ELEMENTS ON THE WORLD SCENE

I had noted to begin with some of the dire elements which, taken together, give substance to the expression "a world in crisis". Let me now suggest some counter elements on which hope for humanity can be based, provided there is commitment and common effort. First, let us look at some of the remarkable achievements of developing countries, despite their extraordinary handicaps and lack of resources.

Since World War II, they have doubled their average per capita income; cut the rate of infant mortality in half, high as it still is, increased life expectancy from 42 to 54 years; the average literacy rate from 30 to over 50%, enrollment in primary grades has increased from 47 to 64%; and the proportion of children with severe or moderate malnutrition has been reduced. There can, of course, be no complacency about these achievements because, while rates of illiteracy, malnutrition, and infant mortality have been reduced, the numbers are larger than ever, due to population increase.

Nevertheless, the directions are extremely significant and give grounds for hope that marked improvement in conditions of health and well-being can be achieved, given world co-operation, and the commitment not only of the governments in developing countries but of nations throughout the world.

Second, I have referred to the campaign concerning breastfeeding and marketing of infant foods. It is an example of an issue that, while well known for a long time in health circles, was catapulted into international prominence because of the advocacy of citizen groups in many countries. The dynamic of enthusiasm and pressure from the wellspring of citizen concern, rooted in spontaneous, voluntary efforts, often through non-governmental organizations, is a source of hope for constructive change. It can be fairly said that this same mass pressure of citizen concern helped push governments, which might otherwise have been hesitant and temporizing, into the unprecedented support of the magnificent international rescue effort during the past two years in Kampuchea.

In his paper on "The Moral Imperative in Mental Health", Keith Yonge says that the ominous diagnosis for our present cultural condition is moral deficiency, with a confounding of moral distinctions, and quotes a statement that "there is ground for declaring that modern man has become a moral idiot". There is unfortunately much truth in this, but there is also truth in the capacity of mankind to make moral distinctions and to act upon them. The evidence in the case of the two movements I have just cited illustrates this. If more is needed on a worldwide scale, one may point to the overwhelming response in scores of countries all over the world to the International Year of the Child, with new dedication, new legislation and follow-up mechanisms to consolidate and continue the efforts given such impetus during the Year.

Case Western Reserve University,
436 Pardee Hall,
Cleveland, Ohio,
U.S.A. 44106

NOTE

* I am indebted particularly to Drs. David Ratnavale, Peter Kim, Martin Gittelman John Livingstone, Peter Neubauer, Aaron Ifekwunigwe and Alfred Freedman, among others, who gave us their insights and, in some cases, their unpublished papers. I also wish to acknowledge the unpublished papers of Dr. J. P. Hiegel, ICRC Medical Co-ordinator for Traditional Medicine, on his experience in the camps on the Thai-Kampuchean border, as well as the insights I received in Nong Samet from Personnel attached to the Centre for Traditional Medicine.

REFERENCES

Baasher, T.
1900 Mental Health of the Pre-School Child: Problems and Needs, Seminar on the health needs of the pre-school child, Karachi, EM/SEM.HLTH.CHILD/9, 15/1/68.

Baasher, T.
1978 Mental Health Services for Children in the Eastern Mediterranean Region. International Journal of Mental Health Vol. 7, No. 1–2, pp. 49–64, M. E. Sharpe Inc.

Beiser, M., Krell, R., Lin, Tsung-Yi, and Miller, M. (eds.)
1978 Today's Priorities in Mental Health: Knowing and Doing. Symposia Specialists, Miami, Florida.

Chintu, C. and Hayworth, A.
1900 Mental Health Services for Children in Zambia. Prepared for WHO/UNICEF/WFMH Meeting 14/7/79.

Galtung, J.
1981 Global Processes and the World in the 1980s: Prolegomenon I for a GPID World Model. United Nations University, Japan.

Gittelman, M.
1978 Child Mental Health: The Need for Alternatives to Modest Proposals in International Journal of Mental Health Vol. 7, pp. 5–17, M. E. Sharpe Inc.

Hasan, Z.
1977 Effects on Child Mental Health of Psychsoçial Change in Developing Countries. International Journal of Mental Health Vol. 6, No. 3: pp. 49–57, M. E. Sharpe Inc.

Hasan Z.
1900 Child Mental Health in Primary Care. Assignment Children. 47/48.

Kapur, M. and Cariappa, I.
1978 An Orientation Course for Schoolteachers on Emotional Problems of Schoolchildren. Indian Journal of Clinical Psychology 6: 75–80.

Meegan, M.
1981 The Reality of Starvation and Disease. The Lancet.
Olatawura, M. O.
1978 Mental Health Services for Children in the African Region. International Journal of Mental Health, Vol. 7, Nos. 1–2, pp. 34–38. M. E. Sharpe Inc.
Posvar, W.
1980 Expanding International Dimensions. Change Magazine. Vol. 12, No. 4: p. 23.
Sondhi, P. R.
1978 Issues and Priorities in Services in Developing Countries. International Journal of Mental Health Vol. 7, Nos. 1–2, pp. 102–105, M. E. Sharpe Inc.
State of the World's Children
1981 James P. Grant, Executive Director of UNICEF.
Tan, Eng Seong
1978 Mental Health Services for Children in the South-East Asian and Western Pacific Regions. International Journal of Mental Health Vol. 7, Nos. 1–2, pp. 49–64, M. E. Sharpe Inc.
WHO
1980 Minutes of Joint Meeting on Early Detection of Severe Developmental Disabilities among Children.

Discussant: MILTON H. MILLER, M.D. (U.S.A.)

THE WORLD IN CRISIS: IMPLICATIONS FOR MENTAL HEALTH

PASSIONATE ADVOCACY BEYOND CLASS AND BEYOND ONE'S OWN PROFESSION

Dr. Stein has outlined in a measured yet clear manner what we need to contend with, even though each of us is but one person and the totality or threat is beyond comprehension. Dr. Stein has also given us hope that we, as individuals, can make a difference in a world where problems are so overwhelming, so complicated and so seemingly out of one's reach. What he has not done in detail, because he is a gentleman – a gentle man – and because he does not wish to start our meeting in a querulous manner, is to raise the question: Can we in the mental health movement say that we're doing a good job ourselves in efforts to end the crisis in our own fields? What would happen if we did our basic job well – really well? Would it make a difference in this world? I believe the answer is yes.

Let me define the job that I think is the main responsibility of the World Federation for Mental Health and no less the responsibility for all of us entrusted with knowledge about mental health and mental illness, and their importance in the lives of human beings. That job is to provide passionate, brave advocacy for those who suffer illnesses, for their families and for those who are at high risk – passionate, brave advocacy that goes beyond class and is not limited by ordinary professional barriers. Without a staunch, strong, ever-watchful, determined and strategic group of advocates, those who suffer mental illness and their families, and those who are at risk, have no chance. They will fall victim to the ravages of prejudice that exist in rich *and* poor countries, in cities and villages, among the sophisticated as well as those who have little education. This is what Rosalind Carter told us in her address to the World Federation Congress in Vancouver. She said she was astonished and horrified by the depth and meanness of prejudice against the mentally ill, and she felt that our most important task is to fight that prejudice and the devastation it produces everywhere.

I've been a psychiatrist for over thirty years, and in my current post as a professor of psychiatry and a director of public mental health services for 2.5 million people in the coastal area of Los Angeles, I'm astonished every day. It would be hard to over-estimate the damage done by prejudice – prejudice and fear that turns up in most unexpected places. I feel that, unfortunately, we sometimes attempt to succeed through the provision of dispassionate advocacy for the mentally ill and, when that happens, we regularly fail. "Reasonable advocacy", advocacy diluted by our understanding of the problems of other professions, the limitations of resources, appreciation of how the national

Richard C. Nann, Dorcas Susan Butt, and Lourdes Ladrido-Ignacio (eds.), Mental Health, Cultural Values and Social Development, 17–20.

leaders work – that kind of restricted advocacy doesn't work, can't work, perhaps doesn't deserve to work in complex societies where there are many demands, some of which will not be met. I think many mental health professionals worry too much about being viewed by their peers and leaders as reasonable, rational, moderate people, when what they – we – should be worried about is what is happening to our patients, or more accurately, the people who need and deserve to be cared for in a competent health care system. They moderate their passion. They wait. They hope. They grow old. The young are impatient with them, and for good reason.

I was a consultant recently to one of the developing nations of South Asia, a nation that has only a handful of psychiatrists, nurses, social workers and advocates for the mentally ill. The 100 mental health professionals in that nation were themselves also assigned a low priority. There were 180 professors in the universities' medical schools, but no psychiatrist was a professor, and of course, their patients and the patients' families fared much poorer. Because of my presence, the psychiatrists got together, held a banquet and managed to gain the attendance of the Ministers of Health and Welfare. After the festivities, one of the psychiatrists rose to deliver the strongest, most touching, meanest, most passionate and most unmistakably personal address I've ever heard. He said: "Honourable Ministers, I am not a brave man. My hands are trembling as I stand here, so I cannot use notes, but I am so ashamed of the miserable condition of our patients and their families, and by the low status in which they are held in our country, that I will overcome my fear of your disapproval of me. I respect you greatly. I believe in our government. I love our country. I must tell you the terrible thing that you are doing by allowing these tragedies to continue."

I sat nervously through his speech. I couldn't believe my ears. In this nation, respect for the powerful is the first rule, yet this doctor was standing by a commitment to heal, to help, to love his patients and their families with no concern for himself. And do you want to know what happened? He won. We won. The leaders respected him as they feared him. He inspired his colleagues and, inspired me, his consultant. He taught me, his consultant. He gave me courage and when I went home, back to Los Angeles, I was the better for it – braver and stronger, and less worried about my own standing and safety, and more worried about my patients. In addition, I discovered that my chance in attitude inspired my colleagues as well. And so it spread from South Asia to Los Angeles. Someone showed us how to be passionate, unafraid and willing to do the right thing, and I felt better in my work, and my work seemed better. Gandhi said that one's personal fear is the result of corruption by a wish for popularity, a wish for possessions, a false pride and preoccupation with one's own body. I need to say again that average passion, reasonable passion, average perseverance by those in the mental health field is insufficient and, frankly, I've been told by Ministers of Health in more than one nation that people who work in our field are wonderful, understanding people and that we are far less aggressive than surgeons. But can you imagine a group of surgeons operating an emergency room with the kind of limitations that we in the mental health field accept? Not really.

One of the problems that haunts all of us in the mental health professions is that we tend to do poorly in developing care systems for people who are not of our social economic class. Whether we look at mental health care in rich cities or poor cities, those who are poor, under-educated, those who are minorities, and those who suffer the most severe of mental illnesses fare poorly at our hands. Now, I'm proud of the various individual projects that psychiatrists and other mental health workers in many nations have developed to demonstrate the need and the ability to serve in poor areas. But what we need nation-wide, profession-wide, and world-wide is a commitment to systems of care, a linkage of health professionals, citizens and teachers who intend to serve beyond their class. Our educational systems in the West, and some in the East, need to address the fact that our biggest problems can't be solved without the joint effort of educators, leaders of government, leaders of the professional organizations, and the inspiration of citizen participation in the creation, monitoring and reporting on system efficiency. Throughout the world, we've allowed ourselves to believe that one can have individual merit as a physician, nurse, social worker, even if the system of care in which we work is unfair and inadequate, but this is a great lie. It violates the golden rule. We are no better, none of us, than the worst part of the system that delivers care in the place where we live and work. Fortunately that's a moral problem that is open to remedy.

What is the bridge between the world in crisis, of which Dr. Stein has so eloquently spoken, and our presence here, in this meeting of the World Federation for Mental Health? Why have we come? What should we do here? Or more important, what should we do when we return home? Could it come to pass that in the lives of each of us, our having been here will lead to a change for the better in the life of at least one person in the world where we work? I tend to be optimistic and my favourite joke goes something like this: Two explorers have been captured by a group of angry aboriginal people. They've been stripped, they've been tied to a pole back to back, fire has been started around them to incinerate them, and for as far as you can see there are thousands and thousands of angry people with spears pointed at the hearts of these two men. One leans over his shoulder and says to the other: "I have a plan."

I think my most deeply held belief is that an individual can make a great difference, and that a group of individuals can make a still greater difference. Many in this room are outstanding people who have made a difference at the world level. Dr. Kusumanto who sits at this table has accomplished miracles in his country. Dr. Tsung-Yi Lin, my astonishing colleague of so many years, has endured so much because of the dream of inspiring a group of people who in turn serve and inspire others. My dear friend Estefania Aldaba-Lim who helped make the Year of the Child such a wonderful and moving period in our history. And Dr. Norman Sartorius, who travels the world and makes a difference, believe me. I know first-hand the difference they make, and here in the Philippines where I have been a frequent traveller and guest, I've seen what a difference Lourdes Ignacio, her projects in the community, and Justice Concepcion who, without concern for his health, works on our behalf. And Edita Martillano and Balthazar Reyes. I have seen here how important individuals can be, and that's true of all of you – all of us – who work with compassion and passion. What I'm saying in part is that we need to inspire each other to work with still more compassion and with much, much, much more passion as advocates in our labours.

We're here in this beautiful land that is struggling to achieve so much for its people, and I would like to close by recalling the ideas in the words of Jose Rizal, whose hope and courage sustained him through his final ordeal and now inspires his countrymen and all of us. It is from a poem of hope. "My dreams when a lad, when scarcely adolescent, my dreams when a young man, now with vigour inflamed, were to behold you one day, jewel of eastern waters, griefless, dusky eyes, lofty, the upright brow unclouded, unfurrowed, unblemished." And for us, with regard to our future efforts, to be passionately what we are and unshamed.

Department of Psychiatry
Harbor – UCLA Medical Center
1000 W. Carson Street
Torrance, California
U.S.A. 90509

CHESTER M. PIERCE, M.D. (U.S.A.)

MENTAL HEALTH AND SOCIAL DEVELOPMENT

Our task during this week is to consider mental health, social development and cultural values. All of these terms relate to the same issue. Persons who are content, happy, efficient, effective and contributing are probably mentally healthy. Such qualities can be reached only within the boundaries of permissable behavior sanctioned by one's culture. The person who is satisfying to himself or herself is likely to be satisfying to others in the culture. Also, the culture is likely to assess that individual as being one who is promoting the general good of the community. In this sense, such a person attends to the social development of his or her own culture, while at the same time providing an example of that culture's mentally healthy person. Such a person practices positive mental health.

I propose that we dwell today on how to get more people to practice positive mental health. Our goal is clear: we must get more people to live longer and to live better. We as a group can examine some of the features of human existence, as recognized by mental health experts, that keep us from attaining the goal. We, as a group, can suggest pathways, distilled from our clinical experience, that would lead us more quickly and more directly to the goal.

To accomplish these twin objectives, we can review and catalogue our own fraction of truth. There will be some universals upon which probably all of us agree. Nearly everyone at an international meeting might be inclined to recognize the paramount necessity of humankind doing all it can to contribute to moving towards global co-operation, which is planetary citizenship. Secondly, most participants here realize that such global fellowship will depend on the willingness and ability of citizens all over the earth to modulate and compromise on things to which they feel entitled. Thirdly, these entitlement negotiations around crucial aspects of existence will require increasing knowledge and delineation of what is human specific. We need to be attuned to feelings, ideas, perceptions, ambitions, hopes, desires, and the fears that all humans possess regardless of when, where, or how they have lived on this planet. Finally, I submit that our concerns today must be so comprehensive that we attempt to frame our charge by understanding events ranging from the extra-galactic to the sub-molecular. This is the reason that mental health and social development demand cosmopolitan behavior as the evidence of planetary citizenship.

It seems human specific that the minimum most people would want for themselves, is the best available health care, the maximum control of their time and space, and a modicum of creature comforts. Several concerns can be mentioned that must be maneuvered on a cosmopolitan basis in order to achieve something approaching global mental health and global social development.

Richard C. Nann, Dorcas Susan Butt, and Lourdes Ladrido-Ignacio (eds.), Mental Health, Cultural Values and Social Development, 21–28.

These concerns are ecological, sociological and cultural. Respectively, they present tasks of understanding climates, containing costs and improving life styles.

The Ecological Concern: Can we have healthier surroundings?

Repose, tranquility and security are features of mental health. Overall surroundings persuade these features. Our surroundings extend from extra-galactic forces, such as cosmic rays coursing through the earth to submolecular chemical reactions that may determine our feelings of joy or grief. On the one hand, this means that we have an excitement and enthusiasm about marvelous potentials to control weather or banish pain. On the other hand, there are other ecological aspects, all well understood, which promote violence, fear, and contention.

There is a world-wide pattern in which over one-half of deaths occur in children under age five. This pattern may be the world's most disturbing limitation to repose, tranquility and security. It is especially gruesome because the state of the art and the technology of medicine could reduce drastically, if not eliminate, most of the diseases culpable for this loss of children. The conditions of poverty, ignorance, crowded living, poor housing, inadequate diet, insufficient food, unsatisfactory water supply and ineffective waste disposal account for a bulk of the morbidity suffered on earth. Lamentably, vaccines and drugs needed to prevent or treat these diseases are available but not accessible to those who need them most (Simon, 1981). Any climate of trust and support is overwhelmed by hostile elements of fear, indifference and selfishness. In addition, a near ubiquitous climate of opinions about these matters nurtures the view that we are all paralyzed with helplessness to resist these hostile elements.

As a model toward thinking about removing this paralysis, it may be useful to look at our surroundings, which can be labeled micro-, meso-, and macroclimates. Each of us lives in his own microclimate warmed by effective and efficient love and work relationships, chilled by mini-disasters, which are characterized by the unexpected, the uncontrollable and the unpredictable. There has now been amassed a plethora of data regarding the biology, sociology and psychology of stress. These data make it clear that as individuals we can reduce the chill and increase the warmth of our microclimates by well-known, well-studied means (Institute of Medicine, 1979).

A microclimate can be improved by each individual having more skill, autonomy and decision making in his everyday existence. It has been found, too, that security, safety, and the opportunity for diversified and socially-rewarding interpersonal interactions is conducive to mental health. Likewise, the mentally healthy person, who in turn contributes to the social development of his community, is found to be certain about whatever roles he must fill. This individual accepts his share of responsibility and functions best when background circumstances provide him with proper resources and a minimum of interpersonal conflict.

The latter point is most important to emphasize, for it says that it is not status nor abundance of facilities or magnitude of problems that makes one happy or unhappy. Mental health depends more on comfortable background circumstances than gross events. Thus, it is easier to absorb a bereavement or serious financial loss than it is to adjust to chronic problems such as family bickering or a strained daily work atmosphere.

Moving to mesoclimates in which we all operate, one can list situations which range beyond the individual to great regions of the world. This, of course, embraces the whole of general political interaction among all people. More specifically, it includes such natural disasters as earthquakes, floods, volcanic eruptions. Both the general and specific mesoclimates can reinforce problems secondary to violence and fear. They are of such scope, grandeur, importance and urgency that their solutions demand world-wide co-operation. The threat to mental health at a municipal level from excessive noise or removal of sewage sludge are but simple, uncomplicated examples of damage to mesoclimates, which produce and reinforce fear and violence. The environmental impact of manufacturing nitrates, the promiscuous emission of aldehydes, the health consequences of aerosols or automotive fuels, the effects of pesticides or antibiotics on food supplies, the problems in sustaining viable aquaculture are all examples of tension-producers on a mesoscale.

Finally, on a macroscale, there are extant problems that are already antithetical to mental health. Few persons can single out these problems as having direct influence on their own lives. These problems proceed from a global to extra-galactic boundary. The official, international efforts to improve long-term weather prediction is an example. Communication systems, military planning, agriculture projections, transportation missions all depend on such efforts. Their success or failure trickle down to the microclimate of each citizen on earth and thereby influence everyone's chances for mental health. For those who consider global mental health, an awesome example to contemplate is that between now and the year 2000, it is expected that at least 20 countries will experience devastating water shortages. Extensive fear and violence could reign if this macroclimatic condition materializes.

The optimistic portion of the cosmopolitan concern about ecology is that we know enough to overcome many of the frustrations, obstacles and hardships. In essence, the solution depends on synthesizing what is known. This means that in some fundamental ways, new information is not required. What is needed is for us to locate and bind, synthesize and utilize existing data banks. In doing this, civilized social development proceeds along with the improvement of the individual mental health of tens of millions of people.

The Sociological Concern: Can we contain costs?

Once we are sensitized to the various climates infringing on mental health and social development, the next concern is to get people to act together for their own self-interest. The self-interests of various aggregates of human beings will differ widely.

For mental health experts, however, there do seem to be some arenas for action which include extremely large aggregates of human beings. At present, nearly everywhere on earth there is an assumption that family interactions somehow contribute to alcoholism, delinquency, child neglect, and drug abuse. Whether in Europe or the circumpolar regions, people are concerned about accident rates, diminished capital and distant markets. All of these intensify the route to mental health. As a generalization, the sociological concerns may be most limited by the forces of world-wide inflation.

Social demands for access to and availability of health care place a burden on already overcommitted exchequers. Each community must decide how much and which of its resources to allot in order to best approach its standard of ideal mental health for each of its citizens.

A recent study in the U.S.A. argues forcibly that a routine battery of tests, which is more broad than is usually done, would help markedly to contain costs in mental health hospitalizations (Hall, 1981). Health cost effectiveness will demand all sorts of experiments to obtain efficient use of funds for the improvement of mental health. Intuitive thinking might regard the reduction of services or the elimination of tests as the best way to do this. Yet, sometimes as the study cited indicates, short-term spending could result in long-term savings.

The solution to the cosmopolitan concern about sociological issues resides in making health delivery systems more effective. In theory, programs that effectively treat and prevent illness should help give all citizens in that community better mental health. Such a condition, by definition, would describe the socially-developed community. Flexibility and adaptability must be even more a part of delivery system experiments.

Thus far in the deliberations about planetary issues influencing mental health and social development, the various surroundings humans operate in and the need for them to act co-operatively have been mentioned. Yet, in whatever surrounding and with whatever degree of collaboration and co-operation, there is still a third component in the establishment of mental health. This component is the perspective and perception the individual and/or community brings to the definition of what constitutes ideal social development.

The Cultural Concern: Can we help people to improve their life styles?

In any given community, mental health and social development are defined by what that society judges to be a wise way for individuals to organize and dispose of their time and energy. The search for human specificity implies that there are large areas of overlap among all human societies. The areas of underlap, however, provide an abundant latitude for all persons in their own culture.

Accordingly, every individual brings to bear his own philosophy and code of living within the structure and framework of his society's rules, i.e. how the society regards and views things. The medical model would hold that either too much or too little conformity to the rules of one's society would bring dis-ease. Increasingly sophisticated thought about disease would go on to state that this dis-ease can be both the cause and effect of even lethal disruptions to one's biological, sociological or psychological systems.

Most of the effort of health workers is devoted to the interface of interaction between the individual and his society. Traditionally, mental health specialists have labored in this way with problems arising from cultural disorganization, family life, age-related difficulties and the impact of media. In all these efforts, the focus is on how people elect to live their lives. The expert attempts to help the patient toward life choices which promote health and prevent illness.

Recently, from all over the world, there are more reports that speak to the demand by consumers to have more input into their health care. This means that part of mental health is being a more active and better informed participant about one's own health. Cultures world-wide are reviewing the quality of their health care, the appropriateness of the care and its availability (Koplow, 1979). Patients' rights are being scrutinized, modified and guarded with extreme sensitivity (Hodge, 1979).

It would follow that such fervent community activity would mean that ethical issues become more prominent (Wright, 1979). Ethics, or what one chooses to do in a given combination of circumstances (relative to one's own health) becomes a more focused part of the definition of mental health. Most of us here, I expect, would consider this aspect of mental health to be a distinct and important social development.

For once choice becomes a more studied and deliberate part of mental health, other cultural modifiers of health may be influenced. For example, people victimized because of skin colour or sex or age may decide that it is in their own life interest to take steps to remove their oppression (Harfouche, 1979; Pierce, 1974; Pierce, Allen, 1975). Of course, this would be followed by some societal disruption until new relationships could be negotiated and stabilized. In the meantime, childrearing practices, education, economics, social life and politics may all be strained and oblige an increase in stress in many peoples' microclimates.

There is a positive side to the increasing awareness of the equation, "What do I owe to others versus what do others owe me?". This positive side is illustrated by the ever-mounting scientific evidence that states that individuals can indeed elect to augment their own longevity. In the U.S.A., actuarial data show that if one elects to reduce drinking, eliminate smoking, keep one's weight in control, sleep seven hours per night, eat breakfast, exercise regularly and not eat between meals, then substantial augmentation to longevity can result (Institute of Medicine, 1979).

Therefore, the solution to the cosmopolitan cultural concern about cultural variability seems to be to develop solid educational and communication methods to help people in each society to choose those healthy life styles, which are within their power to control. Ideally, over the years, more people will have more power to use such information in the service of helping themselves to live better and longer. The accomplishment of this ideal would seem to be congruent with the aims of the World Federation for Mental Health.

CONCLUSIONS

I have discussed the importance of tolerance, sharing, knowledge systems, education and communication in the promotion of mental health and social development. Already universities, governments, and international organizations are working in this field. A variety of approaches from self-help groups to computerized communication networks already are helping us to achieve the aim (Krishnamurti, 1979; Institute of Medicine, 1981; Cornish, 1981).

We can expect far-reaching scientific discoveries that will give us more resources to promote health and prevent illness. These discoveries add to everyone's development and shape everyone's mental health. A state of the art advance in immunochemistry may aid mental health workers in their function as "genetic counselors". A clinical or statistical insight may lead to better development of manpower and more crisp delivery of service. Reevaluation and redeployment of manpower may help us to gain better access to those populations most vulnerable to mental illness (Pardes *et al.*, 1979).

Although there is much need for us to better understand the human-specific qualities of our existence, we must, as always, give over much attention to special needs of each society. For instance, a world-wide concern is the increasing drift to urbanization that has occurred, especially over the past 200 years. Yet, even in the most populous countries, the hundreds of thousands of villages means that rural definitions and concerns about mental health and social development must occupy much attention.

In my own country, perhaps the greatest microclimate difficulty of the future will be loneliness. Another issue of enormous cultural implication is the demographic projection that has been given to our federal government that within 100 years, white people will be in the minority in the U.S.A. The ramifications that loneliness and a colored majority population could have on mental health and social development in the U.S.A. are mind boggling.

Finally, I will end by mentioning that there is available in the world, vast technological and scientific development. Humans routinely change the course of rivers, study polar ice caps on Mars, and have virtually eliminated dread scourges such as smallpox.

Yet, I wish you to be sure to differentiate technological and scientific development from social development and mental health. For the grisly fact is that, during the time you have listened to me, someplace in the world someone has died of starvation, someone else has been murdered, perhaps others have been taken hostage by terrorists and, almost surely, a number of people have been raped (Schiff, 1979; Farley, 1980). This dramatizes the gap between social development and scientific/technical development.

Peace is a prerequisite as well as the end result for mental health and social development. Peace will elude us as long as we confuse technology and science with social development. We must close the gap. Only then can we become cosmopolites, true and peaceful citizens of the universe.

Professor of Education and Psychiatry,
Graduate School of Education,
Harvard Medical School,
Nichols House, Appian Way,
Cambridge, Massachusetts,
U.S.A. 02138

REFERENCES

Cornish, E.
1981 The Coming of an Information Society. The Futurist 25: 14–21.

Farley, R.
1980 Homicide Trends in the United States. Demography 17: 177–188.

Hall, R. *et al.*
1981 Unrecognized Physical Illness Prompting Psychiatric Admission: A Prospective Study. Am. J. Psychiat. 138: 5, 629–635.

Harfouche, J.
1979 Health Care Problems of the Young Child in a Developing Ecological Context. Bulletin of the World Health Organization 57: 387–403.

Hodge, M.
1979 Social Forces, Ideology and The Domain of Mental Health Services. Psychiat. Quart. 57: 280–293.

Institute of Medicine
1979 Healthy People: The Surgeon General's Report on Health Promotion and Disease Prevention. U.S. Government Printing Office, Washington, D.C. 20402.

Institute of Medicine
1981 Stress. To be published U.S. Government Printing Office, Washington, D.C. 20402.

Koplow, L.
1979 Consumer Demands in Mental Health Care. Int. J. Law and Psychiat. 2: 263–270.

Krishnamurti, C.
1979 The Active Involvement of the People: Exploring Unconventional Approaches. Int. J. Med. Educ. 22: 143–149.

Pardes, H. *et al.*
1979 Psychiatry in Public Service: A Challenge to the Eighties 30: 756–760.

Pierce, C.
1974 Psychiatric Problems of the Black Minority. In: S. Arieti (editor in chief), American Handbook of Psychiatry. 2nd ed., 2, 512–523, Basic Books, New York.

Pierce, C. and Allen G.
1975 Childism. Psychiatric Annals 5: 15–24.

Schiff, A.
1979 Statistical Trends in Rape. J. Forens, Sci. Soc. 19: 95–106.

Simon, H.
1981 Pharmaceuticals for Developing Countries: an interface of science, technology and public policy. Pharos 44: 9–15.
Wing J.
1980 Innovations in Social Psychiatry. Psychological Medicine 10: 219–230.
Wright, P.
1979 Some Recent Developments in the Sociology of Knowledge and their Relevance to Sociology of Medicine 6: 93–104.

HEND ABDEL-AL, B.Sc. N., Ph.D. (Egypt)

MENTAL HEALTH AND SOCIAL DEVELOPMENT, THE RESPONSIBILITY OF HEALTH PROFESSIONALS

INTRODUCTION

The theme of this morning's session is Mental Health and Social Development. Being a nurse, I am concerned about effective action. If we are going to talk about Social Development and Mental Health then we must know what we can do, not only in terms of outcome, but more specifically in terms of process, i.e., how do we arrive at the outcome we hope to achieve? I am interested not only in the concrete outcome, but also in the immaterial outcome. In this presentation, I intend to accompany you through a reflective exercise in an attempt to clarify our thinking.

I believe that man is a unity and woman is a unity; we do not live in nature and the environment, but are part of nature and the environment. Knowing this will help you understanding what prejudices my perception and way of thinking. I intend to talk about how perception and thinking influence behaviour, decision for action, and action.

The objectives of this Congress are: (1) To identify and clarify mental health concerns in order to provide a perspective for the 80s and the years to come; (2) To identify various social and cultural factors and their relevance to mental health; (3) To determine mental health priorities in the 80s; (4) To identify strategies for mental health concerns in the field of health, education, social services, justice, advocacy and labour.

We cannot start to do anything about any of these objectives until we clarify what we mean by social development and by mental health. Such clarification will guide us in defining our responsibility as health professionals in these fields.

CONCEPT OF SOCIAL DEVELOPMENT

What do we mean by *social development*? Is development a direction? If we have 'more', is that development? Is the breakdown of some social institutions development? When would I call a phenomenon or an event a development? For instance, considering marriage as a social institution – did it develop? The concept and fact of marriage seems to have lost some of the traditional values attached to it. Is that development? The relationship between man and woman is basic to life. The attitude of man toward woman and woman toward man determines what sort of life we have. Whether it is an attitude of respect and love, or a consumer type of attitude, will influence the implications that ensue. From one's experience, observation and research reports, one can see how relationships lose a little bit of their depth. People don't want to get 'involved'

Richard C. Nann, Dorcas Susan Butt, and Lourdes Ladrido-Ignacio (eds.), Mental Health, Cultural Values and Social Development, 29–35.

or else they are going to get hurt. What does this do to their 'living' experience and mental health? Divorce is more frequent; the duration of marriage is shorter. I don't think divorce is a negative thing in itself, but the rate of divorce and duration of marriage in some societies make one wonder: why do people get married to start with? What is their idea about marriage? What are their expectations? What feeling of commitment to each other and to their children do they have, if any? We all know by experience and by reading research papers published on the subject that a child's disturbance, and later on, the adult's disturbance is very much related to how he/she has been brought up, how much love, understanding, care and attention he/she has received. If a human being does not feel worthwhile, the purpose of life becomes shaky.

Let us examine other aspects of social life, for instance the advance of technology. What has it done to our life? What has television done to our life? In some communities, people go to work and come home to television. Family interaction is restricted and channelled through television. Such a state of affairs must affect the relationship within the family, and the children who receive their role models, socialization and information mainly through television and less through the family and immediate environment. In some developed countries television programs present mainly violence e.g. thrillers, cartoons, information. This high exposure to violence and aggression on television somehow seems to be related to the degree of violence and aggression in their society. How does this affect the mental health of people and their attitude and perception of 'living'? As mental health professionals, we have a responsibility towards this; we can no longer stand back and say this is society's decision. We have a responsibility as citizens and as health professionals, who conduct research into behaviour, perception, attitude, etc.

What about the social phenomenon of population growth? This is the worry of many, among them ecologists. The logic of ecology says that "the creature who makes its habitat unlivable destroys itself". What can we as health professionals do? Are we to encourage birth control indiscriminately? What are the alternatives? I think we have a responsibility to understand, to inform and to educate.

What responsibility do mental health professionals have in relation to phenomenon like drug addiction, violence, crime, and decrease in the spiritual values? How can we delineate such responsibility? We need a great deal of thought to answer such questions.

Claude Olivenstein (1977), a French psychiatrist, in his book "Il n'y a pas de drogué heureux" (*There is No Such a Thing as a Happy Drug Addict*) makes two very important points which show the relationship between social life and mental health, the first being:

Qu'il suffise de donner pour reçevoir, cela serait trop simple: celui qui a eu une enfance et une adolescence massacrées il a pratiquement tout perdu, parfois même la goût de se sauver." (p. 289) (To think that it is enough to give in order to receive would be too simplistic. The person who had a most unhappy childhood and adolescence has practically lost everything, sometimes even the desire to be saved.)

The other point relates to a person in crisis and should illuminate our insight and understanding as health professionals:

"et ce qui émerge alors, c'est justement l'angoisse engendrée de toutes pièces par la famille, les institutions et toute cette masse de spécialistes qui obéissent à une vision prétendument scientifique du devenir des gens, en omettant d'écouter ce qui, en chacun, se dit de profond, d'intime, de viscéral, bref d'essential. C'est à cette angoisse que renvoie la drogue, laquelle surgit comme une réponse aux conflits vécus par un individu dans son unité propre, dans son existence particulière." (p. 268) (What emerges then is precisely this anxiety caused by the family, the institutions and all the mass of specialists acting according to a supposedly scientific vision of what people are to be, omitting to listen to what is in everyone of us said most intimately, deeply and viscerally; i.e. what is essential. It is this anxiety that the person taking drugs is experiencing, which appears as an answer to the conflict experienced by the person within himself, in his particular existence/being . . .)

CONCEPT OF MENTAL HEALTH

Olivenstein leads me to ask: "What do we mean by mental health?" Is mental health the opposite of mental illness or is it much more than that? If I consider mental health as the lack of mental illness then my field of vision is very restricted. If I consider it to be much more than mental illness, I envision a field of action that is much wider. When I talk about mental health, I am talking, among other things, about joy, about expectations, about suffering, about disappointment, about perception, about hopes and aspirations, about isolation, about experience, about interaction with others and with nature, about living, about values; in one word about 'being' in all its dimensions and aspects, about our inner being and our outer being. The richness we have, each one of us, inside, is a vital factor. If I as a health professional want to help the person, I cannot ignore this richness, without seriously failing in carrying out my responsibility. Who am I, as a health professional, to ignore what people experience in their everyday lives in their moments of happiness and in their moments of difficulties? Who am I, as a health professional, to reduce this richness of this person and his life experience under one label of 'schizophrenic' or 'neurotic', or any other label? Am I really helping if I do that?

Here lies the importance of clarifying our concepts. People usually shrink from anything to do with concepts or philosophy, but clarifying concepts is not a useless intellectual exercise, it is an absolute practical necessity. What I mean by mental health directs me to knowing who is involved in mental health and what is involved in mental health. If we examine honestly what we actually mean by mental health at present we find that, even though we talk of mental health, we really mean mental illness, because whenever we talk of mental health we always talk of psychiatric hospitals and psychiatric illness. We regard psychiatrists and, sometimes but rarely, psychiatric nurses, as the ones involved in mental health.

If mental health is rightly considered in its wider perspective and conception then those involved are, among others: lawyers, social workers, economists, teachers, politicians and citizens, as well as health professionals. We need to explicitly interchange what we mean by mental health so that we can start to communicate effectively, and delineate the responsibility of each person or group involved. Responsibility is whole and total and cannot be shared. It is a serious matter. It is up to us to choose whether we consider responsibility as a vacuous concept or as a concept that is binding, meaningful and pertinent to our everyday life and practice. I hope we choose the latter.

RESPONSIBILITY OF HEALTH PROFESSIONALS

What is our responsibility as health professionals in relation to Social Development and Mental Health? I have already mentioned briefly some of our responsibilities in that context. Now, I want to talk more specifically about responsibility of health professionals, within the limits of our field of action. One obvious responsibility is that of education, i.e., education of the 'person' who is going to come in contact with people in the field of health care. I use the word 'education', rather than 'training', as training is restrictive and restricted. I can only speak of health professionals as they are within the context of my domain. I can talk about what nurses ought to be doing and, if the medical profession will allow me, a little bit about what it should be doing.

Each health profession as a distinct discipline has its own identity and its own frame of reference that should be accepted and respected by all health professionals when working together. Such a frame of reference guides health workers' perceptions of the specific situation and hence, the action to be taken. Health is a state of being, and life situations and health situations are complex sets of interacting variables to which each health discipline brings its understanding and needed contribution and action. If I work in a setting where I feel I should tell doctors what to do, or what is, unfortunately, more common, that doctors think they have to tell nurses what to do, this is a problem. The doctor in this case is denying the fact that nursing as a discipline has its own identity, its own frame of reference and, therefore, its own and different contribution to health care. It is much more satisfying for all concerned, doctors, nurses, patient, etc., if health professionals respect each other's frame of reference; this adds to the richness of perception of the situation and consequent action. Expecting everyone to work within the same frame of reference, i.e., that of the doctor, is wasteful of potentials, restrictive, not cost-beneficial, confusing, and simply defeats the purpose of having different disciplines.

Some of the abilities we need to develop in health workers are thinking and dealing with situations in their totality. Edward de Bono (1976) believes in the teaching of thinking; he believes that our system of education does not allow for flexibility in thinking. Teaching people how to think means you are giving them alternatives; it goes against narrowing their perception to one solution/direction. Thinking with greater flexibility opens up possibilities, an ability very much needed in our world today. We should teach future health workers to deal with situations in their totality; and never to lose sight of the context of the whole situation, as isolation of variables results in fragmentation and division.[1]

Our responsibility towards service refers to the quality of care we give. If we say that we are committed to the goal of health care for all by the year 2000, we have to stop and ask what quality of health care we want to give people by the year 2000? Are we really giving quality care if we are propagating the proliferation of new categories of personnel who are ignorant and illiterate? Are we helping people to improve? Have we evaluated the work we are doing? Is teaching a community health worker a few signs and symptoms, or a few skills really an answer? Does it raise the health of people to a higher level?

The health worker who first comes in contact with patients, and who is going to perceive the health needs of people, is the one who would make a difference in the quality of care. Perceiving needs is not a mere process of recognition, or of matching symptoms with predetermined action. All of us know the dangers of this. Perception is a professional skill, on the basis of which, the decision for action follows. In what context I would like to quote Piet Hein, a Danish philosopher, who writes what he calls grooks/rhymed verses. He says:

We leave wisdom to starve and thirst
When we cultivate knowledge as such
The very best comes to the very worst
When ignorants know too much.

I think to be responsible means that we honestly evaluate and reconsider whether the immediate answering of needs hampers our future progress; whether, in the long run, our immediate action causes more damage than good. Another point we need to consider is the mental health of these new categories of personnel that we are creating. The system does not provide a structure for their promotion and they cannot go back, because, once they 'know', they cannot revert to a state of not-knowing. This is beyond the administrative burden caused by their presence within the health care delivery system. We have to rethink many things if we are serious about our responsibility to render a quality of service worthy of the people we are caring for, as the quality of care we deliver reflects our respect for those people.

We also have a responsibility in health care policy. What is our role in favouring hospital care, or community care, as appropriate? What is our influence in pushing people into 'sick' roles, as Parsons says or, as Scheff and Parsons say, in 'labeling people', which invites behaviour to fit the label? Those of us who have worked in psychiatric settings know how, when we labelled a patient 'aggressive', for instance, he never failed us because that is what we expect of him. Labels make us miss a lot in our patients; they make us look for the problems, the negative and what is wrong.

Perhaps one of our major responsibilities as health professionals is to orient our observations and perceptions towards the positive, towards what is going right. Such a change of direction might open up possibilities and help us reach alternative solutions which would be more gratifying for everybody concerned.

Research is a vast area of responsibility for health professionals. I shall not deal with it here but only point out that the research question is framed by our own way of perceiving things: if we perceive narrowly, we shall carry out research narrowly. If we perceive within a wider perspective our research question will give us more meaningful and relevant answers. Let us respect the scientific methodology but not forget that we are human beings and that '*educated subjectivity*' is respectable and essential to our understanding of others. Peters (1973), in his book *Reason and Compassion*, explains the inseparable link between cognition and affect. Mischel (1974) edited a book entitled *Understanding Other Persons* in which such linkage is also apparent.

Health professionals are not only doctors, nurses, social workers, etc., they are also citizens and, like any other citizen, they have rights and duties. I believe one of these duties is to provide information in such a way that it is understandable to others, e.g., publishing results of research to show the public how science contributes to everyday life. Health professionals also have a responsibility to participate in the community.

What I am hoping to encourage is more flexibility and the development of a positive orientation. Let us try to see if such an approach would not take us further than a problem-oriented outlook. Let us see if we do not have more to gain if we look at the positive and the successful. Let us evaluate our concept of help and care. Sometimes help is considered only in terms of concrete outcomes and we forget that 'caring' is equally important. I give you the following quotes for reflection:

Gibran (1926), in the *Prophet*, said

> You give but little when you give of your possession. It is when you give of yourself that you truly give.

Jean Giono (1935) in his book *Que ma joie demeure* (Let my joy last) says

> They have told you that it is what you have that makes you rich and I am telling you it is what you give that makes you rich.

CONCLUSION

What I have been talking about is the importance of clarifying our concepts or our way of thinking for the sake of improved communication and a better service, as the quality of service we give depends on the quality of our perception, thinking, feeling, values and action. I talked a little about the importance of unity of feeling, thinking, values and action, the importance of caring and the importance of educating health professionals. I hope that through education we can foster understanding, respect and consideration for the self and for others. What I have presented is a brief outline on how to serve mental health by respecting man's unity. It is our responsibility as health professionals, for which we should be held accountable.

I would like to close with a quotation from Alan Watts' book, *Nature, Man and Woman* (1958), hoping that we can achieve the ability to:

> . . . see an individual leaf in all its clarity without losing sight of its relation to the tree.

c/o International Council of Nurses,
37 Rue de l'Ancien-Port,
CH-1201, Geneva,
Switzerland

NOTE

[1] An approach to teaching on the basis of complex situations and developing the inferential ability of the student to deal with such complexity was the subject of a research study by Abdel-Al, Hend (1975), *Relating Education to Practice within a Nursing Context*. Unpublished Ph.D. thesis, Edinburgh University.

REFERENCES

Altschul, A. T.
1980 Hints on Maintaining Patient-Nurse Interaction. Psychiatry under Review. Nursing Times Publication, London. pp. 12–14.

de Bono, E.
1967 The Use of Lateral Thinking. Pelican Book.
1967 The Five-Day Course in Thinking. Pelican Book.
1979 The Mechanism of Mind. Pelican Book.
1976 Teaching Thinking. Pelican Book.

Gibran, K.
1926 The Prophet. London: Pan Books Ltd.

Giono, J.
1935 Que ma joie demeure. Bernard Grasset livre de poche.

Hawley, A. H.
1950 Human Ecology. New York: Ronal Press.

Mischel, T. (ed.).
1974 Understanding other Persons. Oxford, Basil Blackwell.

Olivenstein, C.
1977 Il n'y a pas de drogués heureux. Laffont.

Peplau, H.
1980 The Psychiatric Nurse Accountable^ to Whom^ for What^ Perspectives in Psychiatric Care Vol. 18, No. 3: pp. 128–134.

Peters, R. S.
1973 Reason and Compassion. London: Routledge & Kegan Paul.

Piet Hein
1968 More Grooks. London: Hodder Paperbacks.

Watts, A. S.
1958 Nature, Man and Woman. New York: Vintage Books.

Discussant: MORTON BEISER, M.D. (Canada)

MENTAL HEALTH AND SOCIAL DEVELOPMENT

Is the human being a mover or a pawn of social forces? Literature on mental health portrays him or her for the most part, as the latter. While the world changes at a speed we cannot assimilate and while the familiar institutions which would lend stability crumble, the human reacts by developing psychosomatic disorders, neuroses and psychoses. In contrast to this scenario, Dr. Pierce offers us a viewpoint rarely presented in mental health. The mentally healthy person not only reacts to ecological, social and cultural change; he or she acts upon that change.

Social change undoubtedly creates a condition of risk. However, persons in the field of mental health, who usually come in contact only with the casualties of risk, often make the mistake of generalizing from too limited a base. Mounting evidence reminds us of what we probably should have known all along: that there is a difference between risk and inevitability. In his discussion of urbanization, Dr. Pierce gives us an example. Urbanization has been assumed to create a situation of risk by affecting the micro- and meso-climates of individuals. In popular ideology, as well as scientific theory, the movement from village to city in developing countries – a movement which wrenches people out of what is familiar and exposes them to the forces of modernization – is viewed with alarm. Recent studies, however, show that, while some urban migrants do succumb to acculturation stress, most survive in the new environment with little obvious deterioration in their mental health. If, as Dr. Hend suggests, we should be serious about mental health in contrast to mental illness, we should be studying these successes. They contain important lessons about how mental illness can be prevented and positive health promoted in situations of flux.

Before we can seriously study mental health, we need to develop something we currently lack – a vocabulary for concepts dealing with health rather than illness. Dr. Pierce helps us. He does so by suggesting concepts which I find unusual and stimulating – informed decision-making, cosmopolitanism, and acceptance of material restraint.

In speaking of informed decision-making, Dr. Pierce suggests that the more active and better informed a participant is about one's own health, the more mentally healthy he or she can be assumed to be. It is, perhaps, easier to point to examples pertaining to physical than to mental health. Supplied with the information that proper diet, exercise and the avoiding of smoking contribute to longevity, people can make informed choices about their health. Similar mental health principles could be formulated. By way of example, it is probably time for people to be let in on the secret that a micro-climate characterized by a rich social network is more health promoting than one not so characterized.

Richard C. Nann, Dorcas Susan Butt, and Lourdes Ladrido-Ignacio (eds.), Mental Health, Cultural Values and Social Development, 36–40.

The work of Dr. Mansell Pattison and of Dr. Scott Henderson in Australia demonstrate a relationship between restrictive social networks and prolonged mental ill health. Even more strikingly, a recent research report from Alameda County, California demonstrates that, in the case of serious physical illnesses, such as cancer, people with the densest social networks enjoy the longest survival time. Research methodologists will point out, and rightly, that most such studies are correlational. They cannot establish whether people are healthier because they are lucky enough to be provided with socially supportive environments, or because healthier people make it their business to create such environments for themselves. I suspect that it will turn out to be a bit of both. The ability to set up the social network is a sign of mental health: having created it, one sets in motion a spiral of health-reinforcing social interactions. Another case offers an example of how information leads to constructive, health-promoting action. In the 1950s, the work of a number of investigators – notably John Bowlby – which demonstrated the importance of parental contact during the early years of childhood development, began to capture public and professional attention. This, in turn, led to changes in parenting and institutional practices. For example, hospital policies which, at least until the early 1960s in North America, militated against contact between young children and parents when a hospitalization became necessary, have gradually been abolished. The facilitation of parent-child contact during critical periods such as hospitalization has probably been more health-promoting and disability-preventing than many expensive treatment programs mounted in the name of mental health.

Speaking of one's relationship to the human group at yet another level, Dr. Pierce presents the concept of cosmopolitanism – a recognition that what people do affects the lives and well-being of others who may be at a seemingly distant remove. While not a concept familiar to us in mental health, it is one well worth considering. Indifference to the welfare of disadvantaged peoples and disadvantaged nations brutalizes not only the neglected, but also those who choose to neglect.

Dr. Pierce's mental health list includes willingness to accept material restraint. The appearance of this item permits me to underline the importance of devoting serious research attention to mental health as opposed to mental illness. One of the best established findings in mental illness research is that economic disadvantage is associated with a high prevalence of mental disorder. One might extrapolate from this to assume that economic affluence would then be associated with well-being. While the proposition seems logical, research has failed to support it.

How can this happen? How is it possible that mental ill health increases with economic deprivation, but that positive mental health shows no correlation with material prosperity? This seeming paradox can be easily solved by changing a conceptual habit. This habit is, I think, placing mental health on the same continuum as, and as the opposite of, mental illness. Once we abandon this premise, we find, to our pleasant surprise, that we can measure factors like happiness and well-being independently of mental illness, and demonstrate that people without illness (whether this be mental or physical illness) do not necessarily demonstrate well-being. In other words, the absence of the negative is no guarantee of the positive. We can also look with fresh eyes at the finding that, while economic deprivation demonstrates a positive correlation with prevalence rates for mental illness, prosperity does not correlate with feelings of well-being and proffer the interpretation that, while a certain level of economic support is necessary in order to safeguard against the development of mental ill health, beyond that, material acquisition does not contribute to well-being. Recently, the Leisure Development Centre of Japan carried out a study of positive health and human values among national samples of adults living in 13 different countries. One of the results of this important study was that, for men and women of all ages, in all 13 countries, whether eastern or western, developing or developed, the strongest association with feelings of well-being proved to be feelings about one's family relationships. Within the micro-climate, the presence of supportive and satisfying family ties seem to contribute most to people's well-being.

How can we promote mental health? More specifically – if we accept dimensions such as those proposed by Dr. Pierce as patterns of health – what role can health personnel assume in their promulgation? Dr. Pierce's first demand in health is for information, for " . . . more people having more power to use information in the service of helping themselves to live better and to live longer". Dr. Hend cautions us, however, against too quick and too glib acceptance of universals. What may be an effective way to prevent mental illness in one culture may not be appropriate for another. I wonder, though, if she would not agree that the goal of helping to create an informed citizenry making conscious decisions in the light of that information might not constitute one of our few universals in mental health.

How can we arrive at a situation where more people become better informed and assume more control over their own health? Dr. Hend, speaking of the responsibility of mental health professionals, points to the need to educate other health care personnel and also to make useful information available to the general public. Dr. Pierce, speaking of therapy, says it is the responsibility of the expert to help his or her patient toward making life choices which promote health and prevent illness. Both speakers, echoing the same theme, espouse a lofty ideal – but one that is too rarely translated into practice. In order to illustrate our profession's failure to educate, I would like to highlight two concepts – information and choice. I do this in order to differentiate the ideal of educating from something often mistaken for it – the promulgation of technology. What we are talking about goes beyond health care personnel sharing mechanistic skills with a wider citizenry. To share the mechanics of health care without the information necessary to comprehend and to evaluate this technology is to force people to become dependent rather than autonomous.

A personal example will illustrate the confusion between information lending to choice and training leading to a kind of technological slavery. I worked for some time in Senegal, in West Africa, on a series of epidemiological studies which addressed the effect of urbanization upon the people living in that developing country. One of our practices was to go into villages in the bush in order to draw samples of individuals for surveys. During our stays in the villages, people would often come to ask for help with various health problems. One day a man asked me to see his wife, who, he said, was very ill. She was indeed very ill. I was afraid that she was suffering from meningitis and, since we were in a remote village, I did not know what to do. My interpreter asked: "Well, what would you do if you were in a city?" I replied: "We would give her some antibiotics." He then informed me that a bush medical station, equipped with antibiotics, was located within a few hours driving time. We agreed to take our patient there.

The bush station proved to be a low-lying, thatched-roof building with a few beds, a locked cupboard full of medications and a staff of one, a man who had spent three months working as a nurse's assistant in one of the hospitals in Dakar. When I described the patient's symptoms to him, he said: "I think she has meningitis," Having William Osler himself concur in my diagnosis would not have pleased me more at this point. The bush practitioner then instructed the women to sit on a chair, her back to us, her legs straddling the back of the chair. He placed a lumbar puncture needle in a kidney basin, poured alcohol over it, flamed it (thereby disinfecting it), then very skillfully inserted the needle into the patient's back in order to drain some spinal fluid into a test tube. He withdrew the needle and handed me the test tube. Another dilemma. Since there were obviously no laboratory technicians available, no microscopes and no media plates on which to try to grow whatever organisms were in the fluid, I really did not know what was expected. I said: "Why did you do this?" With great equanimity he replied: "We always do that. We always take the fluid and hand it to the doctor." "Well, what do you do when the doctor isn't here?" I asked. "Throw it out." So I handed it back to him and he threw it out. He then gave the lady an injection of penicillin and admitted her to one of his clinic beds.

I offer this story not as an indictment of this bush health care worker's motivation nor of his technical competence. On both counts, he was impressive. Instead, I wish to point to the dangers of ritualizing health care technology. I submit that it is an almost inevitable consequence of too little information. Although in itself no guarantee, information helps insure informed, rather than ritualistic, responses. Not that there is anything wrong with ritual *per se*. We all, after all, practice and seem to need it – as witnessed by our religious rituals, our social rituals, our congress-attending rituals. However, there are times when ritual becomes dysfunctional and, as in the bush health station in Senegal, potentially dangerous.

The danger of making uninformed choices has been addressed by the noted social critic Ivan Illich. Speaking of the movement towards citizen responsibility in health care, he describes a phenomenon that he calls "professionalization of the layman". Illich's concern is that mechanics of care may well be shared but not knowledge. People will be trained to perform certain acts in the service of their own health, but without an appropriate understanding of these activities. Because, under such circumstances, informed choice becomes impossible, we in the health care system run the risk of enforcing dependency rather than fostering autonomy.

Perhaps all my remarks may be looked at as variations around a particular theme. Dr. Sartorius proposes that the success of social development be measured in human terms according to the extent that it contributes to, or detracts from, human mentation. Let us take that one step farther. Within the mental life of man, the quality that I would call centrality is a critical dimension of mental health. The need to feel that one is, to an extent at least, at the centre, rather than at the periphery of events, that one can shape events rather than simply be swept along by them, probably constitutes a universal human need. The satisfaction of this need manifests itself in behaviour such as informed decision-making and the ability to place materialism in proper perspective. Centrality is not the same as selfishness. Clearly, however, it should be tempered by cosmopolitanism, a recognition that choices made in the service of enlightened self-interest affect the welfare and destinies of other occupants of this planet. The feeling of centrality leads to hope, its absence to despair. To the extent that social development can contribute to the development of cosmopolitan centrality, it can be considered constructive, health promoting and desirable.

Department of Psychiatry,
University of British Columbia,
2255 Westbrook Crescent
Vancouver, British Columbia,
Canada V6T 2A1

CARLOS A. LEÓN, M.D., M.S. (Colombia)

MENTAL HEALTH AND CULTURE: SOME VIGNETTES

I would like to share with you some personal experiences accumulated in the course of several years of professional activity. Most are associated with the clinical and epidemiological aspects of mental disorders. I will do this rather than embark upon a formal presentation of a subject which has been extensively studied in previous publications, symposia, seminars and even whole congresses (Mead, 1959; Soddy and Ahrenfeldy, 1967; Dunham, 1976). Most of what I intend to tell you cannot be treated as "scientific" findings determined by theory, method and systematic research. It will rather be a narrative based upon glimpses, impressions and nuances of culture as woven into the fabric of mental health or illness. In one of his essays, Lewis Thomas (Thomas, 1981) refers to things "that human beings can only see out of the corner of the eye", which is a gift, he says, familiar to all children. Even though the following material was elicited in a clinical context, all the while the peripheral vision glanced, almost inadvertently, at certain complementary images, which in a subtle way contributed to color and shape the experience into a meaningful whole.

I would like to present something personal which might reveal my preoccupation with the unsolved, and perhaps never to be solved, intricacies of the states of health and disease, of falling ill and healing as experienced by a sizeable proportion of people in the part of the world where I live. It is hoped that those of you with a receptive eye may discern among these vignettes patterns of some of the major conceptual issues in the study of culture in relation to health. Some of these are: cultural influence on perceptions and feelings; cultural relativity, cultural specificity and cultural expression of mental disorders as well as cultural influence on help seeking and on clinical practice.

Since it is nowadays customary to go back to one's ethnic roots, I would like to start by recalling the feelings of awe and fascination I experienced as a child in the Andean highlands of rural Ecuador about the illness known as "espanto" or "susto" and its traditional treatment "la limpiada" (cleansing). Susto has been described as a "culture bound" syndrome (Gillin, 1956; Sal y Rosas, 1958; León, 1963a; Yap, 1967; Rubel, 1969) and seen as a case of "loss of the soul" brought about by fright or other causes. During a spell of susto, the soul may leave the body and be replaced by an evil force which kills the victim when it reaches the heart. Typical symptoms are malaise, irritability, anorexia, insomnia, fever, diarrhea, restlessness, startle reactions and crying spells. It is believed that in small children the soul is loosely attached to the body and hence, the problem is more frequent among them. The traditional method of treatment is known as "cleansing", which is aimed at wiping out the "espanto" and bringing back the soul to its dwelling place. At the climax of the ceremony the healer or cleanser

Richard C. Nann, Dorcas Susan Butt, and Lourdes Ladrido-Ignacio (eds.), Mental Health, Cultural Values and Social Development, 41–51.

exclaims: "the soul is now back in the body" right after he or she has forcibly blown a jet or liquid upon the patient's back causing a startle reaction to occur. The prevalence of "espanto" is (or was) almost universal in rural areas of the Andean plateau of Ecuador and there is a sharp contrast between the apparent inadequacy of scientific medicine for diagnosing the ailment (or modifying the symptoms) and the success when it is treated by an experienced healer.

Having fallen ill and been cleansed several times during my childhood, I can still remember how fearful and wretched I felt during the illness and the anxious expectation while going through the healing ritual. I experienced the progressive lassitude and sleepiness whilst the cleanser performed her rhythmic rubbing and murmured incantations in a monotone. I remember the sudden startle caused by the jetting of wine on my back which evoked a mixture of fear and anger accompanied by trembling and screaming. Then, there was the soothing sensation of being dried and wrapped in clean linen and affectionately tended by my mother, pampered in a most solicitous manner, and offered a cup of aromatic tizane, which seemed to bring about an agreeable heightening of all perceptions. Following was a beatific state of somnolence which gradually became deep sleep.

As for a subjective image of "la limpiadora" (the cleanser), she always appeared to be a very pleasant and calm person, self-assured, kind and good natured. In my fantasies, she at times was endowed with supernatural characteristics of magic, omnipotence and strength, always using them to fulfill protective functions. Each one of the treatment ceremonies was taken as a beneficial experience, and the cleanser regarded as a maternal, protective and benevolent figure. This retrospective view, when submitted to deep probing and validation during my personal psychoanalysis, did not undergo any substantial change. It may not be entirely unwarranted to regard these poignant experiences as a central core upon which a nucleus of receptiveness for cultural phenomena was built in my personal development. One may see them as some sort of early conditioning or imprinting, which perhaps rendered me more sensitive to the influence of culture in matters of health and disease.

In the early 1950s as a young Intern at Hospicio y Manicomio "San Lázaro" in Quito, I was confronted with one of the most perplexing cases I have ever seen in my entire psychiatric career. A middle-aged Indian farmer from the mountains was brought to the hospital in a state of catatonic agitation, which had progressed to exhaustion and who, before falling mute, complained in a frenzy that he had been possessed by the rainbow! This belief, of course, was shared by the awe-struck relatives, who felt utterly helpless to deal with such a rare, but by no means unheard of, ailment. Several elders in the group confirmed the case as one of "Kwichi-hapishka" (being-caught by the rainbow) and lamented the tragedy, the more so, because the only person capable of treating such a condition was an aged healer who had died a few months ago. The "Kwichi" (rainbow) in the Quechua folklore is a powerful force embodying the reproductive principle in nature and partaking of the fecundative power of both the sun and the rain. When it appears on the sky, you should never point at it with a finger lest it wither and fall off. If it touches you superficially, your skin becomes covered with blotches. Worst of all, it eventually may enter your body if, for instance, you inadvertently step over a puddle where it is reflected. Since the patient did not respond at all to the treatment given in the hospital, I was forced, in desperation, to try to learn as much as I could about the means used by traditional healers to treat the condition. The only clue I managed to discover, through a series of enquiries made to knowledgeable people in the region where the patient lived, was that the rainbow could be forced to leave the body of its victim through the urine. In addition, I found out that the rainbow, as everybody knew, had four colours: purple, red, yellow and green. Armed with these two valuable pieces of knowledge, I returned to the hospital and worked out an impromptu therapeutic plan. First, I informed the mute and altogether unresponsive patient that I had brought with me a powerful medicine used by the late healer and obtained through great efforts to rid him of his trouble. To this, he did not show any reaction but, when I mentioned that I intended to give it to him in four consecutive days so that he may eliminate the "kwichi" out of his system by urinating out one color each day, his eyes suddenly lit up and a fleeting expression of interest replaced his constant apathy. Under a regime of three sealed capsules a day, containing dyes of a different hue for each day plus a diuretic the patient regained speech. On the third day, having voided copiously in four different colors in succession, he was back to normal. On the sixth day he went through the effects of a strong laxative, given at his own request, in order to complete the process of elimination (catharsis?). I am sad to report that my ignorance of epidemiological methods at the time prevented me from conducting a follow-up. Yet, I basked for days in the marvelous feeling of having worked a really magical cure. Many a time in later years I had occasion to reevaluate this instance of youthful hubris.

One of the first confrontations with the puzzle of identifying effective therapeutic factors was put to me shortly after having finished my psychiatric training by an intelligent and well-educated Colombian lady whom I had treated, or so I thought, for an anxious-depressive condition. After feeling free of symptoms for several weeks, she told me that she was grateful to me for having helped with her problems but she confided, rather hesitantly, that she was puzzled as to *what* had *really* produced the cure. She admitted that she appreciated my concern and interest in listening to her troubles and my non-judgmental and supportive attiude, as well as the apparent efficacy of the prescribed medication. But she said that during the treatment period she had also decided to go to a priest and make a general confession. Following this, she went to a medium who read her past and future in the smoke of a cigar and prescribed her to wear a chinese magnetic wrist-chain brought from Hong Kong. I replied, as best as I could, that the important thing was that she had recovered and for that we both should be glad . . . yet, her question still intrigues me.

In the course of a training program on Mental Health Care for Primary Health

Workers (León, 1981), I had the opportunity to spend some weeks with a group of rural students attending a young Peasant's Home. This is an institution that selects children and adolescents from remote rural areas and awards them a scholarship to live as interns in a communal home while attending high school in a rural centre. A workshop held with these students on the characteristics of the mentally healthy persons proved to be, for me, a most instructive exercise. They reached spontaneous consensus about the following:

A mentally healthy person:

(a) "puede aguantar lo que venga . . . "
(can stand any thing that may come up . . . or is able to put up with any hardship);

(b) "es alegre y se rie con ganas . . . "
(is cheerful and laughs with full desire . . .);

(c) "tiene las pilas puestas . . . "
(has the batteries on).

A discussion of each of the answers revealed a wealth of cultural notions linked to the expressed concepts. For the first concept, the emphasis was on coping, on how healthy people can withstand hardship without complaining or cracking under stress, no matter how heavy it may be. It was fascinating how, as a result of admitting that both men and women indiscriminately could show this quality of coping, the group acknowledged that "machera" (a term for courage, derived from "macho") could be an attribute shared by both sexes. About laughing with full desire and being cheerful, the group underlined spontaneity, being genuine, the ability to express oneself and again, the ability to enjoy life as it comes, even in the face of hardship. It is interesting to remark that in describing the characteristics of the *Culture of Poverty*, Oscar Lewis identified as two of its positive assets the capacity for coping and for enjoyment of the sensual (Lewis, 1966). The expression that characterizes a healthy person as one "who has the batteries on" also provided rich material related to culture. The emphasis here was on readiness, speed, efficiency, such as that of a well functioning machine, a well running motor and other images which through associations and similarities brought the group to talk about robots and the "Bionic Woman", seen in a current television series. In a psycholinguistic study on the popular terms for crazy person conducted in Cali (Micklin *et al*., 1974), the corresponding opposite associations were found, but it was surprising to elicit comparable material in a strictly rural group. Further probing on the subject of batteries, ways of charging them and fuel used for the machines, brought on a great display of information about drugs, psychic energizers and mood enhancing substances. The sources were traced back mostly to popular magazines and television. It certainly became apparent that most members of the group felt great admiration for the fast life style of the jet-set beautiful people exalted by mass media all over the world.

Perhaps this is a good moment to reflect on the overpowering stereotype of a glamorous hedonistic-narcisistic life style predicated on the use of intoxicants and consciousness-altering drugs and sustained by gigantic business enterprises of a truly multinational scope built for the production and (illegal) distribution of such substances. It is conceivable that the impact of the massive multi-media promotion of such trade may contribute, as a "great equalizer", to modifying the discrete qualities of the "modal national character" and to generating a new and ubiquitous subculture found, at least in its explicit aspects, everywhere in the "global village". On the other hand, the phantasmagoria evoked by psychedelic drugs seem to have facilitated the emergence of forces that were once repressed but are now activated and beginning to rise with a vengeance. In fact, we seem to be amidst a wave of ever increasing interest and involvement in magic, the supernatural, the occult, the esoteric, eastern mysticism and all of their variants, approximations and substitutes.

The recent upsurge in Colombia of cases of persecution and possession by evil spirits afforded us a unique opportunity to explore certain pathways of expression of psychopathology which are sanctioned by tradition and adopt a cultural mold outlined by community forces (León, 1976). Witness, the case of Ursulina, a 14-year-old girl, orphan, living with her aunt and uncle, who suffered the persecution of a "duende".* It started with throwing of rocks and noise-making, but very soon progressed to physical and sexual attack, which culminated in raping and constant harassing and assault.

The relatives first approached the parish priest who advised them to go to the bishop and ask him to appoint an exorcist for the case. The bishop sent two nuns to investigate, which made the "duende" furious and his attacks doubled in intensity. It was decided that Ursulina should go to confession and communion, but that night all hell broke loose: the "duende" dragged her by the hair through the house; he whipped, scratched and bit her all over and never ceased to torment her with threats and blasphemies throughout the night. She was in such a state the following morning that the priest refused to confess her and urged her relatives to take her to the psychiatric hospital. At the hospital, the case was diagnosed as one of temporal lobe epilepsy and put on anticonvulsive medication. She stayed for 20 days and experienced a gradual disappearance of her troubles, but they began again shortly after returning home. In desperation, her relatives took her to a brotherhood of spiritists and a new and fascinating chapter opened to her life. The leader of the group explained to all present that the girl had extraordinary qualities as a medium and proceeded through a series of séances to instruct her in the ways to communicate with the spirit world, seeking contact with spirits of light and building a "protective shield" against evil spirits.

The group was impressed with her quality as a medium and she began to hold public séances. During these, she was able to go into trance and make "astral trips"; she visited several countries, the sun, the planets, and the stars. In sum, she developed great familiarity with all aspects of the spirit world and became a bona fide member of the circle of spiritists, where she worked regularly under the name of María. As time went by, spirit manifestations started to decrease and only became active during the séances; spontaneous "trances" stopped together and Ursulina felt herself free from any form of persecution. She gradually reduced the intensity of her practices, married, had a child, and for all purposes seems to be leading an uneventful, "normal" life.

In this, as in other more or less similar cases, very often there seems to be as a starting point an interpersonal conflict that gradually becomes unbearable, in a social context with no opportunities for correction or repair and a surplus of destructive emotions such as rage, fear and guilt is generated. If, in addition, because of structural damage of faulty learning, the brain is incapable of carrying on its integrative functions, dissociative states begin to occur. Dissociation affords an opportunity for symbolic expression of unacceptable feelings and the process is facilitated by the adoption of a traditional pre-established model through which inner experiences become incorporated into a culturally sanctioned pattern. The adoption of this culturally determined pattern is first stimulated and facilitated and later reinforced by group beliefs and interpretations. It can also be modified and re-channeled for therapeutic purposes provided that the therapeutic interactions occur within a shared and meaningful cultural frame, such as seen in the spiritist group practices.

One of the hard-to-die myths about mental disorders is their supposed scarcity among populations of primitive and developing countries. Clear evidence on the contrary notwithstanding (Murphy, 1976), there is still heated controversy about the matter. Several studies conducted in Colombia and other Latin American countries (Rotondo *et al.*, 1963; León, 1967; León *et al.*, 1970; Adis-Castro *et al.*, 1970; Micklin and León, 1976) show rates of mental disorder comparable to those in developed countries. In fact, one study conducted in a semirural location showed prevalence figures similar to those found in mid-Manhattan (León *et al.*, 1970). Furthermore, surveys of the general population with standard questionnaires such as the Health Opinion Survey (León and Climent, 1970) and the Langner 22 items (Micklin-León, 1978) revealed that our informants scored higher than other surveyed populations. These findings are in keeping with studies conducted in Latin American populations (Langner, 1962, 1965; Dohrenwend, 1966; Fabrega and Wallace, 1967; Haberman, 1976). The important and, so far, not definitely answered question is whether our informants do indeed have more pathology or are just more expressive and show a higher disposition to admit the presence of symptoms. Expressive behaviour has been traditionally considered to be a cultural characteristic. Dr. Clouston, a Scottish physician and quoted by William James (James, 1927), regarded (North) Americans as "too expressive", which is to say using-up all their reserves, vis-à-vis the "cold, detached, stolid attitude of the British". Now, for any Latin-American observer, it would be the North Americans who appear "cold and detached" compared to their neighbours of the south. In a meeting to prepare a glossary for certain terms used in the International Pilot Study on Schizophrenia, a British psychiatrist characterized expressive behaviour as "something foreigners do".

A unique opportunity for observing the interaction of personal and cultural factors and the effects of transculturation was offered by the study of a series of (North) American housewives who developed psychiatric disorders while living in Cali, Colombia (León, 1963b). Their core symptoms were anxiety, boredom, somatic complaints, feelings of guilt, worthlessness, insomnia, irritability and suicidal ideation. Since these symptoms were found in almost all cases regardless of other clinical characteristics, it was tempting to call the picture "a syndrome of American housewives in Latin America . . . " All of the patients dated the onset of problems at the time they left their country of origin and those who had lived in other countries previously experienced an exacerbation of symptoms in Colombia. Several factors could be identified as associated with the problems, among which the most important seemed to be: lack of information about the country, failures in communication (i.e., the absurd expectation that people should be able to speak English), drastic changes in the domestic situation (i.e., the opportunity to have servants), change in martial relations, changes in social level, keeping a fictitious identity and a deficit of inner resources. A very frequent complaint was not knowing what to do with all the available time, which led to guilt, self-reproach and all sorts of miscarried repairs, such as alcoholism and abuse of hypnotics. Although they invariably perceived themselves as inferior or worthless at an individual level, they seemed able to gain some relief from these feelings by degrading and despising the local culture and thinking of themselves, as a group, as more "civilized", "cleaner", "honest", "industrious" and, above all, "richer". Eventually, in the course of therapy, some patients developed a negative identity with their culture and decided to "go native". The patient-doctor relationship was punctuated by strong feelings of ambivalence, a constant need to degrade the therapist, suspiciousness and distrust explicitly related to the fact that the therapist was a Latin American. On basis of the observation that the severity of symptoms was higher in patients unable to speak the local language, a therapeutic strategy was built by encouraging them to take daily language classes. This, and the finding that engaging in voluntary social work was clinically beneficial, led us to clearly correlate a good outcome with increased proficiency in Spanish and active participation in voluntary work of a humanitarian nature.

In regard to outcome of mental disorders as possibly related to socio-cultural factors, one of the most remarkable findings of the International Pilot Study on Schizophrenia is that on the average patients in centres located in developing countries (Agra, Cali, Ibadan) had a better course and outcome over a two-year period than those in developed countries (Sartorius *et al.*, 1977; WHI, 1979). Approximately 67% of patients in developing countries had a favourable outcome, compared to 41% in the industrially developed countries. Analysis of the available data reveals that the total variance is explained only in a small proportion by factors usually studied as predictors. It has been suggested that the "predictors identified in European and North American cultures are not necessarily relevant to other cultures" (Sartorius, 1977). This emphasizes the need to search for appropriate socio-cultural variables as possible predictors. Follow-up studies at five and ten years and an ongoing specially designed study on the Determinants of Course and Outcome of Severe Mental Disorders in Different Socioeconomic Settings (WHO, 1977) may offer further elucidation of the problem. My personal feeling is that key factors for recovery and a favourable outcome in our population may be a high degree of family cohesion and cultural tolerance for mental disorders.

In a survey conducted in Cali (Micklin and León, 1972), to evaluate the tolerance of the general population for mental disorders, informants were asked: "If a person becomes mentally ill (loco) and gets well after being treated at the Psychiatric Hospital, once he is discharged, would you accept him (a) as your next door neighbour; (b) as a work-mate; (c) as your spouse?" The responses showed a clear pattern of acceptance with variation according to the degree of social interaction involved. Ninety-four percent of respondents would accept the ex-patient as next door neighbour, 87% as work-mate and 40% as spouse. These proportions are higher at all levels of interaction than those found in other similar studies. Comparable findings were obtained from a sample of relatives of patients seen at the time of their initial examination at the Psychiatric Hospital and again eighteen months later (Micklin and León, 1977). It is important to notice that even among a group of respondents who recently had a direct experience with a mentally ill relative, about 75% of them did not show a more stigmatizing view of the mentally ill on the follow-up. A closer look of the data revealed that, in most cases, changing reactions to the mentally ill were related to conditions surrounding the illness itself, rather than to largely unalterable characteristics of the reactor. The results suggest that programs emphasizing treatments that do not involve hospitalization, that deal effectively with reducing disruptive behaviour and that encourage patients to continue treatment, will generate greater acceptance of the mentally ill.

Having presented a somewhat scattered vista of some of the issues related to culture and health as glimpsed at in the course of personal and professional experience, I would like to sketch a few intuitive insights shaped through consensual validation.

First and foremost, one must realize that both the way in which people experience mental disorders and how they express them vary according to characteristics of the culture. From this it follows that in order to identify and treat a condition adequately, there is a need to understand the cultural context in which it occurs. To this we add that isolated efforts of a single discipline are painfully insufficient for grasping the complex problem of transmission of experiential and behavioural patterns and their role in health and disease. Mental health cannot possibly be the province of one profession or even of one type of profession. There is need for a broad and intensive interdisciplinary effort to reach this goal.

Secondly, one must recognize that the emphasis of scientific medicine seems to have been consistently placed on disease and symptoms rather than on development of individual potentials and better ways of coping or adapting. Alternative approaches such as those practiced by traditional and other types of healers may make better use of human potentials and even enhance them. They also seem to make full use of group forces sustained by credibility derived from culturally meaningful and relevant interventions. The understanding of these mechanisms and their eventual incorporation into current therapeutic practices may be a significant contribution to mental health care.

Thirdly, even admidst the severe material limitations that characterize life in the developing countries, there may be some active cultural forces that help to mitigate the impact of mental disorders. There is a great need for studies focusing on cultural tolerance, coping ability and the role of social networks, as well as for the substitution of local theoretical models for theoretical models which ignore cultural realities.

Finally, there seems to be a need to share mutual experiences and to engage in close technical co-operation. Such co-operation will help all to overcome undesirable hegemonies and to reach new insight and self-determination.

Apartado Aereo 1418,
Cali, Columbia

NOTE

* El "duende" is an incubus in the form of a goblin, quite prevalent in Latin America. For a comprehensive description see León, 1975.

REFERENCES

Adis-Castro, G., Hernandez, R., Viquez, C., and Alvarenga, F.
1970 Prevalencia de problemas de salud mental en Costa Rica. En Mariategui, J. y Adis-Castro, G. (eds.). Epidemiología Psiquiátrica en América Latina.

Dohrenwend, B. P.
1966 Social Status and Psychological Disorder: An Issue of Substance and Issue of Method. American Sociological Review 31: 14–34.

Dunham, H. W.
1976 Society, Culture and Mental Disorder. Arch. Gen. Psychiat. 33: 147–157.

Fabrega, H. and Wallace, C. H.
1967 Working Class Mexican Outpatients. Arch. Gen. Psychiat. 16: 704–12.

Gillin, J.
1956 El temor magico en la cultura indigena de Guatemala. Ensayos en Antropologia Social, Ministerio de Educacion, Guatemala.

Haberman, P.
1970 Ethnic Differences in Psychiatric Symptoms Reported in Community Surveys. Public Health Reports 85: 495–502.

James, W.
1927 Selected Papers on Philosophy, E. P. Dutton & Co., New York.

Langner, T. S.
1962 A Twenty-Two Item Screening Score of Psychiatric Impairment. Journal of Health and Social Behaviour 3: 269–276.

1965 Psychophysiological Symptoms and the Status of Women in Two Mexican Communities. In: J. M. Murphy and A. H. Leighton (eds.). Approaches to Transcultural Psychiatry. Ithaca, N.Y. Cornell University Press, pp. 360–392.

León, C. A.

1963a El espanto: Sus implicaciones psiquiátricas. Acta Psiquiat. Psicol. Arg. 9: 207–217.

1963b Problemas adaptativos de un grupo de amas de casa norteamericanas en Latinoamérica. Acta Psiquiat. y Psicol. Argent. 9: 114–121.

1967 Prevalencia de trastornos mentales en un sector urbano de Cali. Revista Colombiana de Psiquiatrían 2: 24–36.

1975. "El Duende" and Other Incubi – Suggestive Interactions Between Culture, the Devil and the Brain. Arch. Gen. Psychiat. 32: 155–162.

1981 Investigadores "descalzos": Papel de estudiantes rurales como promotores de salud mental en un estudio de prevalencia. Bol. Of. San. PanAm. 90(5): 377–385.

León, C. A., Climent, C., Estrada, H., and Jaramillo, R.

1970 Assessment of Instruments for Studying the Prevalence of Mental Disorders. Soc. Psychiat. 5: 212–215.

Lewis, O.

1966 La Vida (P. XLIV, LI) Random House, New York.

Mead, M.

1959 Mental Health in World Perspective. In: M. K. Opter (ed.). Culture and Mental Health, The MacMillan Co., New York.

Micklin, M. and León, C. A.

1972 Rechazo al enfermo mental en una cuidad sudamericana: Un análisis comparativo. Acta Psiquiat. Psicol. Amer. Lat. 18: 321–329.

1976 Perceptions of the Distribution of Mental Disorder in a South American City. Sociol. Work Occup. 3: 273–302.

1977 The Stability of Reactions to the Mentally Ill. Presented to the VI Congress of Psychiatry Honolulu, August 28, September 3, 1977.

Micklin, M., Durbin, M., and León, C. A.

1974 The Lexicon for Madness in a Colombian City: An Exploration in Semantic Space. Am. Ethnologist 1: 143–156.

Murphy, J. M.

1976 Psychiatric Labeling in Cross-Cultural Perspective. Science 191: 1019–1028.

Rotondo, H., Aliaga, P., and García, C.

1963 Estudios de morbilidad psiquiátrica en la población urbana de Mendocita. En: Caravedo, B., Rotondo, H., Mariategui, J. (eds.), Estudios de Psiquiátria Social en el Perú. Ediciones Sol, Lima.

Rubel, A. J.

1969 El susto en Hispanoamérica. Caribbean Studies 13(4): 457–76. Universidad de Puerto Rico.

Sal y Rosas, F.

1958 El mito del Jani o susto de la medicina indigena peruana. Rev. Sanidad Polic. 18(3): 167–210.

Sartorius, N., Tableusky, A., and Shapiro, R.

1977 Two Year Follow-Up of the Patients Included in the WHO International Pilot Study of Schizophrenia. Psychol. Med. 7: 529–541.

Soddy, K. and Ahrenfeldt, R. H. (eds.)

1967 Mental Health in a Changing World (Vol. I) Mental Health and Contemporary Thought (Vol. II) Mental Health in the Service of the Community (Vol. III) Tavistock, London.

Thomas, C.

1981 View from the Corner of the Eye. Discover 2: 68–69.

Yap, P. M.
1967 Classification of the Culture-Bound Reactive Syndromes. Austr. New Zeal. J. Psychiat. 1: 172–179.
World Health Organization
1977 Medium Term Mental Health Programme of the World Health Organization 1975–1982 (Project 04–01–05). WHO (Offset publication).
1979 Schizophrenia. – An International Follow-Up Study. John Wiley & Sons, Chichester.

Discussant: JOHN SPIEGEL, M.D. (U.S.A.)

MENTAL HEALTH AND CULTURE

Dr. León presented us with a series of vignettes as concrete examples of how one delivers mental health services and how one is influenced by and collaborates with a set of beliefs and perceptions which are culturally molded. This leads me to a criticism. Too often, at this conference, we have heard vast and somewhat empty generalizations about the state of the world as it applies to the mental health movement. Some of these generalizations have been full of doom and gloom – the world is going to pieces and poverty is spreading all over the place and we will never have enough resources and we have to be terribly, terribly concerned. That raises our anxiety and, although anxiety sometimes moves people to action, sometimes it moves them to inaction. On the other hand, some of the generalizations we have heard have been full of promise. As Dr. Pierce said yesterday, we know enough. All we have to do is roll up our sleeves and apply ourselves, and we will be able to put the mental health movement forward wherever we are working. We have swung between pessimism and optimism at this conference. What I have missed are concrete examples of what you do for wherever you are in relation to whatever culture you are working in. I thought that Dr. León's examples of what he has done and what he has experienced are the kind of examples that we need, so that we can function in a way to advance things, particularly in under-developed countries. I admired Dr. León's reference to his own experience as a child in the treatment of "susto", that is, his experiencing "susto", which is the loss of soul, and his treatment by a native healer, the "limpiadora". This personal experience is extremely important, so that we know the sort of background from which the person delivering mental health services in a cultural context comes.

At Harvard University and at Brandeis University in Boston, Massachusetts, I teach a course in culture and mental health, ethnic groups and mental health. I also have a training program for mental health professionals, mostly WASPs, to deal with the subcultural ethnic groups that exist in the Boston area. These consist of Hispanics from Puerto Rico and Central America, Haitians, Portuguese newly arrived from the Azores, of some newly arrived Italians, and various other what we call "ethnic" groups, whom one cannot deal with through the standard pattern of training, which is based upon psychodynamic principles. I am attempting to provide trainees with a specific knowledge of the culture of the homeland from which these people have emigrated and I insist upon several things. One is that they learn the language. If they're dealing with people from Portugal, they must learn Portuguese. If they're dealing with Hispanics, they should learn Spanish.

The other thing I do in my training program, right from the very beginning,

Richard C. Nann, Dorcas Susan Butt, and Lourdes Ladrido-Ignacio (eds.), Mental Health, Cultural Values and Social Development, 52–59.

for not only my trainees but also students taking my course in mental health and ethnicity, is to insist they begin by talking about their own cultural background, by talking about their family history, by talking about how they grew up, so that they can see for themselves and we, the others, can see how it is that they hold certain attitudes, that they hold certain biases, that they have certain belief systems. As Dr. León told us, his personal experience as a child gave him a sensitivity to cultural differences and an acceptance of alternative methods of healing, particularly those provided by native healers. This turns out to be a very difficult thing to ask people to do. It's embarassing in the large group for someone to get up and say, "Well, I was a black born in the south and I had certain of these experiences". Or, "I am from Central America" or "I'm from Puerto Rico". Even those members of the class who are Jewish find it difficult, and they usually feel that everybody knows what it is to be Jewish because we have so many films, so many books, so many things about Jewish life in the United States that they don't need to explain it. Nevertheless, even they are sometimes embarassed and sometimes refuse. I had one student who said, "I spent three years in psychoanalysis overcoming that, and now you're asking me to go back into it". I begin to model how one can do this by telling about my own childhood, by telling how I was born into a Jewish family – the only Jewish family in an all-Gentile, all-WASP little town outside of Chicago – and always feeling like outsiders, living in this all-non-Jewish community, and I always felt I had to cross cultural boundaries. That sensitized me, as a psychiatrist, to the differences because I always felt different. Not unaccepted, because being the only Jewish family in this community, we were not feared – there was not going to be any Jewish invasion – but nevertheless I always felt that.

From the point of view of religion, which I also want to bring up today, a very peculiar thing happened in my family. Although we were Jewish, my family became Christian Scientists. I don't know how many of you here know what the religion of Christian Science is, but it happened this way. My oldest brother had a severe head injury and he was taken to the most prominent hospital in the area. The doctors said, "If this boy is lucky he will die, because if he lives, he will either be an idiot or he will be completely paralyzed". It so happened that my mother had a friend who was a Christian Scientist, who have what they call absent healers. You put the absent healer – he doesn't need to see the patient – on the case, and he prays and thinks the right thoughts and so forth, for the person who is sick, and if successful, the healing takes place even though at a great distance, almost as if by magic. Well, at any rate, the diagnosis was wrong. My brother didn't die, my brother wasn't paralyzed, my brother wasn't an idiot. It was just a misdiagnosis and I think if it had happened today, my family would have sued the doctor for malpractice. But, as a result of this experience, they became Christian Scientists, and so I was raised to believe that people can be healed if they only think correctly, that the healing takes place in the mind through a process of correct thought.

Later, because of my interest in science, I decided to be a doctor, and when I told my family this they climbed the walls, because Christian Scientists are not even supposed to see a doctor, and here they had a son who was going to be one. But it helped a little bit when I said, finally, that I was going to be a psychiatrist, because at least that had something to do with the mind. At any rate, I do tend to model such experiences from my own personal life for the students to help them be more forthcoming about their own ethnic and family background, and how that influences their own attitudes. One of the things I've missed at this conference, if I go down my list of critical reactions, is the fact that people who have stood up and talked and made contributions, have not said enough about their own ethnic and religious backgrounds. People will say "I'm from Africa", "I'm from Zambia", I'm from this, I'm from that, "I'm Malaysian", Indonesian, whatever, but that doesn't tell us very much unless they also tell us – a member of what subcultural group in that country, what religion, a little something, so that we can know more about them than just their overall national characteristics. That is the first point from Dr. León's paper. The second is his willingness to invent or use alternative methods based upon the native belief system. The way he treated the person who had been captured by the rainbow spirit was a very clever and very innovative way of proceeding. But the point I want to make here – the general point – is that Dr. León acted as his own anthropologist. He did not really know the origin of the rainbow spirit, or the cure for the rainbow spirit but, nevertheless, he had the courage not only to use his medical training, but also to go out and ask the elders of the tribe "How is this thing, how does it happen, and what is the way to cure it?" He then had the courage, having gotten this information, to innovate, to institute some sort of a procedure that would be within the thought system, within the belief system, within the values of the person from a somewhat different culture, in his own country.

In my training program, we also have the opportunity to do that. In fact, we need to do that because of the nature of the people from the Azores, from the Caribbean, and so forth who have belief systems that are not in accordance with mainstream Boston belief systems. I want to give two or three examples of just how this happens within our own classical university teaching system in Boston, Massachusetts. We had a black patient from the Caribbean islands who had a delusional system. She was quite psychotic. She had the delusion that someone had driven a spike through her vagina, it had come out through her head and she had a hole on top of her head, and nothing could be done for her until this hole had healed. She thought it had been done as a result of a curse placed upon her in her native island due to the fact that her father's body was buried incorrectly. I don't remember all the details now about the particular burial ritual way, but she would not respond to any form of medication or psychotherapy as long as she was under the influence of this belief system. Now, what do you do? In the past, we have collaborated with native healers if the native healer was also a part of the community, as is the case for Puerto Ricans. But, how could we deal with a black woman from the Caribbean who was really isolated from her community? We could not find a native healer from that particular island, but we did locate a black root worker. Root workers from black communities in the south are like native healers in many respects. We managed to find a young, intelligent person who was a root worker, the black form of native healer, brought him into the house, and told him about this woman's condition. He did the research on the belief system in her native island and familiarized himself with how it needed to be corrected, how the particular things around the grave needed to be restored and various ritual methods to be corrected in order for her to be relieved of the curse that had been placed upon her. To bring this root worker into the hospital to deal with an inpatient, we had to overcome the resistance of the department – even, the Chairman of the Department of Psychiatry. But, because I happen to have some clout, having been President of the American Psychiatric Association, I said this was the only way to proceed and we brought the root worker in, he conferred with the patient, and convinced her that all these things about the burial were going to be corrected. The patient did not then entirely lose her delusional system, but she no longer was strongly under its influence. We were then able to talk to her about the interpersonal problems in the family and problems she had at home. The delusional system was a response to interpersonal problems that she had in the community at Boston, but until we could correct that delusional system, we could not even get her attention to talk about these local interpersonal problems. So, that's an example of how we had to perform as our own anthropologist in order to start helping persons within their own belief system.

Another example has to do with a Portuguese girl. We have discovered, as a part of our anthropological research, that if a young woman's mother dies (or father – but particularly mother), it is routine and expected that she will experience an auditory or visual hallucination of her mother's presence. So strong is this expectation that sometimes, if a young woman does not have such an hallucination, she is seen as an unfeeling, uncaring child, not sufficiently grief-stricken. We were presented with a case in which a young woman, whose mother had died about a year previously, had jumped out of a window. Fortunately, it was on the first floor of an apartment building, it was the summer-time and the window was open, and she did herself no great harm. Nevertheless, she was brought into the emergency room as a suicide. She said the reason that she jumped out of the window was because she saw her mother standing on the street, and her mother said: "Come here, I want to talk to you." She went out the window. Now, our question was: Is this really a suicide or is this what a person under the influence of Portuguese belief, Azorean belief system, would ordinarily do? How do you make such a differential diagnosis with respect to what is a psychopathology or what is a norm of a particular culture? Here again we had to function as our own anthropologist. We went to her relatives, we talked to various people in the communities, in the community in which she lived, the Azoreans, and we said: "Do you have to jump out of the window if your mother beckons to you because she died about a year ago", and they said, "No." You, of course, will be seeing your mother, but you don't have to jump out of the window." So the diagnosis – the differential diagnosis – was made for us. But again, we had to act as our own anthropologist.

Finally, I would like to touch on the point that Dr. León made, as have others, about spontaneity, particularly among Hispanics. It's very difficult for people trained as therapists in the Western tradition to be spontaneous, as you know. We tend to be restrained, not to say much about ourselves, to ask the patient or the client a lot of questions. If the patient or the client asks us questions, we say, "No, we ask the questions, you don't ask the questions." We are technically proficient at what we do; we are not supposed to act like just any person. But, because we are working with Hispanics, part of our training system is that, if a therapist is going to be working with Hispanic patients, he or she has to be willing to be somewhat spontaneous. We were presented with a Puerto Rican woman who suffered from depression and a cultural syndrome known as ataqué. I don't know if ataqué occurs here in the Philippines, but among Hispanics, ataqué is something like an epileptic fit. A person becomes very active, sometimes very violent, and then falls down unconscious and later doesn't remember what happened. In this patient, it had not responded either to medication – it wasn't epilepsy – nor to psychotherapy. Finally, the patient was brought to us, because we were running this cultural program, to talk it over with a trainee who spoke Spanish.

We decided to try two things with this patient. One was a paradoxical technique. As you know, paradoxical techniques are becoming more popular in the United States, particularly with respect to family therapy, but also in individual therapy, and it involves saying something very unexpected to the patient, usually something like a task assignment. So the therapist said to this patient: "I want you to have an ataqué by the time I see you next time, you know, a week from today, and tell me all about it. Please have an ataqué." Well, of course she didn't have one. She was unable to have one under instruction because what the therapist had done was to co-opt her resistance by ordering her to have an ataqué. So she then said, "Alright, try again. I'll see you next week. Between now and next week, you'll have an ataqué and then we'll really be able to talk about it." Well, of course, the next week she didn't have an ataqué either. She'd been cured, so to speak, at least for two weeks. But that, nevertheless, did establish a certain confidence on the part of the patient in the therapist that there had been an exchange of some spontaneity and some validity with respect to the symptom. The therapist then, seeing that the woman was quite depressed, said: "Well, you haven't had an ataqué, you haven't been able to get out your feelings, why don't we stop – start jumping up and down and screaming and yelling and just having some fun?" So they both started jumping up, screaming and yelling and having some fun. You might think that was artificial spontaneity on the part of our therapist, but she was a therapist who was very easily able to exhibit such a behaviour. As a result of the spontaneous jumping up and down, screaming and yelling and hollering, the woman's depression lifted. It really did lift, and she was in a better mood. And as a result of the change of mood, she began to be able to talk about the problems in the family that were really affecting her.

Now, fourthly, I drew from Dr. León's paper a very important point to do with a woman who seemed to have a possession state, and was then identified as having a special gift and as a result of entering into the community of spiritists, became a successful medium and lost some of the symptoms – I think, all of the worst for her – of being in a possession state. With respect to this, I want to make a distinction that I don't think has been raised here before, between the "emic" and the "etic." Anthropologists, particularly the medical anthropologists, are more and more making this distinction. An emic explanation is one that occurs from within the culture, a culturally appropriate way of explaining the behaviour. An etic is the outside-of-the-culture way of explaining, particularly based upon scientific western models. Dr. Léon did begin to explain this on both grounds. He explained on an etic ground that this trance state, this possession state, that the woman was in could be the result of repressed feelings. That's the etic – outside of the culture, western scientific – way we would explain it. She probably was raised in a culture where there was a great demand for obedience, politeness and respect for parents and very little opportunity for aggression, hostility, rebellion. In the trance or possessed state, being possessed by evil and the evil probably being her angry feelings, inside her, she was able to release her feelings in the poltergeist sort of fashion. That's an etic, an explanation from outside of the system based upon our western psychodynamic ideology. But it could also be explained, as I think he described, from within the system as this woman possessing a special gift. It isn't everybody who can go into a trance, be invaded by outside spirits and, therefore, be in touch with the spirit world. So, from within the system, it could be identified in a positive way. Because it was dealt with as a gift, that gift was transformed into something that made a contribution, both to the individual and to the community.

Dr. León has also raised a question, both with respect to this case and another. What is it that cures? And, how can we tell what it is that cures? I would like to propose an answer to this because I've also had some of those same experiences. What is it that cures? Is it that we are so clever in providing culturally appropriate experiences, or because some of our patients are seeing native healers? I have to say that we have found that Puerto Ricans are quite apt to be seeing us, the psychotherapists, at the same time they're seeing native healers. Where health is concerned, one wants to use everything there is in the system, and so one plays all sides of the street. We have no criticism of those people who want to use our way of working and, also, combine it with that of a native healer. But, how do you answer the question of what it is that helps? As in the first case I described, we found that if we started with native healing methods and removed what it was that was making the patient ill in an unrecoverable way, we could then follow it with our psychotherapy. I have the feeling that both systems work, that is, something from within the native belief system together with something from without. As to which it is that really helps, I don't think we have to make that decision now. I call it the relativity of knowledge. I don't claim for any of my students or any of the people who work with me that we know everything from the etic, or western point of view. There are more things in heaven and earth than are considered by our knowledge, as Shakespeare said. So, I accept both the explanations that come from within the culture and the explanations that come from outside as appropriate, my preposition being only that we have to understand both from within and from without and try to put those two systems together. This, I thought, was at the core of Dr. León's presentation.

I think my discussion has gone on too long. But, I do want to raise one question about religion, because we have heard so little of it. We are here in the Philippines, which has been conquered by the Spanish, the English, the Americans and has had several different layers of culture imposed upon it. I was hoping that we would learn what it was like to be a member of one of the ethnic groups and how the religious component in this country is put together. Is it integrated or is it not integrated? I would like to give you one example that comes from our own experience with the Catholic religion at home. We deal with Irish Catholics and Italian Catholics, and we have found out there's more than one version of the Catholic religion. We say, and in order to make this very simplified – over-simplified – the Irish have their fast days and the Italians have their feast days. That's the difference between them. The Irish version of Catholicism is very strict, with a very sharp recognition of sin and temptation. Whereas, Italians take it easy, a little here, a little there, and a mixture of both. This makes a difference medically and that's why I'm asking about how it is in the Philippines. We find that the Irish are very reluctant to talk to you about their symptoms. They're stoical, they don't tell you if they have pain, and you have to work very hard to get the story of their illness from them. Why? They're not stoical simply because of courage, although they do have a lot of courage. They're stoical because they believe that illness is a result of God's punishment for their sins. For Italians, it's just the opposite. Ask an Italian about how he got sick or what happened, you'll get a story that goes on for half an hour. Thus, the particular version of the Catholic religion makes a difference in how one begins a relationship with a patient.

I would hope that at this Congress, we could learn more about what happens in the Philippines, particularly with respect to the Philippine version of the Catholic religion. I would also hope that, in the future when we hold Congresses like this, they could be more specific, more comparatively cultural about the countries in which they are being held and about the countries that are being discussed, because comparative services based on culture are something we need to know about.

Florence Heller School,
Brandeis University,
415 South Street,
Waltham, Massachusetts,
U.S.A. 02154

AYO BINITIE, MD, DPM, MRC Psych, FMC Psych, FWACP (Nigeria)

MENTAL HEALTH AND THE THIRD WORLD: MENTAL HEALTH IN AFRICAN SOCIETIES

> Life is the gift of nature
> But beautiful living is the gift of wisdom
> GREEK ADAGE

MENTAL HEALTH AS A PROPOSITION

The term "mental health" is of comparatively recent origin in medicine and related disciplines, but it has always been the concern of philosophers. The concept of Utopia by Plato (427–437 BC) in the Republic is an attempt to construct and develop optimal social conditions for the development of mental health. Aristotle (384–322 BC) defined the soul thus:

> The soul is the entire vital principle of any organism, the sum of its powers and processes. In plants the soul is merely a nurtritive and reproductive power; in man it is as well the power of thought. The soul as the sum of the powers of the body cannot exist without it; the two are as form and wax, separable only in thought but in reality one organic whole . . .

He then postulated the conditions for mental health, recognizing that the aim of life is happiness:

> For we chose happiness for itself and never with a view to anything further. Whereas we choose honour, pleasure, intellect . . . because we believe that through them we shall be made happy.

Aristotle went on to a prescription for happiness. Assuming that physical necessities were available, he suggested that *reason* was the royal road to happiness since virtue, self-control, clear judgement, etc. were dependent on reason, and for reason to achieve its purpose, it must pursue its objectives with moderation – "the golden mean".

After the Greeks came the Romans. They were practical, imperialistic, men of action who borrowed their philosophies from Plato and Aristotle. The legacy of Roman civilization is not philosophy but law, administration and public construction. Nevertheless, in so far as the Romans maintained and translated into Latin many of the Greek works, we are their debtors for the work of preservation they so ennobled.

In the middle ages the direction of philosophy following the break up of the Roman Empire concerned the nature of divinity, and the Bible became the foundation of philosophical thought. The Renaissance (14–18 cc.) witnessed the return to Greek and Roman literature and gave birth to a flowering of ideas in all fields of human endeavour – architecture, science, art, engineering and

Richard C. Nann, Dorcas Susan Butt, and Lourdes Ladrido-Ignacio (eds.), Mental Health, Cultural Values and Social Development, 61–77.

literature. Philosophy was not left behind. Francis Bacon was an important landmark in this field. His contribution to mental health was in the form of observations on nature and intellect:

> Nature is often hidden, sometimes overcome, seldom extinguished. Force maketh nature more violent in the return doctrine and discourse maketh nature less importune; but custom only doth alter or subdue nature . . . But let not man trust his victory over his nature too far, for nature will lay buried a great time and yet revive upon the occasion or temptation.

Philosophy is concerned, among other things, with the ultimate reality and thus, with the nature and form of the human mind and its performance in health. In this task, it studies mind and matter, examining it through reasoning and then goes on to study the inherent nature of reasoning itself. In the process, valuable insights into the functioning of the mind have emerged.

Belief in God has little moral value unless accompanied by belief in an immortality of punishment and reward. As Voltaire said " . . . for the common people a rewarding and avenging God is necessary. If God did not exist it would be necessary to invent him." Man, according to him, is by nature a beast of prey and civilized society means a chaining of this beast, a mitigation of his brutality and the possibility of the development through social order, of the intellect and its joys.

To Helvetus (1715–1771), all action is dictated by egoism. Conscience is not the voice of God, but the fear of the police; it is the deposit left in us from the stream of prohibitions poured over the growing soul by parents, teachers and the press.

Rousseau said: "I venture to declare that a state of reflection is contrary to nature, and that a thinking man is a depraved animal." It would be better to abandon our over-rapid development of the intellect and to aim at training the heart and the affections. Education does not make a good man; it can only make him clever – usually for mischief. Instinct and feeling are more trustworthy than reason.

Writing in his "Treatise on Human Nature" David Hume (1711–1778) stated that we know the mind only as we know matter by perception, though in this case it is internal. Never do we perceive any such entity as the "mind": we perceive merely separate ideas, memories, feelings, etc. The mind is not a substance, an organ that has ideas; it is only an abstract name for the series of ideas. Perceptions, memories and feelings are the mind; there is no observable soul behind the process of thought.

"If we go back to the beginning", says Holbach, "we shall find that ignorance and fear created the gods; that fancy enthusiasm or deceit adorned or disfigured them; that weakness worships them; that credulity preserves them and that custom respects and tyranny supports them in order to make the blindness of men serve its own interests."

The mind of man is not a passive wax upon which experience and sensation write their absolute and yet whimsical will, nor is it a mere abstract name for the series or group of mental states. It is an active organ which molds and co-ordinates sensations into ideas, an organ which transforms the chaotic multiplicity of experience into the ordered unity of thought.

Kant's prescription for mental health may be stated as follows:

The only thing unqualifiedly good in this work is goodwill – the will to follow the moral law, regardless of profit or loss for ourselves. Never mind your happiness; do your duty. Morality is not properly the doctrine of how we can make ourselves happy, but how we can make ourselves worthy of happiness. Let us seek the happiness in others; but for ourselves, perfection – whether it brings us happiness or pain. To achieve perfection in oneself and happiness in others, to treat humanity whether in oneself or in another as an end, never only as a means – this too we feel is part of the categorical imperative. Let us live up to such principles and we shall soon create an ideal community of rational beings.

If mere worldly utility and expediency were the justification for virtue, it will not be wise to be too good. And yet knowing all this, having it flung into our faces with brutal repetition, we still feel the command to righteousness; we know we ought to do the inexpedient good.

POLITICS AND MENTAL HEALTH

It is not only philosophers who have tried to produce an elixir for mental health. The recipe for the enjoyment of mental health is elusive and highly desirable and politicians and political theoreticians, aware of this great need, have attempted to provide a solution. Since Plato's *Republic*, many people have tried to produce a structure for this ideal state, or Utopia, such as Francis Bacon in his "New Atlantis".

> There reigned in this island about nineteen hundred years ago a king whose memory above others we most adore ... His name was Solomon, and we esteem him as the Law-Giver of our nation. This king had a large heart and was wholly bent to make his kingdom and people happy.

Among the excellent acts of that king, one had pre-eminence. It was the creation and institution of the order or society which he called Solomon's House; "the noblest foundation, as we think that was ever upon the earth; and the lantherne of this kingdom". There is not to be found a passage more eminently distinguished by profound and serene wisdom. Bacon pointed out that in this ideal state there are no politicians, only those who have travelled the road of scientific repute sit in the councils of the state. This was government by technicians, architects, astronomers, philosophers and psychologists who were concerned with controlling the forces of nature and expanding the cause of knowledge.

The early citizens of the United States of America, plagued by British imperialism and hampered by the British Crown, were forced to make a stand. On

July 4th, 1778 one of their great leaders, Thomas Jefferson, made a declaration that is now a classic.

We hold these truths to be self-evident: that all men are created equal; that they are endowed by their Creator with certain inherent and inalienable rights; that among these are life, liberty and the pursuit of happiness; that to secure these rights, governments are instituted among men, deriving their just powers from the consent of the governed; that whenever any form of government becomes destructive of these ends, it is the right of the people to alter or abolish it and to institute new government, laying its foundation on such principles and organizing its powers in such form, as to them shall seem likely to effect their safety and happiness.

The sentiments that led to the Declaration of Independence moved the writers of the American constitution to include certain provisions for the common good. The preamble to the U.S. constitution states:

We the People of the United States in order to form a more perfect Union, establish justice, ensure domestic tranquility, provide for the common defence, promote the general welfare and secure the blessings of Liberty to ourselves and our posterity do ordain and establish this Constitution for the United States of America.

Marx and Engels provided the theoretical basis for another new society – a workers' utopia followed later by a people's utopia where no man would be oppressed. The contradictions of capitalism, under which private appropriation frustrates the full development of production to satisfy social needs must lead to socialism, where all means of production are public property and exploitation of man ceases. Production would now be planned to meet human needs, leading to a communist society organized on the principle "from each according to his abilities and to each according to his needs". This would mark the dawn of human freedom. Men would become masters of their own conditions of existence, no longer constrained and limited in their ideas and actions by circumstances beyond their control.

In the place of the old bourgeois society with its classes and class antagonism, we shall have an association in which free development of each is the condition for free development of all.

Encyclopedia Brittanica
Vol. 7, p. 357

You do not change the world, Marx said, by first trying to change people's ideas. It is the other way round. In so far as you are able to change the world, you are able to change man's ideas.

In Africa, politicians have not been left behind in trying to create the ideal structures for mental health. The 1978 Constitution of Federal Republic of Nigeria states:

We the People of the Federal Republic of Nigeria having firmly and solemnly resolved:

To live in unity and harmony as one indivisible and indisoluble sovereign Nation under God dedicated to the promotion of inter-African solidarity, world peace, international co-operation and understanding:

> And to provide for a constitution for the purpose of promoting the good government and welfare of all persons in our country on the principles of Freedom, Equality and Justice, and for the purpose of consolidating the Unity of our people: Do hereby make, enact and give to ourselves the following Constitution . . .

This survey shows that political leaders have been aware of the necessity of creating an atmosphere which promotes the well-being and mental health of the people under their jurisdiction. That they rarely do so, or do so only tentatively, is also a historical fact. There is often much promise but little delivery.

Early in this century, Mark Jaspers, through a systematic study of general psychopathology, determined his concept of the nature of man. Borrowing from the concept of DASEIN or Being from existential philosophy, he concluded:

> Mind and spirit somehow transcend nature and make use of the body to achieve their realization and utterance in the world as well as their own evolution. They are something separate from the body-psyche whole but they do not exist apart; they only exist in their bodily utterance. They acquire the nervous system as it were for their instrument.

Jaspers went on to describe human existence (DASEIN) " . . . we are life in a world as with everything alive. That which encompasses all living things becomes objectified in the products of that life yet – whether these are bodily form, physiological function or the universal hereditary connections of life or on the other hand, specifically human tools, deeds and constructs – life itself is never exhausted in these products but remains that which encompasses whence everything emerges."

He then described many aspects of Being. DASEIN exists as Life, as a tension between matter and form, between inner and outer world; as a SOCIAL Being, as a tension between the collective human will and the individual will, and as a THINKING Being, as a tension between subject and object, self and thing. He suggested that these different aspects of man are difficult to synthesize to produce the concept, BEING. This difficulty is a serious limitation. Jaspers, in fact, believed it cannot be done and, thus, represents the limits of analysis or infinity. Nevertheless, DASEIN exists, but is experienced only as a part: existence is only experienced as a part.

Jaspers regarded morality not as an average, but as a value-standard. This is especially true in the case of psychiatry. In order to judge normality in the psychic sphere, we have to introduce such concepts as social adjustment, capacity for happiness and contentment, integrity of personality, harmony of character traits and a constancy of them, full maturation of the human disposition, a concord of tendencies and drives. This multiplicity of parameters makes the judgement of what is normal difficult, especially when compared to events in the organic sphere.

Normality in the psychic sphere is much more dependent on the frame of reference. It is different for the poor and for the rich. In rural communities, the demands for social adjustment and social skills are much different from those in an urban, sophisticated environment. All these affect the definition of illness.

Cicero characterized health as a state of happy, mutual relationship of the different psychic states. The Epicureans found health to be complete contentment with a measured satisfaction of every need. The Stoics believed that every passion, every sentiment was an illness and their moral teaching was, to a large extent, a kind of therapy designed to destroy psychic disorders in favour of a healthy ataraxia.

The current concept of mental health as a positive state is of very recent origin. In 1908, the Connecticut Society for Mental Hygiene was created, followed in 1909 by the National Committee for Mental Hygiene. The formation of these societies was influenced by the publication of the book, "A Mind that Found Itself", written by a former patient who had suffered the indignities of restraint prevalent at that time. The aim of the movement, apart from treating established disorders in the best possible way, was to maintain public health by using the concepts of hygiene already established. This shift away from the treatment of mental disorder to maintenance of positive mental health represented an important landmark. But, such a major shift in concepts must fall on fertile ground to be effective and, in fact, a liberalizing influence was already at work. Pinel and Bicetre in Paris, Tule in England and Benjamin Rush in America were already in the vanguard of this liberalizing movement, removing the chains and shackles which bound the mentally ill and held them captive.

The term "mental health" slowly began to slip into medical literature and, finally, into legislation. Prior to this, the terms in use were Lunacy (Lunacy Act) and Asylums. In Britain, the Mental Health Act (1959) replaced the Lunacy Law. It is interesting to observe that the Act did not define mental health. Rather, it defined four categories of mentally disordered persons: the mentally ill, the severely subnormal, the subnormal and the psychopathic.

"*Mental disorder* means mental illness, arrested or incomplete development of mind, psychopathic disorder and any other disorder or disability of mind; and 'mentally disordered' shall be construed accordingly.

"*Severe subnormality* means a state of arrested or incomplete development of mind which includes subnormality of intelligence and is of such a nature or degree that the patient is incapable of living an independent life or will be so incapable when of an age to do so.

"*Subnormality* means a state of arrested or incomplete development of mind (not amounting to severe subnormality) which includes subnormality of intelligence and is of a nature or degree which requires or is susceptible to medical treatment or other special care or training of the patient.

"*Psychopathic disorder* means a persistent disorder of mind (whether or not accompanied by subnormality of intelligence) which results in abnormally aggressive or seriously irresponsible conduct on the part of the patient and requires or is susceptible to medical treatment."

The emphasis in all these definitions is on the presence of diease and, by the process of exclusion, infers that all others are mentally healthy. But are they? Consider a case where armed soldiers ravage a neighbourhood and the inhabitants realistically fear of their lives and property. It would be true to say the people are anxious, but do not suffer anxiety state, since the fears are realistic. But in fearing for the safety of themselves, their wives and children, worrying for the protection of limb and property, it would be ridiculous to say that the people of the neighbourhood are enjoying mental health. They clearly are not. Mental health involves much more than the absence of disease.

In this example, an external noxious event raises the manifest anxiety level in the neighbourhood. This, in turn, raises psychic anxiety level and sets up a reaction within the organism, leading to various types of coping responses and varying degrees of success. Some will barricade themselves indoors, purchase guns and set up alarm systems. Others may respond by forming armed vigilante groups with a view to combating the threat whenever it makes itself manifest. A few are frank victims of the raid, a few break down completely, and others move out of the area to less hostile environment.

Objectively, however, the statistics indicate that the number of persons affected is much less than one percent of the population and the proportion of people who develop mental illness less still. Nevertheless, empirically, we feel justified in our original view of the society we have described.

The implication has far-reaching consequences. Mental health is not only a private affair, but a public one as well. In the field of physical health disorders, tuberculosis is both a personal disorder as well as a public health matter. Indeed, in the case of tuberculosis, better control has been achieved by introducing public health measures, such as the tracing of contacts and better environmental sanitation. Mental health, then, involves the organism (self) and the environment. Environment includes other human beings with whom one reacts directly and indirectly, as well as the conditions of housing, water supply, food, electricity, work, climate, and so on. The 'self' is influenced by biological endowment, the will, perception, the fully developed personality, the integrity of the nervous system, the milieu interior. A definition that encompasses all these parameters of mental health must of necessity be very complicated.

Weisaeker described mental health as a capacity to fulfill the natural potential of the human lot. Rogers considers mental health as self-realization with full and harmonious integration into the community. Thomas Szasz (1971), an American psychiatrist born in 1920, set up the controversial point of view that mental illness is a myth and that madness has been manufactured by authorities. He compared today's incarceration in mental hospitals with the witch hunts of the Middle Ages. He compared the Inquisitors of old with latter-day psychiatrists. He compared Sprenger and Urammers book, the Malleus Maleficarum of 1486 (The Witches Hammer) – the handbook for recognizing witches – with modern day works of psychiatrists. He stated:

> ... The good intentions and sincerity of the speakers need not be doubted. Pope, Prince, President – each claims to be trying to help his suffering fellow man. What is chilling is that each ignores the possibility that the alleged sufferer, whether of witchcraft or of mental illness might prefer to be left alone ...

It is clear that Szasz was concerned about the possible abuses of psychiatry. But, neither psychiatrists nor the State invented madness. A schizophrenic disorder is real and occurs in all societies. What is more, all societies have indigenous names for it. Mental illness is a reality. Categories of mental illness have been identified: psychotic disorders, including schizophrenic and manic depressive psychoses, neurotic disorders, and mental subnormality. There are also borderline states, which include psychopathic disorders and personality disorders. These are a source of much controversy. The controversy becomes acrimonious when we leave the realm of individual psychopathology and move into the realm of the community. There is hardly any agreement at all in the area of community mental health. The historical reasons that lead to the development of public health measures have found parallel in psychiatry. As doctors treated individual patients, they found that some of the disorders could be prevented by greater attention to events in the community. Concrete examples of such findings include Lindemen's report on abnormal grief reaction leading to depression; such abnormal grief reaction could be prevented if the patient was assisted to do grief work. Consider the report by Kramer *et al.*, commissioned by the United States Department of Health, on racism and mental disorder.

> Racist practices undoubtedly are key factors – perhaps the most important ones – in producing mental disorders in Blacks and other under-privileged groups, in determining the place where members of these groups receive diagnosis and treatment for these disorders and in determining the quality of such clinical services. Indeed the way in which racism has affected life-style, value system, socio-economic and health status, opportunities for education, work, housing, medical care and recreation of the victimized group accounts wholly or in part for the differences reported . . . Racial stereotypes are a part of white America's world. Whites grow up with them, and we (the whites) need not feel guilty or resentful about admitting it. Racism has been so deeply rooted in our society that it will require new attitudes, new understanding, new will and new tolerance from every American black as well as white if we are to overcome it. If not, America will continue its disastrous drift in two societies separate and unequal, locked in internecine strife. (Quoted by Kramer *et al.* from World Year Book)

The frustrations resulting from such racist practices produce psychological stress, which in turn may be a key factor in the causation of various types of mental disorders. Kramer *et al.* also showed statistical differences in mortality, morbidity and poverty level between the races. If survival tables per hundred thousand are used as a measure, by age 20 differences appear between white and non-white populations, to the favour of whites. A survey of admissions to state mental hospitals shows that the rate of admission was 60 percent higher for non-whites. Birley *et al.* (1970) and Brown *et al.* (1972) showed convincingly that family life does influence the outcome in schizophrenic disorders.

Jablensky (1978) quoting a study by the World Health Organization on apartheid and mental health care found that a stressful psychosocial environment results from apartheid policies and must affect many millions of people in South Africa. Some indications can be derived from statistics on suicide, crime, arrests and convictions, and forcibly broken homes (although no controlled studies have been done).

These findings are similar to Kramer's report from the United States. Cassel and Tyroler (1961), in a study conducted in North Carolina, found that changing from a rural to an urban setting produced morbidity, as measured by the number of absences of more than three consecutive days, and concluded that first generation migrants suffered more emotional and physical disability.

Nearly all (properly investigated) cases of insanity have been found to be the result of a summation of multiple causes, effective in combination, though inadequate alone. It is this that renders all controversy between extremists of the physiogenic and psychogenic schools so futile (Lewis, 1969).

To give meaning to the concept that the mental health of a community is a subject for investigation, we must have some empirical definitions of mental health and define some indices of measuring such mental health in any community.

The characteristics of positive mental health are inner satisfaction, hopeful aspect, financial solvency in order to maintain a decent life, family and social support systems, sexual satisfaction, capacity to manage tension and social pressures, and offspring to succeed in the future.

INNER SATISFACTION

What is this inner satisfaction that is listed as a cardinal prerequisite for mental health? Inner satisfaction is not related to wealth, position in life, or prestige. It is a feeling of inner strength based on an internal knowledge that one has chosen the correct path, that one is achieving it, and one has the psychological and physical energy to maintain this state. There is the further knowledge that nothing can change this feeling. Such a complete state of inner satisfaction often occurs in highly religious persons, some poets and writers, inspired persons and mystics.

The work of Sigmund Freud has produced an understanding of this spiritual state. Freud suggested that the mind can be conceived of as having a part that is in want, which he described as the ID – another part which acts as the conscience, and that between wants and conscience, there is an ongoing battle for supremacy. One's EGO resolves this conflict and enables one to make adjustments to reality.

To illustrate the mechanism clearly, let us assume that you have an examination tomorrow. At the same time, there is the most important dance of the year in your College on the night before (i.e., tonight). Your ID will say to you, "Go to the dance, enjoy life while you are young". Your conscience or SUPER-EGO will say, "This is not good for your work and your prospects at the examination". Your EGO will decide for you whether you have done enough work to be able to go or not.

Returning to the subject of inner satisfaction and considering the example

I have just given, we will find some groups of students who experience inner satisfaction through the avoidance of dances and things of that nature. What is more, they have the energy to sustain this without any conflict. Let me hasten to say that the converse is equally true, that is, some who believe in dances so much that they are convinced they are right and are not troubled by guilty conscience because of attending a dance on a night prior to their examination. These groups enjoy inner satisfaction. This inner satisfaction is a prerequisite to mental health.

HOPEFUL ASPECT

The inner satisfaction we have described implies the righteousness of the cause and the belief that time will show one to be right. Without this, the internal feeling of happiness and satisfaction will soon give way to doubts, later dissatisfaction, and loss of inner security. Hopeful aspect is really an addition to or a component of inner satisfaction.

FAMILY AND SOCIAL SYSTEMS

The maintenance of inner satisfaction is dependent on a system of family and other social support systems. In the face of pressures from these groups, inner satisfaction would soon give way. In the case of a new religion, a new social support system is maintained through regular contact of adherents, frequent repetition and postulation of the faith, and mutual reinforcement of the new ideas. In this way, the faith is maintained and moral support assured.

FINANCIAL SOLVENCY

The importance of this is obvious. But, I would add that the important thing is not the quantity of money or resources but rather, the quantity required to maintain the program of inner satisfaction.

SEXUAL SATISFACTION

Sexuality is one of the most powerful impulses or instincts and is capable of damaging inner satisfaction unless legitimate avenues for expression are found.

OFFSPRING FOR NEXT GENERATION

One always wishes to see the work one has started continue in the next generation. It improves inner satisfaction to know that the work continues thereafter.

FLEXIBILITY TO MANAGE TENSION

Inner satisfaction is enhanced and maintained if one is able to manage stress and assault on one's beliefs and values.

Imokhai (1979), writing about Uzairue society, described the universe as seen by the people of Uzairue. He showed the hierarchical structure of the society in terms of age groups, from birth to old age and death. At the top were the elders, the intermediaries between the present generation and the departed ancestors. The ancestors in turn held communion with God. The citizens of the Uzairue saw continuity between all these forces of nature. This cosmology provides for a continuity with the living world through the elders who act as intermediaries between living citizens and the spirit world.

The immediate departed ancestors keep a watchful eye over the affairs of the present generation – they watch, protect, and guide it. They are the avenging angels for the misdemeanours of breaking taboos and violating customs. Extensive studies of the belief system of Africans have found this to be a common theme.

Radcliffe-Brown and Daryll Forde (1950), Daryll Forde (1954), Fortes and Dieterlen (1965) have published reports from various parts of Africa. They reported extensively on the Yorubas, Biris, Hausas from Nigeria; the Ashanti of the Gold Coast (Ghana); the Fon of Dahomey; the Dogon of French Sudan; Lovedu of the Transvaal; the Abeluyia of Kenya; and the Lele of Kasai. Fortes, writing on ancestor workshop, said:

> One might perhaps generalize and say that they are deemed to be primarily benevolent when social life is running its normal course, but when individual misfortune or threat to social order supervenes, then they are believed to be punitive in the interest of restoring well-being and order. In this connection, one of the more interesting ethnographic facts was the animosity usually attributed to the ghost left out in the wild. Ancestor spirits have to be brought home in the appropriate way for them to be accessible to prayer and persuasion.

We deduce from this that ancestors play an important, even crucial, role in the life of Africans. Ancestors, representing the continuity between God and man, are the agents of communion and continuity between one generation and the next. These ancestral spirits have, as representatives directly on earth, traditional priests, elders and seers who interpret their wishes and minister through appropriate sacrifices to the needs of the spirit world and, hence, to God Himself.

Ancestral spirits are not remote, impersonal gods but rather, they are a living force, omnipresent and constantly watching over the present generation. There is thus a holistic reality to the presence of ancestors within the social fabric. This living presence – albeit invisible – is the main agent for social cohesion and maintenance of law and order.

Piddington (1950) observed that in traditional societies, instead of anarchy and chaos, a well ordered social system in which tradition, taboo and the "cake of "custom" laid down certain rules which members of the community invariably obeyed. Hence arose the misconception of the savages automatically obeying the traditional rules of his society either from his own goodness of heart or because of some mystical quality of primitive social behaviour, such as group consciousness or communistic organization. This perception of the universe is maintained by the realistic misfortune that visits malleasants. The visitation of punishment by ancestors is swift and effective. There is evidence that some of it is contrived by the elders through agents such as masquerades, rituals, placing of curses, recitation of incantations, and so on. Whatever the case, psychological anxiety is created, which reinforces the prevailing social system.

There are clearly other features common to Africans. These include the skin colour and the curliness of the hair, harmony and a sense of rhythm and movement, and a common heritage derived from our previous colonial domination and subjugation, albeit by different metropolitan powers. However, all the colonizers – British, French, German, Spanish, Portuguese and Dutch – in turn derive from one great Western European tradition, and a similar European religious tradition, namely Christianity.

There have been attempts by African scholars to capture this ethos of the African. Leopold Senghor, poet, philosopher and President of Republic of Senegal, coined the term NEGRITUDE to describe this quality:

> Negritude is the sum total of the values of the civilization of the African world . . .
>
> More precisely, it was the communal warmth, the image symbol and the cosmic rhythm which instead of dividing and sterlizing, unified and made fertile.

Leopold Senghor then contrasted this African way of life with European:

> Classical European reason is analytical and makes use of the object, African reason is intuitive and participates in the object.

The ethos I have just described is primeval in the African; it is the root source of our being. It is the milieu which nourishes and permeates our existence. The influence is subtle and pervasive and mainly unconscious. It represents the psychic force in the African. This, in fact, is the racial archetype described by C. G. Jung.

Let us contrast these findings with those of Europe. The European mind is often described as materialistic and mechanistic. It is a mind that thinks in terms of cause and effect, that operates on the principle of contrast to give effect and heighten meaning.

> We are so accustomed to thinking in polar opposites – human beings are not only things male or female, good or bad but they are persons, sick or well, old or young, normal and abnormal.
>
> Margaret Mead

The God of the European is remote and distant and has nothing of the quality of the immediate presence and urgency of ancestors of the African.

He is benign and benevolent and waits patiently until the man is dead before rewarding him with hell fire or heaven. This contrasts with the spirits of ancestors who may reach out from beyond the grave to punish any wrongs. One may not lightly offend the ancestral spirits of the African.

Europeans emphasize individuality, personal responsibility and competition. Africans emphasize harmonious relationships with one's neighbours. Excessive competitiveness or success may cause jealousies and invitation to the spirits of the night to intervene. To be in harmony with one's neighbours and to know one's position in the scheme of things is an African's greatest good. Everyone has a share of power and glory in the community through the kinship networks. In European communities you may find that the millionaire's brother is a pauper. A situation like that would not be allowed in an African society.

Western European culture is an urban culture. The majority of citizens live in urban areas. African culture is still largely agrarian and rural. Western culture is characterized by large-scale organizations and high technology, to satisfy the mass of people living in a relatively small place. The technology of the Europeans can make both bread and guns rapidly and cheaply.

Just over 100 years ago, traditional African culture met in a headlong collision with Western European culture. European culture, backed by superior technology, gained ascendancy at every point of contact until slowly European culture came to be regarded as superior. At every point of contact, the ancestral spirits of the African could not protect Africans from the foreign religion and social system of the European. Ancestral spirits appeared to exert no influence whatsoever on the newcomers. Even when they violated social taboos and desecrated the holy places, the avenging spirits were powerless. The psychological and cultural basis for the protection of African societies was not understood. African culture is what we Africans do naturally. We interpret events through African contact. In religion, the European God appeared more powerful; in politics, the European system, backed by superior communications, was more successful; medicine was simpler and more efficient; technology was vastly superior; life-style was more relaxed and comfortable. Following the Protestant ethic, the European was more efficient and serious in his work; his bureaucracy was supporting and efficient; his power, all-conquering and omnipresent; his king, prince or ruler, almighty and unstoppable. Consciously and unconsciously, Africans said to ourselves, "Let us be like them, let us identify with these Europeans". African culture was in retreat and Western European culture in ascendancy. African culture has capitulated before a powerful, more materially satisfying culture. It must be stated that this change was not without struggle; stiff resistance was put up against the invaders by many princes and leaders. But, whenever necessary, the carriers of the new social order forcefully put down such rebelliousness. The places, time and factors leading to such occurrences have been recorded in the pages of history as COLONIALISM, and need not concern us here. The point is that repeated contacts over the past 100 years or so have set the pace of Westernization. As a result, although African nations have become independent, the course for Westernization has been charted and accepted as a desirable and, both by the people and their leaders. In so doing, we abandon things that we know how to do and take on things we have not yet mastered. Our roots, ethos and cosmology is African. We still see the world in our peculiarly African way but try to think, believe and see the world as European.

The choice we have made and the course we have chosen devolves the following new responsibilities towards us: a materialistic approach to the cosmos, the Protestant ethic in the context of a Christian religion. This is an important instrument in the arsenal of Westernization. As Max Weber pointed out in "Protestant Ethic and the Spirit of Capitalism", the Protestant ethic involves frugality, sobriety and efficiency, and accumulated surpluses of wealth are used to produce more wealth. It promotes individualism and competitiveness, a peculiar life-style of thinking in opposites and acting on the basis of these, good guys for wealth; bad guys for prison. Efficient worker retain, inefficient worker sack. Since there are no punishing ancestral spirits, an efficient law-enforcing agency takes the place of the avenging spirits; a technology develops on the basis of large-scale production.

This is the conscious choice we Africans have made. The evidence can be found in the budgetary provisions of any African nation. There are provisions for building schools, roads, bridges, houses, hotels, medical schools, universities and water supply. Minimal or no provisions are made for family support systems, rural agriculture, local technology or African workship. Similarly (although much ado is made about African traditional medicines), more provisions are made for research into African medicine by Europe and America than by we Africans ourselves.

IMPLICATIONS FOR MENTAL HEALTH

I earlier described the characteristics of mental health in any society and pointed out that mental health is an attribute of the individual, the family and the community. It is possible to use these parameters to judge the mental health of an individual, a family, a neighbour or the inhabitants of any town. It is clear that for any society it is possible for one segment to enjoy mental health and another inadequate mental health, bordering on illness. It is my empirical observation that in any society where more than one third do not enjoy mental health, that society, as a whole, is unsatisfactory and heading for violent revolution. In a non-homogenous society in which there is a majority that enjoys mental health and a minority that is excluded or discriminated against, this minority will either migrate or so disrupt the majority that the majority no longer enjoys mental health and is brought into a situation closer to that of the suffering group.

When we apply these findings so contemporary African society, interesting findings emerge. The conflict between African traditional ideas and newly acquired Western systems produce tensions. Identification with the Western way of life has no archetypal roots and stands in vacuum. The African is nourished on African soil, sustained by African culture but identifies not with African culture but with European. A conflict of identity then ensues. The conflict of identity breeds inner dissatisfaction and with it, self-doubt and self-hatred. This inner dissatisfaction has been produced by identification with a system that is alien but which is viewed as the desired end. This self-hatred shows itself in many ways. Africans who have made it make their homes not in Africa but in Europe. Their friends are Europeans. Even their wealth is invested not in Africa for the upliftment of their brethren but is in Switzerland and other safe havens. These people wish their money to be protected from their African brothers by their "new brother Europeans".

At the lowest level is chronic frustration and complete inner dissatisfaction. Forcible means are adopted to catch up with their more "successful brethren". This may take the form either of armed revolution or armed robbery. The avenging ancestors are in limbo.

Our business and large industries suffer also from the Psycho African Limbo. For one thing, the systems are new and, for another, the Protestant ethic and the left-right reasoning of the West, necessary to ensure success, is also missing. Inefficient workers, especially in high places, cannot be removed.

We are tyrannized and oppressed by a new culture we have identified with. As Franz Fanon pointed out,

> Oppressed people kill each other all the time. Angered by the misery of their lives but cowed by the overt superior might of the oppressor, the oppressed people shrink from striking at the true object of their hostility and strike at their more defenceless brothers and sisters near at hand.

African societies as a whole are not yet mentally healthy. There is an identity crisis which much be resolved before we can free ourselves from our psychological oppressors.

Department of Mental Health,
University of Benin,
Benin City 243619, Nigeria

REFERENCES

Aristotle
1961 Story of Philosophy. Will Durant, Washington Square Press Inc.

Binitie, A.
1976 Mental Health Implications of Economic Growth in Developing Countries. Mental Health and Society 3: 272–285.

Birley, J. L. T. and Brown, G. W.
1970 Crisis and Life Changes Preceding the Onset of Relapse of Acute Schizophrenia. Brit. J. Psychiat. 116: 237–33.

Brown, G. W., Birley, J. L. T., and Wing, V. K.
1900 Influence of Family Life on the Course of Schizophrenia. Brit. J. Psychiat. 121: 241–58.

Cassels, J. and Tyroler, H. A.
1961 Epidemiological Studies of Culture Change. Archives of Environmental Health 3: 25–33.

Encyclopaedia Brittanica

Erikson, E. H.
1950 Childhood and Society, Middlesex, Penguin Books.

Forde, D.
1954 African Worlds Studies in the Cosmological Ideas and Social Values of African Peoples. Oxford University Press.

Forde, D. and Kaberry, P. M.
1967 West African Kingdoms in the Nineteenth Century. Oxford University Press.

Francis Bacon
1961 Story of Philosophy. Will Durant, Washington Square Press Inc.

Freud, S.
1900 New Introductory Lectures to Psychoanalysis. London Hogarth Press.

Hall, S. S. and Lindsey, G.
1957 Theories of Personality. New York, John Wiley & Son.

Harding, T. W.
1977 Mental Health Research in Africa – Preliminary Results of a Questionnaire Survey. Afr. J. of Psychiatry 1, 2: 31–37.

Harding, T., Moser, J., and Raman, A.
1977 Mental Health Training in Africa – Analysis of Information from 23 Countries. Afr. J. of Psychiatry 1, 2.3: 17–30.

Holmes, T. H. and Rahe, R. H.
1967 The Social Readjustment Rating Scale. Journal of Psychosomatic Research 11: 213–218.

Imokhai, C. A.
1979 The Missionization of Uzaire: A Study of Missionary Impact on Traditional Marriage. Ph.D. Thesis, Columbia University.

Jablensky, A.
1978 Mental Health Care in South Africa. Lancet 1: 270–1.

Jaspers, Carl
1926 and 1946 General Psychopathology. Manchester, The University Press.

Kettle, A.
1963 Karl Marx. London: Morison Cubb.

Kramer, M., Rosen, B. N., and Willis, E. M.
1900 Definitions and Distribution Mental Disorders in a Racist Society. Reprinted from, Racism and Mental Health.

Lewis, A.
1969 Edward Mapother and the Making of the Maudsley Hospital. Brit. J. Psychiat. 115.

Lieberman, D.
1971 In Wolf, L. (1971) (ed.). Social and Cultural Factors in Mental Health and Mental Illness, C. C. Thomas, Springfield, Illinois, U.S.A.

Margolis, C.
1971 Socio-Psychological and Ideological Perspectives on the Black Communities. In: K. Wolff (ed.). Social and Cultural in Mental Health and Mental Illness.

Mead, Margaret
1948 Social Change and Cultural Surrogates. In: C. Cluckhorn and H. A. Murray. Personality in Nature, Society and Culture.

1970 Optimum Mental Health. In: Albert Deutsch and Helen Fishman (eds.). Encyclopaedia of Mental Health, New Jersey: Mini Print.

Morris, Desmond
1967 The Naked Ape. London, Corgi Books.

Murphy, E. and Brown, G. W.
1980 Life Events, Psychiatric Disturbances and Physical Illness. Brit. J. Psychiat. 136, 326–338.

Musgrove, F.
1966 The Family, Education and Society. London, Routledge and Kegan Paul, p. 46.

Osahon, N.
1976 Black Power, Lagos, DI NIURO Press.

Paykel, E. S., Emmes, E. M., Fletcher, and Rassaby, E. S.
1900 Life Events and Social Support in Puerperal Depression. Brit. J. Psychiat. 136: 399–346.

Peterson, M. D.
1975 Thomas Jefferson. U.S.A., Viking Press.

Piddington, R.
1950 An Introduction to Social Anthropology. Edinburgh: Oliver & Boyd.

Prince, R.
1976 Culture and Psychosis Among the Loma Tribe of Liberia, West Africa. African J. of Psychiat. 3: 381–3983.

Radcliffe-Brown, A. R. and Forde, D.
1950 African Systems of Kinship and Marriage. Oxford University Press.

Senghor, L.
1976 Prose and Poetry. Translated by Reed and Wahe, London, Weinman.

Szasz, T.
1971 The Manufacture of Madness. London, Routledge and Keegan Paul.

The International Communist
1975 Leninist Theory of Social Revolution and the Contemporary World. Moscow: Progress Publishers.

Weber, Max
1948 Essays in Sociology. Translated by H. H. Gerth and C. W. Mills, London: Routledge and Keegan Paul.

Wolff, L.
1971 Social and Cultural Factors in Mental Health and Mental Illness. Springfield, Illinois, U.S.A., Charles C. Thomas.

Zilboorg, C.
1941 A History of Medical Psychology, New York: W. W. Norton.

LOREN J. AMOR (Philippines)

MENTAL HEALTH AND THE THIRD WORLD: A CHALLENGE TO YOUTH

My primary task today is to speak on behalf of a sector comprising of persons between the ages of 0 to 20 representing a vulnerable stage in a person's life when he or she undergoes the processes of observing, understanding and experiencing the surrounding spiritual, physical and social environment. After absorbing and assessing, the youth slowly adjusts himself or herself in preparation for adulthood in the adolescence period which is considered as a second and final chance to work out the psycho-social problems of childhood before entering adulthood (Banaag, 1980).

Youth share common dreams; common descriptions of love and hate, good and bad; common enthusiasms and common paragons for ambition and strength of character. But never do they share a common means of transition from childhood to adulthood. It is this difference that separates one youth from the other; not religion, political antecedents, social status or language, but the environment he or she was born in, lives to survive for, and aims to assist and possibly eventually lead. It is this difference that separates the youth of the Third World countries from those of the industrialized and developed countries.

When I speak of the *Third World*, I refer to those countries where the process of development has not reached its maximum because although there are numerous resources available, both human and otherwise, they have remained untapped, unproductive or wasted (International Year of the Child, 1979).

When I refer to *means of transition* in the Third World, I refer to my brothers and sisters in Africa whose lives have been a long struggle against hunger, malnutrition and disease brought about by droughts, by the lack of productivity of agricultural lands and by the unavailability of proper health services. My brothers and sisters in Indochina are living in countries stricken with wars and face evacuation to borders where the people and their language are incomprehensible and strange. They face unavoidable and permanent separation from their families, resettlement and adjustment. My brothers and sisters in some countries in the Americas, Caribbean and Asia belong to impoverished families. Modern facilities and trained personnel in urban areas are expensive and not readily available to those in need in rural communities. They are deprived of such benefits by the many miles of rough roads, mountains, rivers and swamps which are accessible only by boat or small bancas. They are also cut off by the diversity of dialects separating one community from another.

Despite this unsettling picture of our countries, we have rich cultures and distinctive traits and traditions that enrich our lives and make transitions bearable and, at times, easy. One such strength is the uniqueness of close family ties and extended families. This has helped us hurdle the difficulties of our

Richard C. Nann, Dorcas Susan Butt, and Lourdes Ladriod-Ignacio (eds.), Mental Health, Cultural Values and Social Development, 79–83.

childhood and deepens our understanding and awareness of human relationships. Familial guardianship and family reunions were no rare treats for many of us. The primary responsibility of older brothers and sisters was the well-being of the younger ones. Aunts and grandparents were always around to lend a hand in caring or spoiling us and guiding our parents on proper and suitable child rearing practices.

A second strength is the spirit of "Bayanihan" or camaraderie among members of the community. I remember well how neighbours would come to knock at our door to share fruits, sweets or viand even if it was not Christmas or someone's birthday. Friends would gather around planning surprise parties for any occasion. One always felt included and needed.

A third strength is the genuine experience of childhood. Many of us would recall the regular visits to our parents' hometowns in the provinces. There were always endless tales of town legends and folklore from relatives and friends, food eaten on banana leaves and baskets, long walks to town. There, games revolved around plants and trees, haystacks and farm animals.

The last strength is the transmission of moral and cultural traditions by each generation to the next. Each village has its own set of traditions that makes each homecoming and village feast a spectacle of pomp, sentimentality and fun. A visitor was always treated as a guest of honour and each home was open to all.

Each family passes on to the next old-time lessons on love, patriotism, fidelity, respect, religion and the many joys and tears of life; values which have always stood on the solidarity of the families, together with the knowledge that, despite all odds, each would come to each other's aid in times of need or would share the bounties in times of plenty. It was always hard for a parent to see their child go and settle elsewhere and for a child to part ways with his parents. The same is shared by the community who feels sorrow for a departing son.

Today, all of these are slowly fading, not by choice or neglect, but by circumstance. In an effort to be economically stable and live up to a set status in society, traditions have been sacrificed for more "practical" means. Thus, children are sent to colleges to learn new ways that are mote practical than traditional. Unfortunately, school instruction and equipment have been patterned after those of industrialized countries. When a village youth returns to his home there is the inevitable frustration of application. Trained with machines available only in urban or industrialized areas, they flock to the cities believing that their skills are not for their villages. Rural migration becomes a cause and a circumstance that tragically leads many youth to the misleading comforts of the modern city. From there starts a long saga of social problems which I believe are the effects of modernization.

There arises a "cultural shock" among our youth when the industrialized countries perpetuate issues such as divorce and single parenthood, homes for the aged, abortion, early sexual experimentation, women's liberation. Such ideas were tagged by Filipino adolescents in a consultation as "Western ideas" (National Seminar on Adolescents, 1980).

I cannot understand how one could suggest putting one's parents in homes for the aged where others would care for them. I believe that just as we are God's gifts to our parents, our parents are to us. Would you disregard their many years of patience and industry in bringing us up, putting us through school, accepting our inadequacies and idiosyncrasies and still love us? I know I cannot and so will those of my Third World brothers and sisters. They are family and we always take care of our own. Besides, the very idea is never thought of since it is against tradition. It, likewise, lessens family ties and promotes insecurities among our people that upon reaching a certain age, society would consider them inadequate.

Another is the tendency of people to prefer living on their own, away from their parents. Many of us look forward to independence but not to the extent of breaking family ties. We look forward to be able to earn and buy things on our own, choose our friends, our career and life partner. We, likewise, expect, despite our independence, advice and guidance from our parents. Though we like to make decisions on our own, we sometimes snatch a side look at whether our parents are nodding or shaking their heads over our actions.

Our parents are to us a morale booster as well as our showcase of achievements, seeing the glow on their faces and the voice of pride whenever we are introduced to friends. Our parents want the best for us and seeing us standing on our own two feet and happy are their primary goals. We rarely call our parents by their names, always the traditional mom and dad in our dialect; the same for grandparents, older brothers, sisters and cousins. A sign of welcome to an elder was always a kiss on the hand, or on the cheek.

Stories of early sexual experimentation have influenced many youth in Third World countries. Still it is uncommon for young girls to be proud of not being virgins. Discretion is still practiced. Should pregnancy arise, alternatives are given, but never abortion, a practice which I regret has spread. How can anyone want to kill an innocent baby all for the sake of one's own person? Mothers who have known how hard it was to carry a child for nine months and then see it through childhood and adulthood would not even consider recommending abortion to their daughters and sons. Even though it has brought dishonour and pain to the family, it has been their advice to let the baby live and almost always the families have them adopted by members of the family. Despite stories of abandonment and family banishment in movies and radios, it rarely happens in real life. To a woman whose upbringing had been respect for relationships and human life, she would much rather suffer bitter words than imagine the cries of a baby whose only fault was that he or she was conceived out of wedlock.

Another issue is the inability of parents to "talk" to their children and vice-versa. Popularly known as the "generation or communication gap" between the youth and adults, I personally can sum it up for two reasons. One, due to the quality of education to which we are exposed, we are sometimes filled with ideas that clash with or confuse our parents. Learning is attributed less to the school, and more to a persuasive mass media and rapid technology. There are more things to see and questions to ask. We are much bolder in asking them outright. Parents whose basic learning were the "3Rs" find it embarrassing when children of elementary age seek their assistance in solving algebraic problems and scientific theories. Pity the parents who have not gone to school at all.

Two, the alteration of priorities, with economic sufficiency coming first and living up to a set status coming second, have forced even mothers to seek jobs. No one is left to care for the children, guide their erring ways and find means to divert their energy to creative and self-learning activities. Family relationships are disrupted and families uprooted due to migration to places where jobs are available. The youth whose childhood orientation has been limited to his or her school, immediate environment and playmates will now find it difficult to express himself to his parents. Likewise, parents will find it difficult to talk to a child whom they have failed to realize was growing up or mature enough to understand the A's from the B's. Both parties then let incidents pass unnoticed or unattended to until a situation flares up. The parents and child blame each other as the culprit. To me, this is a result of the changing times and values, producing such effects that can translate into being unloved, unwanted or unaccepted by both parties.

Such are the issues that confront us today. I feel I am in a position to discuss the values that I can personally delineate on and with which I am familiar. I also believe that values are of a lasting nature and can be instrumental or detrimental in achieving the mental health of each individual.

As we accept modernization we must be aware of the consequences. We, the youth, can only consider the question: How much progress should we accept and how much of the past should we believe in which has guided many then?

If a mentally healthy person is a person adjusted to the conditions of his or her environment and its ever changing patterns, I believe that we should retain those necessary conditions and values despite modernization. To me, these conditions are the traditions inherent in each country – cultural heritage. Culture must be perceived as what it really is:

> It is more than being a passive mirror of societal mores, culture should be conceived as a living instrument for the presentation and enhancement of those values, attitudes and behavioural patterns conducive to nation building as well as the dignity and integral development of each individual . . . much in it protects the interests and promotes the development of our people, in general, and our youth, in particular. (Montemayor, 1980)

Value transmission is a key instrument lost to many but it will, when experienced during childhood and adolescence, provide lasting impressions. This would also ensure that, in spite of the changing times, we will be provided with tools to develop our own principles as adults for self-development and meet the demands of a growing and moving nation. If so, the Third World youth would not be afraid of having that "poverty of loneliness . . . poverty of spirit" as of those in the industrialized countries (UNICEF, 1979). "In the process of development, these values that have kept human relationships viable will not be lost as they have been almost lost in the industrialized nations today." (UNICEF, 1979)

This is a challenge to every youth in Third World countries today. How can we maintain the viability of human relationships, and of spirit? How can we preserve values which will be tools for human development and preservation despite the rapid changes that beset our countries as well as the conditions that fall on us – war, natural calamities, poverty, political expansionism. We, the the youth, have a challenge to meet.

For those of you who are here in the hall, I wish to present a similar challenge – will you as leaders and initiators of progress listen and understand? Can you share your past and our present so that there will be a future? Remember . . . a child is born every second, grows every minute, learns every hour, sees all every day. The child will not wait because it cannot be. His needs of youth are now! At any moment he may already be an adult!

c/o Philippine Mental Health Association,
Post Office Box 40,
East Avenue,
Quezon City 3008, Philippines

REFERENCES

Banaag, Cornelio, M. D.
1980 Health and Values. National Seminar on Adolescents. Part III, pp. 13–18.
International Year of the Child
1979 The Needs of Children in the Third World Discussion Paper on Themes Related to IYC, pp. 1–4.
Montemayor, Leonardo Q.
1980 Socio-Cultrual and Economic Environment of Adolescents. National Seminar on Adolescents, Part III, pp. 19–22.
Presidential Decree 603
The Child and Youth Welfare Code. Article 2.
Where the Third World is First
1979 The Situation of Children in the Developing Countries. UNICEF News Features.
Youth Consultations on the Needs and Problems of Adolescents
1980 Social Issues. National Seminar on Adolescents. Part I, pp. 1–14.

Discussant: BASIL JAMES, M.D. (New Zealand)

MENTAL HEALTH AND THE THIRD WORLD

We have listened to two papers, the titles of which are dissimilar. Yet in spite of these differences, I discern a common theme.

Firstly, Dr. Binitie's paper traced in a most scholarly fashion, the struggles over many centuries to identify the healthful society and the fulfilled individual. Yet it might seem somewhat depressing that so many great minds have been turned for so long to the question of what constitutes that vision. It seems a daunting prospect when we realize that the intellectual giants of the last two thousand years, at least, have produced formulae and descriptions, many of them poetic in their majesty, of that ideal state. Yet we are also aware that material progress has produced as many problems as solutions; and we seem as remote from the answers as any of our predecessors.

Karl Popper, the philosopher of science, addresses himself to the illusions of definition. He would say that there is no such thing "out there" as mental health. Mental health is in itself only a *phrase*. As Humpty Dumpty said, "Words can mean anything you want them to mean". Our definition may be different from place to place, or change over time, but what we choose to call mental health must be *relevant* – to the needs of both the time and the place.

Dr. Binitie was alert to this need. We have, he said, to come up with an empirical definition of mental health and work out some indices so that we can measure it in any community. He went further and gave us a seven item description of what *he* means by mental health. He then gave us some of the flavour of what characterizes the traditional African way of construing the world. In contrast to the European process of analysis which leads to sterility and exploitation of resources, Dr. Binitie presented the African philosophy of life as intuitive and fertile, involved in the cosmic rhythm, unified and in tune with the environment of which *man forms a part*. This was an echo of Dr. Hend Abdel-Al's paper on Tuesday, in which she said we should see ourselves not *in* the world, but part of it. Such a concept seems to me to be central to the human race's very survival, touching as it does on the great issues of the day such as pollution, population and exploitation. We must learn to live as part of nature and abandon the quest to conquer it.

In a beautiful book "The Dream of Kilimanjaro" Rolf Edberg, a former Swedish diplomat, examines the situation surrounding the great Rift Valley, which anthropologists have described as "the cradle of man", in the heart of Africa. Dr. Binitie spared us, which the author of "The Dream of Kilimanjaro" did not, an account of the physical rape of the continent by the invading white tribe. The exploitation of the physical resources, charitably attributed to ignorance as much as greed, profoundly altered the delicate eco-system, so that not

Richard C. Nann, Dorcas Susan Butt, and Lourdes Ladriod-Ignacio (eds.), Mental Health, Cultural Values and Social Development, 84–86.

only is water a more pressing problem than it was before, but the arable topsoil is now prey to the bleaching winds, and disappears in tens of millions of tons a year, being deposited as far west as the Caribbean Ocean. Deserts such as the Sahara grow each year at an alarming rate, and I recall the prediction voiced by Chester Pierce on Monday of the implications for mental health of a severe water shortage in more than twenty countries of the world by the year 2000.

Dr. Binitie, perhaps, thought that Mr. Herman Stein's talk earlier in this conference had been sufficient reminder to us of the dire effects of physical privation upon mental health, and he referred to it only briefly in his third condition for mental health – the wherewithal to manage a decent life. It is, as he says, obvious. But being only too aware of our capacity for denial, I would like to take the opportunity to underscore the obvious. It seems to me that the World Federation for Mental Health might address itself at some future conference to this capacity for denial. I no longer accept it comfortably as a defence mechanism. Already it results in "apocalypse now" for millions. Denial has outlived its usefulness, and now constitutes a major threat to the very survival of mankind.

Before returning to the remainder of Dr. Binitie's paper, I should like to address myself to that of Ms. Amor.

George Bernard Shaw, the great Irish playwright and cynic, once said that youth is such a wonderful quality that it is a pity it is wasted on the young. It was said that Shaw was born before his time; I should like to say that he also died before his time. If he had been alive today, I believe that he would have been the first to say that youth is not at all wasted on the young of our time. Indeed, Ms. Amor's paper was an excellent example of vigour and idealism. Who should be more concerned or more involved with mental health in the third world than its young people? The introduction of the developmental theme sits well in a discussion of developing countries. Whilst the developed world is appropriately concerned with its aging population, the statistics of the age structure of the third world are skewed to the left. Who better to be concerned about the future than the young? There were potentially controversial points in Ms. Amor's paper including abortion, and she had the courage to identify them.

Her paper overlapped with the final theme of Dr. Binitie's – the conflict of value systems and cultural *mores* which occurs when the traditions of an old but materially impoverished country collide with those of technologically more advanced societies. Barry Adams' "The Survival of Domination" deals with the resolution of such conflicts. They include isolation, both psychological and social, identification with a dominant culture, intra-group conflict and controversy. There was implicit in his book a need for pride in one's own heritage if one was to avoid dissonance both within the person and within the family. Ms. Amor's observation on the availability of supportive family and social networks are particularly pertinent. Many of you, like myself, are visitors to the Philippines, and I would like to share with you two personal observations.

Firstly, in my several visits to the Philippines, I have never seen a crying child. In the crowded Rizal gardens on a Sunday afternoon, when the whole of Manila seems to be strolling in the sunshine, the patience and tolerance of parents is remarkable, as is the reciprocal contentment of the children. Perhaps more surprisingly, the same interaction is found in the crowded commercial streets of Metro Manila under far less favourable circumstances. You will be aware that this is in marked contrast with the frustrated parents and tired distress of unhappy children that you will see in any street or in any store in a Western country.

The second observation occurred at a party given by one of my Filipino friends some years ago. At about 10:00 in the evening, he was mingling amongst his guests, carrying his four-year-old daughter. A Western visitor commented that it was very late for her to be up, and our guest replied, "Oh, she just wanted to see what was going on and who was here". "You will have trouble later if you don't teach her some discipline and self-reliance" replied the intrusive guest. "Oh, we don't hurry these things here" was our host's final comment.

Interestingly, it is in Australia that Dr. Scott Henderson has established the value of a supportive interpersonal network as a buffer between the individual and the slings and arrows of outrageous fortune. In Canberra, a series of surveys was conducted using the same population, to determine the prevalence of neuroses. Between the first and second interviews, separated as I recall by some two months. there was a decrease in prevalence of some 25%. Explanation may lie in the reliability of the measuring instruments, but Scott Henderson himself dobts that. The key may lie in the answers to the question "Do you have anyone with whom you can discuss your private troubles and feelings?" On the second occasion, when the answer was in the affirmative, the interviewer then asked who. The subjects looked at the interviewer and said – "You".

This may be a sad comment on the affluent world which not only, as Dr. Binitie says, analyses, but also isolates.

It is clear that mental health workers alone cannot achieve the broad ideals espoused during this conference. Attention must be paid to the social and physical environment. We must address ourselves to the socioeconomic realm, to legislation and politics. Perhaps with this in mind, the great biologist Virchow said "Politics is medicine writ large". It has also been said that medicine is a practice informed by science. We should ensure that social planning, the making of legislation and politics, is a practice informed – and indeed audited – by those concerned with mental health.

Director of Mental Health,
Head Office, Department of Health,
McCarthy Trust Building,
Wellington, New Zealand

MICHAEL H. COOPER (New Zealand)

MENTAL HEALTH PRIORITIES: A SOCIO-ECONOMIC VIEWPOINT

INTRODUCTION

The results of epidemiological and socio-economic research over the past 10 years have led to much questioning of our health care delivery systems. For example, many of the characteristics thought peculiar to mental health are now found to be true, of health in general. Although, at the macro level, we still await an integrated model, there is now a consensus of opinion that, traditionally, the socio-economic variables have been under-valued and the medical over-valued.

The twin notions that (1) health is dependent upon a complex range of inter-related variables and that (2) "need" is largely a matter of informed subjective opinion have had the most serious implications for the organization, planning and financing of health care systems. They have thrown into strong relief the potential role of the individual in maintaining and improving his or her own physical and mental condition. The impetus for reform has been given weight by the current world-wide economic recession and the seemingly popular view that less public expenditure is preferable to more. Indeed, taxation is increasingly seen as confiscation rather than the public price for goods and services.

THE DEMEDICALIZATION OF HEALTH

A growing volume of academic literature suggests, albeit often rather impressionistically, that the history of the post-war health sector is one of more and more health inputs associated with less and less output. During a time when medical science has flourished as never before, and both medical manpower and the health sector's share of the gross national product have grown dramatically, improvements in age-specific mortality rates have tapered away to virtually zero, particularly for those middle aged or older. The very rich nations have spent proportionally more on health care than the merely rich, but appear to live no longer as a consequence. Indeed, as nations have become richer in per capita income, their health care expenditures have risen more than proportionately and yet, there is no evidence, at least in the western world, that there is any marked improvement in health when viewed from the narrow perspective of life expectancy (Fuchs, 1974; Maxwell, 1974; Cooper, 1975; Newhouse, 1975).

The inter-related variables that determine the health status of any given population at risk appear to include income and its distribution, unemployment, welfare provisions, education, housing, public health, climate, genetics, pollution,

Richard C. Nann, Dorcas Susan Butt, and Lourdes Ladriod-Ignacio (eds.), Mental Health, Cultural Values and Social Development, 87–94.

the curative services, preventative medicine and personal life styles. It is not the purpose of this paper to review this voluminous literature, but simply to point out that most of these variables are, in theory at least, controllable. They are, to a large extent, the outcome of past individual and collective choice. Naturally, individual choice is largely constrained and influenced by the environment and is subject to a complex set of trade-off decisions. Both societies and individuals have many objectives of which health is only one, and many of these objectives will be mutually incompatible. Life may be lengthened by turning from alcohol, cigarettes, stress and cholesterol to a diet of bran and flouridated water consumed rapidly during brief breaks from jogging, but at what cost to its quality? Instead of actually adding to life expectancy, life may merely seem longer!

Much work has been undertaken in the attempt to quantify and estimate the importance of socio-economic factors. There is strong and consistent evidence linking those health conditions associated with stress to a range of economic indicators, such as unemployment. Brenner has recently shown that a 1% increase in unemployment that is subsequently sustained for a six-year period, is associated with increases of 2% in the total deaths, 3% in mental hospital admissions, 4% in suicides and 6% in murders in the sixth year (Brenner, 1976). Somewhat surprisingly, a number of econometric studies find formal educational attainment to be consistently the best predictor of life chances, although why this is so remains rather obscure (Auster, 1972, Grossman, 1975). It may be that the well educated absorb more easily health-related information, have lower access costs to, and make more effective use of, the health care system, lead healthier lives, or are simply better at self-diagnosis and more persistent in their demands on the system. Further, rather discouragingly, rising real income levels are no longer (if indeed, they ever were) the unqualified friend of health. There is no evidence that the very rich countries, for example, enjoy better health than the not quite so rich. Regression analysis in the U.S.A. suggests that, at the margin, increases in income may be more life threatening than life enhancing (Auster, 1972).

It must be admitted that much of the evidence for this broad model of health care remains circumstantial. The evidence, taken overall, however, is powerful. It is clear, from historical case studies, that society's faith in medical intervention as a cure-all has been largely misplaced. Over the past century and a half, the reduction in age-specific mortality rates has flowed mainly from improvements in nutrition and sanitation rather than from formal medical interventions. The improvement in life expectancy has come, in the main, from an improvement in the economic lot of the highest risk groups. In 1900, a quarter of the population survived beyond their seventieth birthday, but another quarter failed to reach 23. The last 80 years have seen a levelling of risks although, of course, acute disparities still remain.

The influence of life style and enviornment on mortality data can be seen most clearly from contemporary case studies. There are data comparing different regions of the United States and the national mortality data with that of other countries (Fuchs, 1974). Utah and Nevada, for example, are adjacent states with much the same per capita incomes, numbers of doctors, and climate. Nevada, however, has a 42% higher infant mortality rate and a 54% higher mortality rate for middle aged males. Life expectancy at birth is three or four years less. Cirrhosis of the liver and respiratory neoplasms in middle aged males are both six fold more common. Nevada also has twice the percentage of single households and six times the number of residents born outside the State. It, of course, attracts the "high-livers" in stark contrast to Utah's Mormon population. Similar contrasts can be obtained by comparing the Seventh Day Adventists with the general Californian population. The causes of death linked to smoking, alcohol and stress tend to occur among Adventists at one-fifth to one-half of that prevailing generally.

One of the major impacts of such econometric and case study work has been to highlight the fact that it is difficult, if not impossible, to justify the entire fabric of medical intervention, whatever the specialty, solely, or even mainly, on the claim that it prolongs life. Clearly, all health care is a multi-product business producing in addition to the curative services, reassurance, relief of symptoms (many of which are, in any case, self-limiting), care for those in varying degrees of dependency (the handicapped, terminally ill, very young and old, etc.), and of course, health education. There can be no doubt that despite the attention paid to its life-saving achievements, medicine has made an enormous contribution to both the quality of living and of dying.

THE NATURE OF NEED

The founders of socialized health care systems tended to think of health care as being primarily concerned with the cure of disease. It was assumed that with given medical technology and a given population at risk, the total benefit to be derived from medical intervention (as assessed by professional providers) would be self-evident, finite and readily quantifiable. Further, once the manpower and resources necessary to confer this benefit had been established, the only problem would be to persuade the taxpayer to divert sufficient resources from their next best alternative employment to make the necessary health care available. Access to these resources for those in need was seen as a "human right" and the means of realizing it consisted of nationalizing all existing health care resources, funding the system from taxation and making it available to all those in genuine need at zero prices at the time of consumption. The hope was that once the backlog of need had been met and people were no longer constrained by their inability (or unwillingness) to pay, health care would become a self-eliminating expense. This "miscalculation of sublime dimension" (Powell, 1962) ignored the fact that death is extremely cheap and survival often very expensive since a faulty body must be maintained until death claims it by the same or another means.

Further, it was clearly based upon an incorrect understanding of the true natrue of need and of the variables affecting it.

Need is essentially a continuum ranging from a state of complete physical and mental well-being at one end to death at the other (Figure 1). General agreement is likely to exist only at and towards its extremities (AB and CD) but not in the middle (BC). Need, like beauty, tends to lie chiefly in the eye of the beholder. It is, for a wide range of services and conditions, an opinion and not a medical fact. Questions such as, what levels of blood pressure or emotional distress are clinical conditions or, what consultations, home visits, prescriptions, referrals or hospital admissions are legitimate, in practice attract little in the way of medical unanimity (Cooper, 1975).

Figure 1. The need continuum

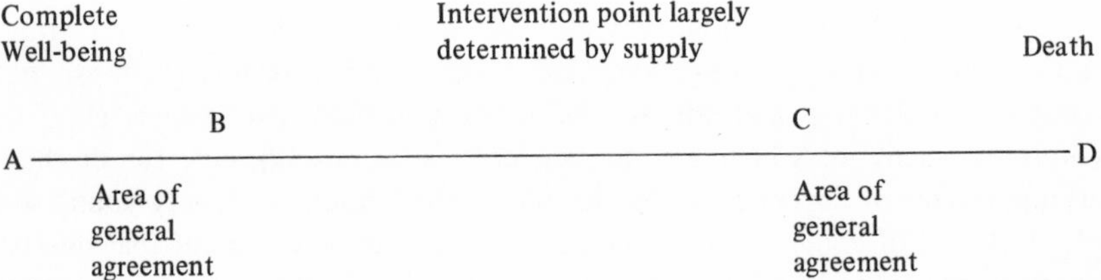

The point at which intervention commences along the range BC is dependent upon a number of variables, the most dominant of which appears to be the supply of resources and manpower. Considerable empirical evidence exists to suggest that the individual's capacity to see himself or herself as unwell is, for all practical purpose, limitless. When invited to recall our state of health over the preceding 14-day period, 90% typically report one to six symptoms of sickness and 9% in excess of that number (Wadsworth, 1971). To conceive of oneself as being ill is clearly normal. The decision to translate such unconstrained "wants" into "demands" by going to the doctor, however, depends upon the intensity of that want relative to the barriers of fees, time costs, fear, and doctor attitudes. The degree of want appears to relate as much to the individual's general state of contentment, reactions of family and friends and so on, as it does to his actual physical condition (Cooper, 1975). With any given level of want, the lower the barriers of fee and time costs, the more the supply side is likely to determine the need cut-off point along the continuum. In a socialized system with zero prices at the point of consumption, "induced demand" is more likely to be a prominent phenomenon than in fee per item of service systems with substantial patient contributions. Further, systems where general practitioners act as gate-keepers to further resources are more likely to be supply dominated than those where patients have direct access to specialist and hospital service.

In all systems, whether socialized or not, the doctor acts as the patient's agent. Subject to the nature of the presenting physical and mental condition and the extent of the barriers to be overcome, the doctor can profoundly influence the quality, quantity and, in non-socialized systems, the price of any service provided. The constraints on the scope for induced demand will, of course, vary with the category of ailment in question. A brain tumour is a finite state as is a broken leg. The resources brought to bear upon such conditions, however, even in these cases are anything but finite. They can be treated in conditions resembling the Hilton or a hostel for vagrants, immediately or after a delay, by distinguished surgeons or the newly qualified, and so on. As, however, the latent demand at zero or highly subsidized prices already exists over at least the range BD, supply tends to be the final determining factor.

In practice, both demand and need are constrained, and the point of intervention determined, by available resources. The more resources that are made available, the more new need floats to the surface. American surgeons manage to find a need for twice as much surgery per capita as in the United Kingdom, where there are more severe constraints in the form of medical numbers, theatre time and beds available. In addition, within the U.S.A., the number of surgeons per capita in any area is by far the best predictor of the surgical intervention rate (Lewis, 1969). In New Zealand, areas relatively well-endowed with general practitioners (1 to 1,700) have consultation rates over 50% higher than those in areas with relatively few (1 to 2,700), a contrast fully reflected in their relative prescribing rates but not in their morbidity or mortality rates. Doctors clearly educate their patients, explicitly or implicitly, into a realization of what they regard as a legitimate call on their time. This will, in turn, be influenced by the time they have available, their system of remuneration and their conception of their proper role. A doctor who takes a wide pastoral view of his role (readily providing reassurance, and advice), makes home visits, treats self-limiting common ailments, expresses doubts as to the wisdom of the self-medication and has low prescribing and referral rates, is likely to be struggling to cope with the needs of 1,500 patients. With a narrower view of his or her functions, he or she could probably quite adequately cope with more than 4,000.

Subject to certain constraints, the supply side creates its own demand. The mechanism by which supply is determined therefore becomes critical.

HOW IS AVAILABILITY DETERMINED?

The realization that need is, to a large extent, a function of supply has led to the almost universal questioning of the current system of delivering health care, irrespective of what that system is.

The major problem within the socialized systems, for example, has been the lack of macro objectives by which to plan, monitor or assess performance. The objective of the individual physician has been to return the patient to as normal a life style as possible as soon as possible, given the constraints on his clinical freedom imposed by available resources and current medical knowledge. The doctor has never been explicitly instructed to practice best-bargain medicine, but rather to do the best for the patient. Faced with two possible treatments, one 10% superior but 20% more expensive, he has not been expected to provide the cheaper. No health economist I know wishes anyone to be told by his doctor that, as the odds of successfully adding two years of life expectancy are only 20:1 at a cost of $20,000, he should go home and die unaided since, in the doctor's view, the money would be better spent on a new heating system for the geriatric wards. Instead, unavoidable rationing decisions have been explciitly resolved by shifts in the intervention point along the need continuum. Priorities, when force upon the system, have been formed away from the work-force and, largely by reference, to the relative immediate threat to life rather than according to the potential benefit or, still less, the net benefit after consideration of cost.

At the macro level, health planning has proceeded by the time honoured "$n + 1$" or two budget (ongoing and incremental) method. Annual allocations from the centre have tended to reflect the previous years expenditure plus (or, more recently, minus) some growth factor. Existing services have been taken as their own justification, the fact of their being used serving to "prove" their absolute need. The growth factor has commonly been linked to the growth in services provided over the preceding year plus an allowance for new capital works completed. Where need related allocation formulae have been employed, they have been based upon population weighted by some combination of age, sex, bed stock and patient "through-put". The problem has been that the weighting factors tend to be determined by reference to current practice, thus perpetuating the status quo (eg. weighting those 60 years old by five because they currently cost five times as much). Systems have proved unwieldy and insensitive to the need for change, their overall shape reflecting history rather than conscious design. Priorities have tended to favour "unavoidable" crisis medicine at the expense of caring for the chronic sick and handicapped, curative institutionally based services rather than preventive community-based measures. Prevention and education are essentially impersonal and statistical and, hence, thought postponeable.

CONCLUSIONS

This paper has made no attempt to separate mental health from health in general because there is, with respect at least to the issues discussed, no essential difference. The need continuum is equally true of all branches of medicine, whether it be surgery or psychiatry. There is no uniquely "correct" allocation of resources. Mental care, however, has suffered badly in most countries from the widespread belief that there is a "necessary" level of spending on other branches of medicine that is scientifically attestable, finite and unavoidable. The mentally ill and handicapped have often been a residual charge after so-called unavoidable death-averting services have been provided for. Priorities in medicine have rarely been made explicit and have often reflected the estimated degree of danger to life represented by a condition rather than the potential for good intervention. Similarly, charges against psychiatry of unproven efficacy or of the vagueness of the need for services, are just as applicable to medicine in general, as are charges that it is susceptible to fad and fashion. Psychiatry is not alone in having its dromomanias to live down (a condition said to have been suffered by slaves who displayed an urge to run away). Health care is in crisis and, as Lord Rutherford once remarked, we have no money left and little option but to sit down and think.

University of Otago,
Department of Economics
Box 56,
Dunedin, New Zealand

REFERENCES

Auster, R. *et al.*
1972 The Production of Health: An Exploratory Study. In V. R. Fuchs (ed.). Essays in the Economics of Health and Medical Care. Columbia University Press.

Brenner, H.
1976 Estimating the Social Costs of National Economic Policy: Implications for Mental and Physical Health and Criminal Aggression. Joint Economic Committee.

Bunker, J.
1974 Risks and Benefits of Surgery. Benefits and Risks of Medical Care, O.H.E.

Cooper, M. H.
1975 Rationing Health Care. Croom Helm, London and Halsted Press, Wiley, New York.
1976 Health Costs and Expenditures in the U.K.. In: Teh-wei Hu (ed.). International Health Costs and Expenditures. DHEW No. 76–1067, Washington, D.C.
1979 The Demand and Need for Dental Care. Social Policy and Administration. Backwells Vol. 13, No. 2.

Cooper, M. H. And Shannon, P. T. (eds.)
1978 A New Health Service for New Zealand. University of Otago.

Fuchs, V. R.
1974 Who Shall Live? Basic Books, N.Y.

Grossman, M.
1975 The Correlation between Health and Schooling. Household Production and Consumption. National Bureau of Economic Research, Washington, D.C.

Lewis, C. E.
1979 Variations in the Incidence of Surgery. New England Journal of Medicine 281, 6, 880.

Maxwell, R.
1974 Health Care: The Growing Dilemma. McKinsey.

Newhouse, J.
1975 Development and Allocation of Medical Resources. Address to the XXIX World Medical Assembly. Tokyo.

Newhouse, J.
1979 The Economics of Medical Care. Addison-Wesley.
Powell, E.
1962 Health and Wealth. Proceedings of the Royal Society of Medicine 55: 1–12.
Wadsworth, M. E. J. *et al*.
1971 Health and Sickness: The Choice of Treatment. Tavistock Press.

SHOICHI WATANABE, Ph.D. (Japan)

MENTAL HEALTH PRIORITIES: A SOCIO-ECONOMIC VIEWPOINT

Two years ago we celebrated the International Year of the Child, and the World Congress on Mental Health in Salzburg, Austria with the main theme "Children and Families – Needs, Rights and Action". On that occasion I had the honour of being a Plenary Session speaker, and said that we were living in a schizophrenic world. The reason was as follows: a couple of years before the whole world celebrated the International Year of the Woman, the main theme of which was how to liberate women from their families. It seemed at that time that the family was almost regarded as the root of all evils. On the contrary, in the International Year of the Child the prevalent concern seemed to be how to make children happy in their respective families, and the family was again being recognized as the root of happy children. In other words, the happiness of mothers is often incompatible with the happiness of their children. This incompatibility, it seems to me, still persists. This curious-sounding observation directly leads us to the very heart of today's main theme: Mental Health Priorities: Socio-Economic Viewpoints. That is: to whose happiness is priority to be given, to mother's happiness or to their children's happiness? Or, whose mental health has a greater priority, mothers' mental health or their children's mental health? Priority problems of a similar kind take place everywhere these days. I should like to quote a couple of examples of frequent occurrence.

On the early morning of August 28, 1974 a middle-aged man of 46 years of age entered his neighbour's flat and killed the housewife and her two daughters, one aged 7 and another aged 4, in a public condominium near Tokyo. The reason why he killed three women, of whom two were only little children, was that he had been troubled by the noises made by the piano-playing of the 7-year-old girl. His flat was situated just above that of his victims. Noises of musical instruments can be really troublesome.

In the above-quoted case, however, none of the other neighbours of the victims had even complained of noises made by the poor girl's piano. She seems not to have played the piano excessively, and all her neighbours, but the killer, had found her playing tolerable. Our natural doubt is whether the killer was normal or not. Investigations into his past have shown that the killer was abnormally sensitive to noises, for example, while he was living in country districts he was so annoyed by the chirping of sparrows early in the morning that he used to make desperate efforts to drive them away. After he moved to the said public condominium, he once complained to a female neighbour about the chirping of a lark she was keeping. He could not tolerate the barking of dogs in the neighbourhood and killed dogs which barked at night. He forced his wife to make no noises in the house, with the result that she formed a curious way of walking noiselessly. Her neighbours say she walked like a cat.

Richard C. Nann, Dorcas Susan Butt, and Lourdes Ladrido-Ignacio (eds.), Mental Health, Cultural Values and Social Development, 95–98.

From these pieces of evidence it is clear that the killer was so abnormally sensitive to sounds and noises that he should not have lived among ordinary people in a public condominium. It must have been impossible, however, to separate him from normal circumstances before he committed murder.

If I may be allowed to be personal, I myself have experienced serious trouble from a neighbour who was abnormally sensitive to sounds. When we, that is, my family and I, went to live in a city in Great Britain, I was fully aware that my children might cause trouble by their musical exercises at home. Well in advance, therefore, I explained the musical situation of my family to my landlord-to-be and had my estate agent make a written contract stipulating the hours in which my children were allowed to play their musical instruments. My landlord-to-be was a shrewd businessman of non-British origin, and I agreed to a specially high rent. In fact, it was the highest rent for a private flat in that city. Thus, we came to live in a flat directly below that of our landlord and his wife.

A few months later our landlord complained to me of our children's music. I pointed out that our children had been playing their instruments strictly within the hours on which we had agreed in the written lease, and added that if he wanted to change the contract, I would be ready to negotiate. Our landlord would not negotiate any change of the contract, but took legal proceedings against us. My lawyer looked confidence itself when he glanced at my written lease. In the civil law court, however, an unexpected fact was disclosed, that is, my landlord's wife had been suffering from severe manic-depression. The document said that her doctors had been administering to her the full dose of a potent antidepressant. I felt as if I were ambushed. The landlord should have told me about the facts and nature of his wife's disease beforehand and before starting negotiations about the article of our lease concerning musical practice.

Finally, I have found in the present law of Britain a pathological viewpoint or consideration of a mental health case is placed above a legal contract. This is really one particular view of value. In a sense it is humanitarian, but another view of value might have been possible, that is, ordinary or average people should be protected from the abnormal sensitiveness of psychopaths. As it was, our children were not legally protected, but the right of a psychopathic woman not to stay in hospital overruled the legal right of our children to do their homework at home.

The above-quoted two cases, one in Japan and the other in Britain, show the fact that people of mental ill-health are living among ordinary people in modern society. The rules and customs of a society naturally tend to be formed in conformity to the average behaviour of average people, that is, the majority. In a society in which the convenience of the majority is the primary consideration the minority tends to suffer, but there are also cases in which ordinary people are physically victimized and supralegally overruled by special consideration for the minority. When the minority means, for example, the racial aspect of a society, the problem of conflict could and should be solved, in most cases, by concession on the part of the majority, but when the minority means people of mental ill-health, the problem cannot and should not be solved by concession on the part of the majority. The majority of people cannot afford to follow the behaviour of psychopaths. In this sense, in the problem of mental health, priority must go to the healthy people. Mentally healthy people must be protected from the influence of mentally ill people. Of the tragic accidents which often appear in today's newspapers a considerable percentage is connected with mentally ill people who are living among ordinary people. The above-mentioned case in which a woman and her two daughters of tender age were killed by a psychopathic man is a striking example.

To separate mentally ill people from ordinary people used to be a common method and it was often done at the sacrifice of those separated ones. At present the swing of the pendulum seems to have gone too far to the other end: is there not any better way? I think there is.

It is not fashionable nowadays to express one's optimistic faith in material and scientific progress, but we must trust and promote it in some areas. I happened to quote two cases of conflict between mentally ill people and ordinary people about the practice of musical instruments. So, I should like to stick to these examples and suggest a solution. The solution I should like to propose is very simple, that is, to make a house or a flat sound-proof; the killer and the killed could have been happy neighbours. If our landlord in the said British city had been provident and generous enough to renovate the ceiling or floor and make it sound-proof, we could have remained good neighbours to each other.

On returning to Japan from Britain, I put that idea of mine into practice, for I knew that one of my neighbours was not quite normal. Modern technology and new products can make a house or room sound-proof with comparative ease. After the completion of our sound-insulating renovation I began to realize that I myself felt much happier and more relaxed. The reason was simple. To give out no noise from the rooms meant at the same time not to be invaded by noises from outside the house. In Tokyo certain clever landlords have built some sound-proof condominiums especially intended for students of music. The rent is higher than usual, but the rooms were filled at once and the tenants seem satisfied.

A careful consideration of these examples should encourage us to a further positive step and try to make all the condominiums in the city sound-proof, whether or not their inhabitants are players of musical instruments, whether or not their inhabitants are abnormally or pathologically sensitive to sounds and noises. The condition of mental health in big cities surely will be improved greatly by this kind of renovation, for a great number of city-dwellers are more or less consciously suffering from noises. They are looking for a quiet private retreat at least unconsciously. What is more, the acoustic insulation of condominiums will be able to make co-existence of a considerable number of mentally ill people and ordinary people more easily realized.

Seen from this point of view every case of mental ill-health could be regarded as a potential indicator to show us which way the progress of human society should be made. Even ordinary people feel happier in a quiet private room than in a room with a noisy neighbourhood. Nobody likes to be molested by unwanted noises from outside. Ordinary people can usually endure them, while mentally ill people cannot. In a case like this we should improve the material condition so that even men with abnormal sensitivity can endure them. It means at the same time making ordinary people happier and more relaxed. This shows, no doubt, the direction of progress we should follow.

In conclusion, I should like to emphasize the two following points. First, we should give top priority to the ordinary people. They must be protected from mentally ill people.

Secondly, that is, at the same time, we should try to perceive in the symptoms of mentally ill people the true direction in which human efforts for progress are to be made and in which social and economic resources are to be mobilized steadily, so that more and more mentally ill people will be able to live together in ordinary society, while at the same time ordinary people themselves will feel happier.

1–10, Seki-machi,
Nerima-ku
Tokyo, Japan

Discussant: K. PATRICK OKURA (U.S.A.)

MENTAL HEALTH PRIORITIES: A SOCIO-ECONOMIC VIEWPOINT

Dr. Cooper mentions the term "de-medicalization" of health, which is something of a new term for me. He also mentions that for choice of a better word, that's what he came up with, but I think I understand what he means. He states that in the post-war period there has been more health input with little or no discernable output, and that this has had a profound effect on the politics and politicians. This may be the economist's viewpoint and I agree with a great deal of what he had to say to you this morning. But as a mental health person, as well as being involved in several other areas of health care, I find it a little difficult to agree entirely. Consider that, prior to World War II, the United States had nearly 650,000 patients in psychiatric hospitals, but with the advent of psychotropic drugs and new psychotherapy techniques, that number has been reduced to less than 120,000 in-patients at the present time, and being reduced daily. At the same time, psychiatrists are seeing many, many more patients each year than ever before. Through the establishment of the community mental health centre system our large psychiatric hospitals are being emptied and patients are returning to their communities. The whole theme of deinstitutionalization seems to be a universally accepted form of treatment. This is not a utopia, but, in many ways, it is far superior to the previous system of institutionalization that existed for the thirty or forty years prior to the war.

Dr. Cooper states that there is no hard data to show that the rich countries enjoy better health than the not-so-rich countries, and regression analysis in the United States suggests that increases in income may be more life-threatening than life-enhancing. However, there are many other variables in this equation besides health that must be considered to substantiate such a statement. He touched on these when he alluded to lifestyle and all the other things that accompany additional income. The comparison he made of Utah and Nevada, with much the same per capita income, much the same number of doctors and climate, provides a good example that these factors do not have the same impact on health. An aside relative to these two States is that the State of Utah, despite its stability and Mormon population, sells more liquor than about 30 other states in the union, including Nevada. The reason for this situation is that you can't buy a drink in Utah. You have to buy a bottle from the State stores if you want a drink, so from the standpoint of selling more liquor the State has a very high rate. Also, the State of Nevada is known as the gambling capital of the world, and most of its residents are out-of-state people who are involved in this kind of life. So, despite the fact that incomes may be comparable, despite the fact that the number of doctors are about the same, there will be different results due to these various extraneous factors.

Richard C. Nann, Dorcas Susan Butt, and Lourdes Ladrido-Ignacio (eds.), Mental Health, Cultural Values and Social Development, 99–102.

Dr. Cooper emphasized the point that it is very difficult, if not impossible, to justify the entire fabric of mental-medical intervention, whatever the specialty, solely upon the claim that it prolongs life. This is particularly true in the specialties, such as psychiatry or the field of mental health. There can be no doubt that despite the undue attention paid to its life-saving achievements, medicine, and again, psychiatry have made enormous contributions to both the quality of living as well as the quality of dying. I think most mental health advocates would agree with Dr. Cooper's point that the issue is not prolonging life, but the quality of life itself. In determining the need – the nature of the need, the health professional assumes that the total benefit to be derived from medical intervention would be self-evident, finite and readily quantifiable. Further, once the manpower and resources necessary to confer the benefit have been established, the only problem is to persuade the taxpayer to divert sufficient resources to make the necessary health care available. He pointed out that we should not be quiet about this if we need more resources. I would further suggest that if a member of every politician's family became mentally ill, you'll get the attention of every politician in the country.

Also, Dr. Cooper, as an economist, uses a supply and demand theory and points out the number of doctors available creates the amount of demand. This is the old theory of expectations. He cites the example of surgeons and the number of surgical interventions. The way "availability" is determined is by where the funding comes from, that is, from privately-funded insurance or the tax-supported system. In the United States, according to Dr. Cooper, 40% is tax funded or federally supported and the remainder comes from private third-party supported areas. In the UK, 95% comes from government or tax-supported funds and only 5% from private resource. In the United States, much effort has been spent for mental health coverage to prove that the cost for such coverage is no greater or more expensive than coverage for physical ailments. Private insurance coverage has slowly acknowledged this fact, and most major medical insurance coverage now includes mental illness. United States Congress has for the past several sessions attempted to legislate a national health benefit package, but this has become a large political issue, with the same basic data being used to prove either for or against such a proposal. The present climate does not look favourable for any kind of national support in either physical or mental health.

The entire amount of mental health service funds provided by the federal government will go directly to the individual states, with a 25% cut in the amount that was provided this past fiscal year through the federal agency, namely National Institute of Mental Health. That means that every state will only receive 75% of the money they now get for mental health services. But, there are many States with very minimal programs and it's our belief that these will eventually deteriorate even further. In fact, some states will probably have no mental health programs whatsoever. However, Congress changes every four years, so we may see this pendulum swinging another way in the next four or eight years.

With the swing to block grants we see a serious need for a strong consumer movement to boldly represent or boldly lobby the respective State legislatures and State governors to provide adequate mental health service programs to meet the needs of their citizens. The National Institute of Mental Health has initiated a program for citizen participation in community mental health centres' programs. We have actively tried to arouse consumers and citizens to make themselves available to advisory boards, since every community mental health centre in the country that is federally supported must have a community advisory board, and people who have an interest in this area should make themselves available. Also, all of the teams that evaluate these community mental health services, as well as committees and other task forces, should be part of the consumers' area of responsibility. For these reasons, we have provided as much technical advisory material as possible to make sure that we have that kind of support on all of these various committees and councils. In this way, we hope that we will bring about the pressure that Dr. Cooper mentions is necessary to ensure the realization that mental health is just as important as physical health.

In his conclusion, Dr. Cooper states that no attempt was made to separate mental health from health in general because there is, in essence, very little difference. The need continuum is equally true throughout all the branches of medicine, whether it be surgery or psychiatry. However, in the United States, the one reason that mental health has received some prominence is because we have designated it as a categorical program with the establishment of a federal agency designated specifically to meet the mental health needs of its citizens. I'm afraid that if we did not have this emphasis, we still would be at the tail end of the whole health spectrum. Without the establishment of the National Institute of Mental Health with its three-pronged approach of research, training and services, many of the advances made in these areas would never have been made. Ideally, we should be able to consider mental illness in the same light as we do physical illness, as suggested by Dr. Cooper. But I think that day is still quite far away.

I find Prof. Watanabe's paper rather difficult to discuss because of his basic approach to mental illness. He comments on the schizophrenic nature of the world and relates it to the way in which we deal with mother and child. He sees this incompatibility as being at the heart of the theme of this session, "Mental Health Priorities: Socio-Economic Viewpoint". He cites two examples to expand his point. The first is of a man who was so sensitive to noise that he committed murder to eliminate the noise that he found intolerable. The second is his own personal experience relative to the intolerance of noise and the predicament he found himself in where the consideration of a mental health case was placed above a legal contract that he had faithfully signed.

The outcomes of the two cases he mentions indicate to him that the mentally ill, who are in the minority, should not be shown any concession on the part of the majority, who are considered normal. He further states that the mentally healthy should be protected from the influence of the mentally ill. He cites today's news headlines regarding the percentage of the mentally ill committing major crimes. He also states that the pendulum has gone too far in the protection of the mentally ill.

The question I must ask is: Why does it have to be one or the other, why can't it be both? Is it not possible for both the mother and child to have good mental health? This does not seem incompatible in my judgement.

I find it quite difficult in 1981, with the knowledge and research data available to us, to agree with Prof. Watanabe's conclusion. In modern society, with the tremendous stresses, pressures, mobility, etc., anyone of us who consider ourselves normal could at any time suffer mental illness. It is a very fine line that separates those who are ill from those who are so-called normal when statistics show that four, five or six persons, depending on where you reside, out of every ten persons sometime in their life span will need psychiatric care. The answer is not segregation of the ill from the normal but a better understanding of the mentally ill and their problems.

The suggested solutions Prof. Watanabe offers, using the two examples he has presented, are rather simplistic and the many ramifications involved are not taken into consideration. Being placed in a soundproof room, with the deprivation of noise, has caused mental illness in children. Many experiments have shown that deprivation of any sensory stimuli has caused serious damage in the normal development of children. Nature and natural noises, the hustle and bustle of the community, are what gives character and colour to our lives. I am not so sure I would enjoy living in a noiseless world.

Prof. Watanabe, in his 1979 paper on Women's Role at the Salzburg World Congress, raised many provocative questions and he seems to be in true form by raising similar questions in his paper today.

6303 Friendship Court,
Bethesda, Maryland,
U.S.A. 20817

TSUNG-YI LIN, M.D., F.R.C.P. (C) (Canada)

MENTAL HEALTH AND THE THIRD WORLD – CHALLENGES AND HOPE: THE MARGARET MEAD MEMORIAL LECTURE

OPENING REMARKS

The singular honour accorded to me as 1981 Margaret Mead Memorial Lecturer simply overwhelms me, for I fully realize that it is beyond my ability to give a lecture of a significance to match the name of one of the great thinkers of our time. I have accepted the distinction only because the theme suggested to me, "Mental Health and the Third World", a field of my own life-long endeavour, was also a subject of great concern to Margaret throughout her life. I vividly recall our conversation when I first met her at the time of the 1957 Copenhagen Annual Meeting. As the President of the WFMH, she welcomed me as a newcomer to the Federation and said, in essence, "Tsung-Yi, we need more people like you from the East and from developing countries to join us. The real work of mental health should be done for the greatest mass of mankind living in that part of the world. I hope you will one day help us to have a Congress in Asia." Since then, I have been trying to follow her example and have been learning from her as a faithful disciple and colleague. This Manila Congress has a special significance in that I have in fact, 24 years later, helped organize a WFMH Congress in Asia as Margaret wished. I only wish she were her today among us.

For me to give an address on the theme of "Mental Health and the Third World", and in the Philippines, has another significance. From my perspective, Manila is among the first rallying points of the mental health movement in Asia and in the Third World. It was in 1958 that the First Asian Seminar on Family Life and Mental Health was held in Baguio under the sponsorship of the Philippine Women's University, the Philippine Mental Health Association, the World Federation for Mental Health and the World Health Organization. It was this Baguio Seminar that set in motion ensuing mental health movements and developments in various countries in this part of the world that have been led by the Seminar participants. It is so gratifying to identify some of the familiar faces, in this auditorium today, of participants of the Baguio Seminar. Estefania Aldaba-Lim who, together with Helen Benites, ably organized the Baguio Seminar; Edita Martillano, a Filipino delegate to the Seminar, who has been instrumental in organizing this Manila Congress; Kusumanto Setyonegoro, an Indonesian delegate to the Baguio Seminar and now a national leader in the mental health movement; and my wife, Mei-Chen. Most significantly, I warmly remember the leadership of our revered Margaret Mead whose wisdom, scholarship and courage led the Seminar to its success.

The title of the Seminar's published report, "Reality and Vision" (Lin 1960), seems to have captured the spirit and the concerns of the meeting. It pointed

Richard C. Nann, Dorcas Susan Butt, and Lourdes Ladrido-Ignacio (eds.), Mental Health, Cultural Values and Social Development, 103–118.

out the enormous gap between the aspirations of the mental health professionals in Asia and the reality of limited resources, manpower and tools available to achieve these goals. Emphasis was repeatedly laid on learning well and quickly from the West in order to narrow the gap, while striving to utilize traditional social and cultural strengths, particularly the resource of family groups in the pursuit of mental health goals.

The prevailing mood of the Seminar as expressed in its report can be summarized as romantic and optimistic; optimistic in the sense that attainment of goals was viewed as just around the corner and romantic in the fervent belief that goodwill, applied persistently and sincerely, would inevitably lead to success. It is this very same romantic optimism, which inspiring its adherents, came to affect most of the mental health movements in the developing countries during the 50s and 60s. It was, at times, unspoken but it was an optimism so firmly and so widely held that it did not need conscious articulation. The strength of its appeal was plainly evident wherever one looked. Perhaps one may even trace the root of romantic optimism to the 1948 London Congress when the founders of the World Federation for Mental Health met and joined forces to initiate a world-wide mental health movement under the theme of "Mental Health and World Citizenship" (World Federation for Mental Health, 1948). The vision was noble, and enthusiasm was contagious. But what is the reality of mental health and the Third World today, after a quarter of a century and what will be the future prospect?

Today, I should like to attempt to find some answer to the above question by discussing the following four topics:

(1) The Third World at a crossroad;
(2) Major mental health issues in the Third World;
(3) Major developments and promising models;
(4) Task ahead: challenges and hope.

THE THIRD WORLD AT A CROSSROAD

The term "Third World" was coined in the early 50s, deriving from the French "le Tiers-monde", referring to those nations regarded as neither members of the developed capitalist nor the communist blocs (Dictionnaire des mots contemporain, 1980). The Third World includes most of the countries of Latin America and the recently independent states of Asia and Africa. Many of these share a colonial past and a strong feeling of resentment towards imperialism. They are poor and economically "underdeveloped" or "developing", compared to the industrialized nations. In foreign policy, following the Indian example, many of them have favoured neutralism. The Third World accounts for about one-third of the membership in the United Nations. The most prominent public event which ushered the Third World into the forefront of worldwide concern was the Bandung Conference in 1955, at which time 29 nations from Asia and Africa gathered, issuing a 10-point declaration condemning Western colonialism and emphasizing the need for economic and cultural co-operation among neutral developing countries (Romulo, 1956; Abdulgani, 1964).

What was happened to the Third World nations in the last 25 years since the Bandung Conference, which was shaped by the vision of their early leaders and, in my view, permeated with romantic optimism? The guiding principles of economic and social development have generally been modelled after Western societies: industrialization, urbanization and, lately, consumerism. Through this kind of development, it was thought that the gap with the Western nations could be narrowed by taking the best that the West had to offer while avoiding some of the mistakes made by the West. The reality today, however, seems to indicate the contrary. In spite of the tremendous national and international development effort and relative success in achieving growth, poverty and inequality have been rapidly increasing in many, if not most, developing countries. Robert McNamara of the World Bank summarized the situation succinctly in 1978:

"The past quarter cenury has been a period of unprecedented change and progress in the developing world. And yet despite this impressive record, some 800 million individuals continue to be trapped in . . . absolute poverty: a condition of life so characterized by malnutrition, illiteracy, disease, squalid surroundings, high infant mortality and low life expectancy as to be beneath reasonable definition of human decency." (McNamara, 1978)

Politically speaking, many nations are ruled by new military or dictatorial regimes; and they are not experiencing political or social stability and have little hope for such in the near future. Furthermore, the influence of the super-powers, compounded by the multi-national corporations' economic strategies, seems to exercise an enormous unsettling effect on these newly independent nations.

The frequent reference made by Third World leaders, politicians among them, to the preservation of traditional social and cultural values of each nation or ethnic group seem to have amounted to little more than lip service. As Paul Harrison states, "With a few notable exceptions, development has been a piecemeal, pragmatic endeavour, aimed for the most part at the multiplication of material wealth. Basic values such as justice, co-operation, charity and respect for nature have not only be subordinated to that, but are often trampled underfoot in the gold rush" (Harrison, 1980). He goes on to say that some of the leaders even acquire the habits of their old colonial masters in their appalling arrogance in the face both of nature and of traditional cultures. The rape of the earth and its wealth has been central to the past progress of Western industrialization: the plunder and waste of irreplaceable resources, the poisoning or destruction of fragile ecosystems, the belief that man can mould nature with no need to take account of nature's reactions to such a violation . . . As a result one development project after another triggered irreversible changes in local habits. And the whole development process did not build on the foundation of traditional society but fell on it like a nuclear bomb, tearing it asunder (Harrison, 1980).

It is abundantly clear from the above that the romantic optimism entailed in "selective adoption" of Western models has not led the Third World to the promised results, but rather, has brought about the opposite, with new and even sharper disparities and inequalities further widening the gap between reality and vision. The imitation of Western models has created new problems while intensifying old ones, at the same time traditional, indigenous models have been sacrificed on that very same altar of Western-style development. Third World nations are today at a crucial cross-road and they should, as some are in fact beginning to do, search for new and constructive guiding principles andstrategies for economic and social development.

MAJOR MENTAL HEALTH ISSUES IN THE THIRD WORLD

The Third World with its absolute poverty, political instability, social upheaval including wars and migration, rapid population growth, and unequal distribution of wealth as summarized above, does not provide living or social conditions favourable to healthy human growth and development. Only 10 to 15% of Third World population have access to basic health services (WHO Technical Report No. 564, 1975). High infant mortality, epidemic and endemic diseases and serious malnutrition sap the vitality of the population and impair the physical and mental development of their children. Mental health aspects of health care or human services universally lag alarmingly behind other services. Assuming that 1% prevalence of seriously disabling mental disorder applies to all communities, "for every working psychiatric there are 80 patients (so afflicted) in the US, 110 in Ireland, 170 in the Soviet Union, and 190 in England and Wales; there are nearly 5,000 in Senegal, 20,000 in Nigeria and 50,000 in Ethiopia" (Harding, 1978). These figures clearly indicate the scarcity of trained personnel and the dismal state of development of mental health services in most developing countries, although it is not my intention to imply that mental health services depend solely on psychiatrists or psychiatric nurses.

The low status accorded mental health in the Third World is commonly attributed to a preoccupation with basic issues of survival and economic growth. Mental health concerns are dismissed with statements such as, "One cannot be bothered with mental health at this stage. We have many more important things to do". There is a certain justification to this kind of reasoning. However, other reasons have contributed to the neglect of mental health in developing countries. The age-old stigma placed upon mental illness in primitive societies remains unchanged, sometimes rather accentuated, by preoccupations with modern technology and science. Psychiatry and mental health have yet to benefit from the tremendous prestige and power which rapidly advancing modern technology has gained in the eyes of both professionals and the lay public. The supernatural character of image attached to mental illness seems to be still very active in the minds of many. Furthermore, a fragmentary awareness of modern psychiatric research suggesting that heredity plays a part in the causation of mental illness seem to have deepened their fear of mental illness. The lack of demonstrable treatment results for mental illness plus the inability of the mental health profession to offer simple preventive measures, such as have been applied successfully in campaigns against acute infectious diseases, have further stained the image of mental health. At the same time, the burden on the family and the public of caring for the mentally ill has increased both in financial and psychological terms, due to the decreasing capacity of the family to care for its sick members in an environment characterized by mobility, urbanization, migration and an ever-increasing emphasis on the nuclear family.

Obviously, poor image and low status have serious effects on all aspects of mental health activities. Patient care suffers not only from lack of resources for service delivery, but also from the resistance of the patients and/or their families to seeking help in the first place (Lin *et al.*, 1978; Lin *et al.*, 1981). Rehabilitation of patients is greatly compromised by the lack of understanding support and co-operation given to patients and their families by the community. Very few bright and ambitious young people are attracted to psychiatry or mental health as lifelong careers, for fear of few opportunities for professional advancement or poor financial remuneration. Support for program development, whether curative or preventive in purpose is seldom forthcoming. As a result mental health remains at the bottom of policy makers' priorities in most governments and remains as an isolated, neglected branch of human endeavour.

Margaret Mead once used the term "psychiatric imperialism" to warn mental health colleagues not to impose one's own cultural values in bringing up children of other cultures (Mead, 1948). The message was that the theory and practice of psychiatry and psychotherapy should have a "cultural fit". Unfortunately, this principle has not been applied with rigor in the ensuing mental health developments in the Third World. Instead, we have been witnessing "psychiatric imperialism" in most everyday practice. Many leaders of mental health in the Third World seem to be intent on practicing or teaching what they have learned in the West, although homilies are offered concerning the adaptation of these methods to fit their own cultures. For example, in most developing countries it is common practice to use Western qualifying standards for psychiatrists, psychologists, psychiatric nurses or social workers, or to blindly accept degrees or diplomas obtained from Western institutions as sufficient qualifications for mental health professionals, without due consideration given to cultural and social applicability of training experiences abroad.

Furthermore, substantially diverse expectations require a psychiatrist to do more than simply act as a good clinician if he is to function effectively in his home environment. In most instances, he is expected to function as a leader, administrator, and teacher, all in one. He must be a researcher, as well, in order to meet new demands or solve new problems, as most of the problems he encounters at home are not likely to be familiar ones, easily solved by applying what was learned during overseas training (Harding, 1978; Lin, 1973). Not one single psychiatric centre in a developed country offers a training program designed specifically for trainees from the Third World for their use after returning to their home countries.

Research has been emphasized as an important, necessary tool for gathering factual data used to develop mental health programs and culturally relevant curative or preventive measures. In fact, however, little has happened in this regard as far as the Third World is concerned, owing to practical limitations on research manpower and resources. Therefore, most of the mental health research in the Third World, with a few exceptions, has been done by Western investigators, with the local personnel playing a secondary role. The majority of even these studies, however, seldom resulted in benefit to the local mental health community in terms of planning or improvement of services, training of research personnel, or development of a continuing research base. Oftentimes, research results obtained have not even been transmitted to either concerned local personnel or policy makers. It appears that psychiatric or mental health researchers from the developed nations often use the people or societies of the Third World as objects or samples of study for their own scientific interest in testing hypotheses without feeding the results back, let alone with a view to benefitting the Third World in its desperate situation.

This leads to the serious issue of the brain-drain that has significantly affected mental health development in the Third World for the last two decades. A host of factors – individual, family, economic, professional or political – act independently or in combination to push a physician into leaving his own country to seek training or employment in a developed country. Many of these foreign medical graduates, or FMGs, however, have never returned to their native countries. The number of such FMGs remaining in the developed countries is staggering; for example, while there are fewer than 100 psychiatrists working in various capacities in Pakistan, the number of Pakistani psychiatrists in the UK and US well exceeds 700. Pakistan is not alone in having such problems of brain-drain depletion of psychiatric manpower.

The draining of foreign medical graduates gravely affects the recipient countries, the FMGs themselves and the countries of origin. On one hand, the presence of a large number of FMGs working in public mental hospitals has an enormous impact on the quality of patient care and the administration and politics of mental health services in the recipient countries. On the other hand the majority of FMGs are not necessarily happy with their personal or professional lives in the host countries. The plight of these FMGs in terms of their emotional and professional dilemma is well documented (Lin *et al*., 1973; Miller *et al*., 1974; Chen, 1981). Fuller Torrey even describes them as "cheap labour from poor nations" (Torrey, 1973). It should be emphasized, however, that the real victim of the brain-drain is a silent victim, the mental health of the Third World. By this I mean not only the well-being of the mentally sick who have been deprived of trained professionals to care for them, but also the serious impediment to mental health development resulting from the critical shortage of trained youthful professionals. Furthermore, it has had an enormous impact on the young professionals who, in the face of this mass exodus of the most talented among their countrymen, feel insecure and hopeless about their own future at home, and feel compelled to seek even a "second-class citizenship" in a developed country fully aware of the price they may have to pay for that decision in terms of unhappiness and discontent.

MAJOR DEVELOPMENTS AND PROMISING MODELS

Against the background of difficulties outlined above, however, a number of pioneers in the Third World have made, and are continuing to make, heroic attempts to promote mental health, both in treatment of the mentally ill and promotion of mental health as an integral part of broader human and social development. In reviewing the developments, one can identify five major models that have been successful in attaining some of the goals set and which also promise to be effective in the future.

The Hospital-Centred Model

The mental hospitals, which had been established largely to isolate "socially undesirable lunatics", were a logical place for the early pioneers in most developing nations to initiate their mental health activities. They endeavoured to improve the quality of care delivered to the mentally ill and also to promote mental health education in the family and community using the hospital as a base. Although there have been successes in certain places, the dire shortage of manpower, extremely limited financial resources and the stigma of mental illness have combined to render much of these pioneers' work without reward. Only those hospitals whose leadership possessed consistent vision and courage have continued to grow and leave a lasting impact on the treatment and care of the mentally ill, either through liaison with a university department of psychiatry or by becoming a base of active community mental health services. It is, though, particularly sad to see that much of the very limited manpower and financial resources of some nations have been gobbled up in the endless tasks of administering gigantic mental hospitals and, thus, neither any significant lasting improvement of the hospital nor any visible development of mental health services can take place, particularly after the departure of the energetic and farsighted pioneers.

The Medical School-Based Model

The department of psychiatry in medical schools, although existing in rudimentary form in most places in the Third World until recently, have been chosen by many pioneers as the base for initiating psychiatry and mental health programs. The potential advantages of this model are obvious; teaching of psychiatry to undergraduate medical students is essential not only for integrating psychiatric knowledge and skills into the training of future physicians and public health officers, but also in helping to recruit able and motivated students for future specialization in psychiatry and mental health. A few departments of psychiatry have developed further in offering postgraduate specialist training and conducting research.

The leadership role of the department is strengthened and widely appreciated especially when the scope of their activities goes beyond academic psychiatry or clinical psychiatry. For example, affiliation with a mental hospital or with mental hospitals, community mental health programs, school mental health programs or government mental health services serves to strengthen medical school-based mental health programs (Kusumanto, 1977). Furthermore, in a few instances, efforts have been made to develop interdisciplinary teaching and training programs with social workers and public health/mental health nurses, which have contributed to community mental health programs and the mental health education of the public (Lin, 1961). One must, however, not overlook some of the disadvantages of the medical school-based model. There is a danger of developing a rigid medical or biological model of psychiatry. In fact, we witness many such examples in various parts of the world, which deter development of broadly-based interdisciplinary mental health activities, culturally relevant teaching and training programs and public health approaches to mental health.

The Community-Based Model

Tigani el Mahi, who was succeeded by T. A. Baasher in Sudan, may be regarded as a pioneer in conceiving and initiating this model in the Third World (el Mahi, 1957). With neither a mental hospital nor a university department of psychiatry in existence, he singlehandedly started a small clinic in the city of Khartoum as the centre for psychiatric care. In addition, involving the religious healers and folkloric medicine practitioners as allies, he developed a network of mental health services for the community which was well-accepted and well-utilized by the populace.

Another pioneer, T. A. Lambo, established the well-known community program in Aro village in Abeokuta for Nigerian patients. Through this program he initiated a bold effort to bring psychiatric treatment to the villagers in their own setting, while making the best use of family and community resources. All the treatment and care, including many recreational and rehabilitational activities, are carried out within the context of the same standard of living as the patients' home environment in order to maximize the therapeutic effects (Lambo, 1960).

The philosophy and method of this approach are worthy of our fullest respect and have been well publicized. We still await well-documented results attained through systematic and objective evaluative research in order to assess its feasibility and applicability for treatment and care of patients in other social/cultural settings. WHO has recently initiated a project to promote this approach by organizing regional conferences (WHO Canberra Conference, 1980).

The Voluntary Organization Model

In countries where non-medical professionals or volunteers assume leadership for promotion of mental health, they either work on specific issues or form an organization to address general mental health issues, or both. The Philippines and Zambia are prominent examples of this. Emphasis is placed on working in education, welfare and judicial activities and also functioning as a lobbying group to ensure that policy decision makers take mental health principles and skills into account within overall development priorities. One possible weakness of this model as it has occurred must, however, be mentioned. With a few exceptions, most mental health associations in the Third World either fail to work closely with delivery of mental health services, or go to the other extreme of serving mainly to offer organizational support for psychiatrists' care of the mentally ill.

I should like to point out one significant feature common to all four of the above major development models: all of them have been started by a man or women or a small group of people with vision, interested and committed to the cause of mental health. It is the matching of the personality and the professional background at the time that produce the model developments. Furthermore, one can see that unless the program he or she created has become an integral part of the total health care system, most of the accomplishments come to an end soon after he or she disappears from the scene. It is this aspect of the institutionalization of the pioneer programs that seems to be a decisive element in the longterm success of a given model.

It is painfully evident that the above developments, with all their significant achievements, have not been able to provide large scale effective mental health services to the masses, especially in rural areas. In other words, the "number problem" in the Third World has not been dealt with in a significant way. By the "number problem", I refer to perhaps the most serious issue confronting the Third World, where a small number of trained professionals are overwhelmed by a bewilderingly large number of complicated needs and problems felt by the suffering masses.

I would like to mention another important development model which in my view, holds a great promise for the future. It is our fifth model.

The Primary Health Care Model

A prominent example of this model comes from the People's Republic of China, which in 1965, introduced four major principles for nationwide mental health programs: (a) Mental Health in Primary Care – the integration of mental health services with general health services, by the use of non-specialists and the so-called "barefoot" doctors from the onset of illness to the return of the patient to home and his rehabilitation; (b) Continuity of Care – integration of services in hospital wards, outpatient clinics and patient homes; (c) Self-Reliance –

participation of the patient, his relatives and the community in the care and rehabilitation of the sick; (d) The combined use of traditional medicine and modern medicine – in all phases of mental health programs including services, teaching and research (Worth 1973).

From what has been reported by visitors to the People's Republic of China, this particular model has been put into effect with certain impressive results (Leung *et al.*, 1978); Allodi *et al.*, 1978; Xia *et al.*, 1980; Xia *et al.*, 1981). Ilza Veith noted in 1978, "The (mental) patients are not lost sight of until they have been reintegrated into their family, their community and the type of work that they can handle best" (Veith, 1978). Kleinman and Mechanic observed in 1981 that, "The simplicity of Chinese agriculture and industry, the strong family network, and the tight system of social organization provide considerable flexibility in managing patients in the community. Family members and commune officials are involved in patient planning and co-operate in arriving at work assignments patients can manage" (Kleinman *et al.*, 1981).

TASKS AHEAD, CHALLENGES AND POSSIBILITIES

Delivery of effective mental health services still remains a major task for the Third World. The serious constraints are painfully evident. The bulk of populations, especially in the rural communities, are still uncared for. This poses the greatest challenge to the still too few mental health professionals – to come up with a realistic, economic and effective system of delivery that will be accepted by the public and the policy-makers alike. The dilemma facing mental health leaders in coming to grips with this immense challenge is shared by general health planners. This concern with the issue of "Health for All" in the Third World has recently resulted in a policy decision by WHO and UNICEF, which was expressed in the Declaration of Alma Ata, 1977. The Declaration included mental health as one integral element of general health for all, the attainment of which is a responsibility for all nations by the year 2000 (Report of the International Conference on Primary Care, 1978).

I personally believe that the future of the delivery of mental health services in the Third World depends largely on how well mental health care can be integrated into primary health care delivery. This will require the involvement of non-psychiatric or non-medical health manpower in the treatment and care of the mentally ill, the maximum utilization of community resources including traditional medical practices and, most importantly, the maximum participation of patients, their families, and the community in the system. The precious few trained psychiatrists and mental health professionals would be required to perform the kind of tasks that go far beyond those taught in most post-graduate courses of psychiatry. They would need a public health orientation and the ability to administer, supervise, and teach within a widely dispersed health-care system that is heavily reliant on auxiliary health workers (Harding, 1978). In other words, we need new leadership that will plan, design and administer a socially relevant mental health system for the Third World.

Social relevance can be achieved by mental health services which are closely tied to the family and social system. An understanding of health behaviour and social interaction among one's own people, as well as the socio-cultural resources of one's own community is essential for developing relevant treatment and care for the mentally ill. Recent studies comparing the prognoses of schizophrenia and other psychoses in developing versus developed countries repeatedly point out that communities in developing countries seem to have favourable conditions resulting in better prognoses of the mentally ill (Rin *et al.*, 1963; WHO International Pilot Study of Schizophrenia, 1973; WHO Schizophrenia: An International Follow-Up Study (1979); Murphy *et al.*, 1971; Waxler, 1980; Jilek *et al.*, 1970). Discovering what constitutes these favourable conditions should be a major and immediate task for Third World mental health researchers. Is it due to differences in family structure, family emotional interaction or family expectation for the patients? Or is it due to differences in the social network prevalent in the village or communal life or the extended family of the patients? Our clearer understanding of such issues would greatly enhance the chances of developing relevant delivery systems of mental health services in the Third World. The time has come, I believe, for cross-cultural research to be carried out, testing some of the promising hypotheses based on such theories as social network or intrafamilial emotional interaction (Bott, 1971; Brown *et al.*, 1966; Brown *et al.*, 1972).

The role of mental health in the Third World should also be focussed upon the larger context of human and social development. As Margaret Mead pointed out in 1955, "In all technical change, even when it seems to be concerned with tools, machines and other impersonal objects, the individual person is both the recipient of change and the mediator or agent of change. His integrity as a person, his stability as a personality, must be kept ever in focus as the living concern of all purposive change" (Mead, 1953). Unfortunately, however, her farsighted advice has not been heeded, with tragically destabilizing results visible across the globe. Robert Giel refers to the "process of detribalization", which occurs as the sense of identity and of belonging are lost and the traditional cultural norms disintegrate while the social supportive system becomes ineffective (Giel, 1978). Individuals in this state of social disintegration become psychologically vulnerable and confused due to shifting standards and expectations.

Mental health programs which aim to cultivate and promote human development should, in my view, take the family and the school as strategic targets, for these two social institutions represent the foci of the most intensive human interaction where conduct and learning are fostered and modified. With the growing trend toward universal education, the schools are increasingly influencing aspects of human development which heretofore have been within the domain of the family. It is important, therefore, that mental health efforts should focus on these two institutions simultaneously in order to influence young people in their formative years. It is particularly important that they learn how to cope with technical change and accompanying social change. They should be taught how to acquire new knowledge, while not losing what is valuable from the traditional life, usually transmitted through their family and the elders. According to research published by Rin, Chu and Lin, those who are willing to acquire new knowledge and skills, while retaining the traditional cultural values are least vulnerable to developing psychophysiological reactions in rapidly changing Taiwan (Rin *et al.*, 1966). The WFMH project on Children in Stress, which has just had its first meeting in May 1981 undertakes to analyze the complex psycho-social factors related to children in stress and the problem of how to reduce the stress while helping children to grow with a clearer sense of their place in a changing world (Krell *et al.*, 1981).

The patterns of international communication and co-operation which have prevailed until now deserve examination, for the flow of information and spread of technical know-how have so far been a one-way street flowing from developed, industrialized nations to the developing nations. This pattern has its advantages, as well as some serious flaws. As described above, progress in development by the Third World has never been accomplished through simply learning and copying. With the ever-increasing accumulation of information and experience, the time has now come for the developing nations to mutually share their views and experiences with each other, to take advantage of the similarities in their social development and cultural background. Naturally, a constant interaction with the developed nations is essential to introduce new ideas and technological advances for the forseeable future. Incidentally, in designing The International Pilot Study on Schizophrenia, it was felt essential to include five developed nations and four developing countries working together closely in all aspects of the project, starting from research design and data collection through data analysis and reporting (WHO International Pilot Study on Schizophrenia, 1973; Lin, 1967). This project has already done a great deal to stimulate the growth of psychiatry in the developing world and will continue to assist in future growth.

CLOSING REMARKS

In closing, I am sure that most of you share my uneasiness in the face of this difficult and challenging future for mental health and the Third World. Much of the romantic optimism voiced a quarter of a century ago has faded. Ronald Hargreaves, the first head of mental health for the World Health Organization, once said to me in Taiwan in 1955, "I feel so excited about the mental health developments in the developing world. In 25 years I am sure we will be sending students and trainees to the psychiatric centres in the developing countries to learn from you". Such prophecy provokes, at best, a sad smile in light of what we have seen and experienced in the course of those 25 years.

We should, however, never fall victim to despair. Looking at the history of human civilization, 30 years is a short period indeed for accomplishing any new, useful and longlasting human endeavour on such a massive scale. As a person who believes in human ingenuity and resilience, I am hopeful that our experiences during the last three decades have given us the material to build our future mental health. What I am afraid of is that we will fail to learn from our past mistakes or will not be flexible enough in our approach as we cope with the changes brought about by the new technological civilization.

It seems essential that we should see to the roots of basic issues to understand the goals of our endeavour, and to develop tools that will use fully the resources latent in our own socio-cultural heritages in order to build relevant mental health programs for our own societies. To achieve this, we must make sure that our prospective leaders are equipped with the required new skills and perspectives. We must make sure that our policy makers include mental health as an integral element of social development. We must also be sure that the public becomes active participants in this evolutionary process. If we all can view our future tasks in this light, then, there is hope. On precisely this point, the subject of hope, I would like once again to quote Margaret Mead, writing in her autobiography "Blackberry Winter".

"I speak out of experience of my own lifetime of seeing past and future as aspects of the present. Knowledge joined to action – knowledge about what man has been and is – can protect the future. There is hope, I believe, in seeing the human adventure as a whole and in the shared trust that knowledge about mankind, sought in reverence for life, can bring life." (Mead, 1972)

Department of Psychiatry,
University of British Columbia,
2255 Wesbrook Mall,
Vancouver British Columbia,
Canada V6T 1W5

REFERENCES

Abdulgani, H. Roeslan
1964 Bandung Spirit: Moving on the Tide of History. Badan Penerbit, Prapantia.

Allodi, F. and Dukszta, J.
1978 Psychiatric Services in China: Or Mao Versus Freud. Canadian Psychiatric Association Journal 23: 361–371.

Bott, Elizabeth
1971 Family and Social Network. Second edition Tavistock Publication, London.

Brown, G. W., Bone, M., Dalison, B., and Wing, J. K.
1966 Schizophrenia and Social Care. Oxford University Press, London.

Brown, G. W., Birley, J. J. T., and Wing, J. K.
1972 The Influence of Family Life on Schizophrenic Disorders: A Replication. British Journal of Psychiatry 121: 241–258.

Chen, Ronald (ed.)
1980 Foreign Medical Graduates in Psychiatry: Issues and Problems. Human Science Press, New York.

Dictionnaire des mots contemporain
1980 Paris, le Robert.
el Mahi, Tigani
1957 Personal communication.
Giel, Robert
1978 Psychiatry in Developing Countries. Psychiatric Annals 8: 92–99.
Harding, Timothy W.
1978 Psychiatry in Rural-Agrarian Societies. Psychiatric Annals 9: 74–84.
Harrison, Paul
1980 The Third World Tomorrow: A Report From the Battle Front in the War Against Poverty p. 40.
1980 Ibid. pp. 38–39.
Jilek, W. G. and Jilek, L.
1970 Transient Psychoses in Africans. Psychiat. Clin. 3: 337–364.
Kleinman, Arthur and Mechanic, David
1981 Mental Illness and Psychosocial Aspects of Medical Problems in China. In: Kleinman, Arthur and Lin, Tsung-Yi (eds.). Normal and Abnormal Behaviour in Chinese Culture. D. Reidel Publ. Co., Dordrecht, Holland/Boston, U.S.A.
Krell, R. *et al.*
1981 Symposium Children in Stress at APA Annual Meeting. To be published.
Kusumanto, Setyonegoro
1977 Culture and Mental Health in Indonesia. Presented at World Congress on Mental Health, August 21–26, 1977, Vancouver, Canada.
Lambo, T. A.
1960 The Village of Aro. In: King, M. (ed.). Medical Care in Developing Countries. Nairobi, Oxford University Press.
Leung, Sophia M. R., Miller, Milton, and Leung, S. Wah
1978 Chinese Approach to Mental Health Service. Canadian Psychiatric Association Journal 23: 354–360.
Lin, Tsung-Yi (ed.)
1960 Reality and Vision: A Report of the First Asian Seminar on Mental Health and Family Life. Philippine Women's University, Manila.
Lin, Tsung-Yi
1961 Evolution of Mental Health Program in Taiwan. American Journal of Psychiatry.
1967 The Epidemiological Study of Mental Disorders by WHO. Social Psychiatry 1: 204–206.
1973 Search for Relevancy for Overseas Training in Psychiatry: A Case for Leadership Training. In: de la Fuente, Ramon and Weisman, Maxwell R. (eds.). Psychiatry. Proceedings of the Fifth World Congress of Psychiatry, Mexico, 1971, Excerta Media, Amsterdam, pp. 1543–1549.
Lin, Tsung-Yi and Lin, Mei-Chen
1981 Love, Denial and Rejection: Responses of Chinese Families to Mental Illness. In: Kleinman, Arthur and Lin, Tsung-Yi. Normal and Abnormal Behaviour in Chinese Culture. D. Reidel Publ. Co., Dordrecht, Holland/Boston, U.S.A.
Lin, Tsung-Yi, Miller, Milton, Workneh, Fikre, Brody, Eugene and Lewis, David
1973 Foreign Medical Graduates: A Symposium in: American Journal of Psychiatry Vol. 130.
Lin, Tsung-Yi, Tardiff, Kenneth, Donetz, George, and Goresky, Walter
1978 Ethnicity and Patterns of Help-Seeking. Culture, Medicine and Psychiatry 2: 3–13.
McNamara, Robert
1978 IBRD World Development Report.

Mead, Margaret
1948 International Congress on Mental Health. The Lancet p. 303.
1953 Cultural Patterns and Technical Changes, Paris, UNESCO.
1972 Blackberry Winter: My Early Years, 1966. William Morrow, New York.
Miller, Milton, Lin, Tsung-Yi and Lin, Mei-Chen
1974 Foreign Medical Graduates: A Panel in: Bulletin of the Menninger Clinic 38, p. 1974, Topeka, Kansas.
Murphy, H. B. M. and Raman, A. C.
1971 The Chronicity of Schizophrenia in Indigenous Tropical People: Results of a Twelve Year Follow-Up Survey in Mauritius. British Journal of Psychiatry 118: 489–497.
New York Times
1980.
Personal communication with Professor Mohammad Rashid Chaudhry.
Personal communication
1955.
Report of the International Conference on Primary Health Care, Alma Ata, U.S.S.R. September 6–12, 1978 ICPHC/ALA/78.10.
Rin, Hsien and Lin, Tsung-Yi
1963 Mental Illness Among Formosan Aboriginese as Compared with the Chinese in Taiwan. Journal of Mental Science 108: 134.
Rin, Hsien, Chu, Hung-Ming, and Lin, Tsung-Yi
1966 Psychophysiological Reactions of a Rural and Suburban Population in Taiwan. Acta Psychiatrica Scandinavica 42: 410.
Romulo, Carlos P.
1956 The Meaning of Bandung. Chapel Hill, The University of North Carolina Press.
Sivard, Ruth J. (ed.)
1980 World Military and Social Expenditures.
Torrey, Fuller
1973 Cheap Labour from Poor Nations. American Journal of Psychiatry 130.
Veith, Ilza
1978 Psychiatric Foundation in the Far East. Psychiatric Annals 8: 12–41.
Waxler, Nancy
1980 Is Outcome for Schizophrenia Better in Non-Industrial Societies? The Journal of Nervous and Mental Disease 167: 144–158.
WHO International Pilot Study of Schizophrenia, World Health Organization 1973 Geneva.
WHO Technical Report No. 564
1975 Organization of Mental Health Services in Developing Countries. Geneva.
1975 Ibid. p. 14.
WHO Schizophrenia: An International Follow-Up Study, John Wiley and Sons, Sussex,
1979 England.
WHO Canberra Conference
1980.
World Federation for Mental Health
1948 Mental Health and World Citizenship. Report of Interprofessional Preparatory Commission for Third International Congress on Mental Health.
World Bank Report
1980.
Worth, Robert
1973 New China's Accomplishments in the Control of Diseases. In: Wegman, Myron, Lin, Tsung-Yi and Purcell, Elizabeth (eds.). Public Health in the People's Republic of China. Josiah Macy Foundation, New York.

Xia, Zhenyi and Zhang Mingyuan
1981 History and Present Status of Modern Psychiatry in China. Chinese Medical Journal 94(5): 297–299.

Xia, Zhenyi, Yan Heqin, and Wang Changhua
1980 Mental Health Work in Shanghai. Chinese Medical Journal 93(2): 127–129.

E. MANSELL PATTISON, M.D. (U.S.A.)

TOWARDS A PSYCHOSOCIAL CULTURAL ANALYSIS OF RELIGION AND MENTAL HEALTH: THE MARY HEMINGWAY REES MEMORIAL LECTURE

It is with humble honor that I present this memorial lectureship on religion and mental health. For me, the topic is relevant because of both my personal life-long religious commitments and some 20 years of professional research in this area. For you, an audience of mental health personnel, I hope to offer cogent evidence for us all of the relevance of religion to mental health.

In this address I wish to show the historical relationships that have been obtained between mental health concerns and religious concerns. I wish to illustrate that although secularization has produced a marked separation, such a separation is more apparent that real. Evidence will be presented of the mutual relationship of religious issues and mental health. This will be illustrated in an examination of religion and mental health interactions in terms of culture, social networks, family, and individual behavior. Finally, I shall present an analysis of religious philosophy as a major influence on mental health concepts and mental health delivery systems.

I. HISTORICAL ATTITUDES

There is a striking paradox in the historical attitudes between the academic human sciences and the mental health disciplines toward religion. The psychology of religion, dating from William James' *Varieties of Religious Experience* in 1902 onward to the current empirical studies, has been a robust and ever increasing sophistication in the analysis of religious beliefs, attitudes, values, and behaviors. The sociology of religion was a central concern of the pioneer sociologists such as Durkheim and Weber, and continues today as a central sociological theme. In anthropology, religion is a central aspect of almost all ethnography.

In contrast, in my recent review of the mental health literature on religion, I found virtually no theoretical work published and little more in empirical research. What is published in the mental health literature is mostly case reports of psychopathology or psychoanalytic discussions of religion in terms of intra-psychic conflict (Pattison, 1978).

Yet, if we look back over the development of the western mental health movement, it is immediately obvious that religion and mental health were deeply intertwined. The first modern textbook of psychiatry published in 1563, *De Praestigiius Daemonum*, by Johan Weyer was, after all, a treatise on the proper interpretation of religion in relation to mental illness. The first modern treatment methods in psychiatry, that of "moral therapy" instituted by the Tuke family at the York Retreat in England in the 1700's, was founded on Quaker religious principles. However, by 1850 a scientific neuropsychiatry

Richard C. Nann, Dorcas Susan Butt, and Lourdes Ladrido-Ignacio (eds.), Mental Health, Cultural Values and Social Development, 119–151.

had taken hold. Thomas Kirkbride, a founding father of the American Psychiatric Association and Superintendent of the Pennsylvania Hospital, challenged the principles of moral treatment in the name of spurious statistics. A psychiatry of the brain replaced a psychiatry of the person. Meanwhile, the psychoanalytic movement contributed to a philosophy of man grounded in the western intellectual history of rationalism, naturalism, and empiricism, which led to the flowering of logical positivism and a skeptical agnosticism, that passed into the mid-twentieth century as a mild-mannered, humanistic, progressive social evolutionism, accompanied in measured tread by a western Christian theology of an amorphous social gospel of human redemption through the good works of social welfare. Thus, by 1950, the mental health disciplines in the western world had become virtually separated from religion.

Since 1950 there has been a curious amalgamation. The community mental health movement called attention to the clergy and churches as community resources for the mental ill. International mental health movements have brought western mental health professionals into personal contact with traditional and changing religious cultures where religion is very much part of mental health concepts, quite unlike the secularized western cultures. And western culture itself has undergone fascinating revivals of religious interest, forcing western mental health professionals to reconsider religious issues.

Let us now consider these developments in western culture in some detail, since they afford some insight into the common dilemmas of the human in history.

II. RELIGION IN WESTERN CULTURE

Religion has always loomed large in human affairs, and continues to do so even in western 'secularized' society. A full century after the conventional scientific and philosophic wisdom of the day declared the idea of God a "costly and unnecessary hypothesis", conventional religious movements are alive and well in contemporary America (Zaretsky and Leone, 1974). Even more striking is the tremendous upsurge of 'new religions' whose devotees vehemently reject traditional and conventional religious beliefs and practices (Needleman, 1970; Needleman and Baker, 1978). To a significant extent, this renewed religious concern is neither a surfacing of continued conventional religion nor a revival of traditional religion, but a "new religious consciousness" in the culture (Glock and Stark, 1976; Wuthnow, 1976).

To understand this current religious consciousness, we must hark back to the prevailing consciousness of mid-19th century western thought. The notion of "cultural evolutionism" was the reigning zeitgeist: whether we turn to biological, philosophical, or social thought, all was of the same fabric. In essence, human culture was viewed as a process of cultural evolution. Culture was ever developing toward new and higher forms of social organization. Older social beliefs, forms, and practices were giving way to a new social order based upon rational scientific data. Western civilization was the apogee of such evolution – leading toward the utopia of a rational scientific society.

Among the intellectual cognoscenti of that time, conventional wisdom held that religion had been a necessary and useful force for social cohesion in primitive societies. But now progressive evolution of the social order rendered religion obsolescent. Religious faith and belief was perceived as atavistic, anachronistic, magical, and naive. Religious structuring of behavior was viewed as coercive, constrictive, and obstructive of the continued development of a society based on rationalism and scientism. In sum, religion was viewed with perhaps benign tolerance, beyond the merit of skepticism and, above all, an epiphenomenon scientifically demonstrated to be irrelevant to a mature human society.

As historian John Dillenberger (1960) has clearly described, there was a 500-year debate in critical western thought over the constitution of an overarching "weltanschauung" or world view. The issues were more profound than a simple battle of science vs religion, extending into the definition of reality, meaning, matter and substance, the essence of society, and the nature of man. And above all, it was a debate over where the locus of grounding for human behavior was to be found. As Dillenberger points out, the religious assumptive weltanschauung gradually gave way, and by the last of the 19th century the scientific weltanschauung held intellectual sway. This is not to say that popular and conventional religion did not remain, particularly in America; but rather that a superficial patina of "civil religion" (Bellah, 1975) remained. This patina of religiosity, however, did not command the commitment of life and action, serving more to obscure to the common mind the radical degree to which a scientific consciousness now informed western behavior.

Not all of the intellectual world took these changes in western consciousness with sanguine and enthusiastic acceptance. With remarkable and foretelling prescience Jean-Paul Sartre (1957) explicated the problems for the new human society:

> The existentialist is strongly opposed to a certain kind of secular ethics which would like to abolish God with the least possible expense. . . . The existentialist, on the contrary, thinks it very distressing that God does not exist, because all possibility of finding values in a heaven of ideas disappears along with Him: there can no longer be an *a priori* Good, since there is no infinite and perfect consciousness to think it. . . . Indeed, everything is permissible if God does exist, and as a result man is forlorn because neither within him nor without does he find anything to cling to. . . . I find myself suddenly along without help, engaged in a world for which I bear the whole responsibility. (pp. 21ff.)

Sartre saw the fabric of society rent apart by the loss of religion, and not stitched together again by the seamstresses of science. The themes of existential angst, the philosophy of the absurd, the sociology of the lonely crowd, the ennui of the workless week-ends, all manifest the central notion of the existential man of freedom. Man is totally free. The consequence is social isolation, aloneness, the loss of meaningful social bonds.

This leads us to a central tension: existence in human relationships involves commitment, compliance to the demands and expectations of others, the willingness to submit to personal and social demands. The excesses of social coercion are set in bas relief by the excesses of lack of social relationships.

The sociologist Philip Rieff (1966) describes the ebb and flow between social commitment which becomes constrictive, and social commitment which is nourishing. He describes *negative* communities that require no commitment and offer no symbolic integrative values in contrast to *positive* communities which demand commitment and offer symbolic integration. He concludes

To speak of a moral culture would be redundant. Every culture has two main functions: (1) to organize the moral demands that make men intelligible and trustworthy to each other, thus rendering the world intelligible and trustworthy; (2) to organize the expressive remissions by which men release themselves in some degree from the strain of conforming to the controlling symbolic, internalized variant readings of culture that constitute individual character. The process by which a culture changes at its profoundest level may be traced in the shifting balance of controls and releases which constitute a system of moral demands. (p. 28)

Note that Rieff does not subscribe to a progressive evolution that will cut the Gordian knot of tension between controls and releases. Rather human society reflects a fluctuation between the need to provide more control and the need to alleviate such.

These basic cultural processes are at the center of religion. Indeed, anthropologists have seen religion as a central organizing process of culture. The late Harvard anthropologist, Clyde Kluckhohn (1966) comments:

There is a need for a moral order. Human life is necessarily a moral life precisely because it is a social life, and in the case of the human animal the minimum requirements for predictability of social behavior that will insure some stability and continuity are not taken care of automatically by biologically inherited instincts, as is the case with the bees and ants. Hence there must be generally accepted standards of conduct, and these values are more compelling if they are invested with divine authority and continually symbolized in rites that appeal to the senses. (p. iv)

Sartre challenged the scientific consciousness on philosophical grounds, but he also writes after two world wars and genocide. Can the scientific weltanschauung hold a society together? Is such a grounding of being sufficient – not just on logical grounds, but in terms of human experience and action? Or is it possible that both tough-minded logical empiricism and obdurate philosophical existentialism are manners of rationalization – while in everyday life these very exponents of non-religious groundings exemplify in their lives the rootings in the dirt for nourishing substance?

I suggest that the current new religious consciousness is just such a manifestation – a growing sense of the need for groundings, which are experienced in meaningful commitments and symbolized in shared religion. This interpretation is supported by the recent observations of religious historian Martin Marty (1977):

> The age-old dogfight between science and religion is entering a strange new phase – strangest of all, in place of the ancient set piece between belief and unbelief, we are now seeing internecine warfare between old school religionists and a newer breed of theologians cautiously open to scientific advances, and between hard core, slide rule scientists and their colleagues who are open to the new findings about mind and consciousness. Both the theologians and the scientists are warring among themselves .... Scientists and theologians of conviction, whether they be conservative or liberal, positivist or not, now do link in subterranean ways, or they meet in alliances across party lines in what once was no-man's-land. (p. 25)

The struggle over the "consciousness of our world" is spreading to the man in the street. We have witnessed the immense popularity in the past decade of movies, plays, and books about magic, mysticism, and supernaturalism. The western man in the street no longer has a consciousness committed to the infallibility of science. Even if that man on the street is not religious in the conventional sense, surely many consider the mystical, the transcendental, the cosmic, the supernatural, and even the the religious as not incidental to their lives.

A number of social scientists have interpreted this return to a supernaturalistic cosmology in a secular western culture much along the lines already described.

S. K. Pande (1968), a non-western psychiatrist, noted that the scientific western cosmology created

> deficits in the Western way of life ... negative psychological implications ..., and Western psychotherapy, especially the psychoanalytic model, as a symbolic and substantive undertaking to correct them. (p. 432)

This theme is underscored by Henri Ellenberger (1970) in his history of western psychotherapy, where he notes that psychotherapy was a response to cosmological problems of the educated elite.

> By the end of the nineteenth century the upper classes could no longer be content with the existing method of hypnotic and suggestive therapy and demanded a new, nonauthoritarian psychotherapy that would explain to the patient what was going on in his own mind. (p. 887)

The problem, of course, is that we now live in a post-modern age in which people no longer find the cosmology of the western scientific ethos satisfactory. The current rise of supernaturalism in western culture – belief in demonology, possession, exorcism, and the gamut of supernaturalistic cosmologies now popular – is not unpredictable. Social conditions were ripe in the western world for the re-emergence of supernaturalism. These conditions include a society perceived as oppressive, trust in social institutions has disintegrated, social protest has been realistically dangerous, and a mood of hopeless impotence has emerged. Such social conditions certainly typified the late 1960's when the wild hope of social activism faded and people withdrew into person privatism and supernaturalism.

The Spanish anthropologist Baroja (1964) notes that the breakdown of western rationalism has brought us full circle back to medieval supernaturalism because:

> Ours is no period of calm, with an optimistic view of public morality and religious philosophy and beliefs. It is an age of existentialism and an existential way of life, which leads man to break down the barriers and conventions and face up to his own angst. (p. 257)

The existential consciousness of our day is the stark sense of alienated and singular responsibility for everything. Historian Judith Neaman (1975) finds it not surprising that psychiatry is becoming more biological just at the time when our society is becoming more metaphysical. She recalls that, in every culture, a period of hyperrationalism is followed by a renewal of supernaturalism. For with the rationalism and ultimately the existentialism comes too much responsibility – too much to bear. Psychiatry brought man from outer reality into himself and only himself, and left man there. Neaman concludes:

> The legacy of the Middle Ages was the increasing interiorization of the self and a concomitant increase in responsibility for human action. These ideas were consumated in the twentieth century beliefs that we are responsible not only for our own actions but also for our own guilts, fears, and obsessions. The fantasy of the 1970's has been a wish to return to an age of exorcism. (p. 190)

Similarly, in her study of new religious movements, anthropologist Erika Bourguignon (1973) finds:

> There is a wish to find alternative ways of living, and thus not only modify society, but modify the self. (p. 352)

In summary, western man is the inheritor of an intellectual legacy of the idea of cultural evolution. That legacy interpreted religion primarily in terms of an oppressive and constrictive social force that exacted destructive compliance in the behavior of adherents. From that perspective it might seem puzzling that both intellectuals and the common man might deliberately resurrect the supernatural. However, we have also seen that the intellectual legacy was naive. Thus, in the western world, we observe the search for new religious cosmologies, with new modes of religious healing of mental ills, which have reappeared in new forms, but of the same substance as the traditional religious cosmologies of other traditional religious cultures.

III. THE DEFINITION OF REIGION

To discuss the functions of religions, we must clarify what we mean by religion, for it is a complex phenomenon. It is multivariate in form and function. Consequently, to pose the question of the effect or influence of religion on this or that human behavior is not very productive. Rather, we must define specific religious factors that may influence human behavior. More often, no one religious factor operates in isolation, but in permutations or combinations of multiple religious factors. It is rather like asking how parents influence children. Obviously they do – but through multiple and interactive variables.

The most well-known set of religious variables was constructed by Glock and Stark (1965). They proposed five major dimensions of religion:

(1) Ideological: Refers to commitment to a group or movement as a social process.
(2) Intellectual: Refers to specific sets of beliefs, explanations, or cognitive structuring of meaning and value.
(3) Experiential: Refers to the feelings one experiences, which may be entirely personal, or structured group activities which produce specific experiences.
(4) Sacramental: Refers to participation in symbolic rituals.
(5) Consequential: Refers to religiously defined standards of conduct.

It is obvious that each religious dimension has a different import for human conduct. In different religious cultures there may be primary emphasis on one of the five dimensions to the relative exclusion of all others. Thus, when we say a person is religious, or ask of the influence of religion, we must qualify our inquiry to a specific dimension or combination of dimensions.

IV. RELIGION AND CULTURE

The potency of religion in the influence of human behavior is related to the level of cultural organization and complexity. On the one extreme we have the small face-to-face village which is the existent society and the culture – even if there be similar villages nearby. Here there is a low differentiation of social roles and a relatively homogeneous social existence. In such a society, religion is the culture and culture is the religion. Religion is infused into every aspect of daily life and provides an overarching structure for existence. Here "religion-culture" defines meaning and action to everything. All of life is *ipso facto* religious. In such "small societies" there is relative unformity and conformity. There is early and rigorous socialization into the religious beliefs and practices for they are the warp and woof of existence. One could scarcely function without being religious. Although deviant behavior can and does occur, the limits of deviancy are severely constrained by the survival needs of the society. In turn, substantial deviancy from the "religious-cultural" norms is high-risk for survival – where else can one go and survive?

Somewhere intermediate is the small town phenomena as part of a large and differentiated culture. The small town retains the essential social homogeneity of the village. Religion and culture are one, despite the superficial variations between local denominations. The social history of small towns in America (Lingeman, 1980) reflects the paramount importance of immediate personal interaction and insulation from the pluralistic values and life styles of urban industrialized society. Lingeman (1980) notes that the insular small town society first came under attack at the turn of the 20th century when economic subsistence and viability in these small societies was compromised by larger socio-economic developments on a national scale. Seeking survival in the urban society, the expatriates might feel displaced and long to return to the security and safety of the structured "religious-culture" of the small town. Others, like Sinclair Lewis in *Main Street* and Edgar Lee Masters in *Spoon River Anthology* satirized the coercive social structure of small town "religious-culture". The perceived oppression of small town mores, however, is from the perspective of the cosmopolitan and pluralistic culture of urban society.

In this case, deviancy from the small town cultural construction of reality becomes possible and feasible for two reasons. First, there is an available alternative reality of urban society against which to measure the small town reality. Second, there is an alternative culture to which the small town deviant can flee – and even be non-deviant in the alternative society.

The same process has obtained in urban areas in both Europe and developing countries, in which small town "religious-culture" has been re-created in "urban villages", more often termed shtetls, barrios, ghettos or the "ethnic community". Urban villagers function with the same tensions of cultural collision as their country village cousins. Some members find comfort, solidity, support, and meaning in the urban village; others find it stifling and coercive.

The point is obvious here that the village structure is maintained, whether in country or city, by a uniform "religious-culture" which maintains a viable structure of meaning and demands relatively homogeneous behavior of community members. High commitment is required to maintain village viability in the face of the larger impinging cosmopolitan culture. Personal value is lodged in shared beliefs and values, shared styles of behavior, and shared ideology. Your social role is determined before your birth and remains with you throughout life. Who you are in the established continuity of social order is more important that what you do. Therefore, the social task is to learn your ascribed role and live in it.

In contrast, the urban cosmopolitan culture is not based on continuity or on similarity. This is a highly differentiated society of multiple tasks and roles. Social role is achieved and lost with equal rapidity. Beliefs, values, and ideologies take a distant second place to the immediate utilitarian performance of tasks which anonymously link with the tasks of others.

As a result, the structure and function of the utilitarian culture is not threatened by divergent and pluralistic beliefs, values, and ideologies. Even deviant behavior does not threaten the culture or the individual – "just so long as you get your job done". Thus a "religious-culture" is not necessary for the production of goods and instrumental services. Religion is intrinsically less relevant to the instrumental achievement tasks. Religion and culture can be separated. And for this reason, religion is, indeed, increasingly irrelevant to urban man, and religion is less potent. On the other hand, the very anonymity of the impersonal urban society role performances makes religion all the more relevant to personal meaning and personal social relations. This process leads to highly "personalized religion" – typical western concepts of personal relations between man and God. Yet this option, too, fails to address the need for "social religion", which links fellow man to fellow man. Again, this is reflected in the characteristic nature of religious resurgence, which stresses religious community. In this latter case, we arrive at religious norms of *personal* conduct, but not religious norms which define the *totality* of all events and behavior.

In summary, religion is both strong and central to an agrarian peasant culture. Relgiion is attenuated in the urban or country small town society, whereas religion is impotent and irrelevant to urban utilitarian achievement culture – yet here religion is paramount to personal meaning and interpersonal relations.

To the extent that a religion addresses multiple spheres of life activity, the greater such religious structure will impact on the lives of people The one extreme case would be the religious commune that withdraws from the urban society and establishes a separate "religious-culture". Here there is re-creation of a "total religious community". At the other extreme is the case of "civil religion", which addresses no specific aspect of actual life behavior. Here there are no norms to comply with nor any social religious structure in which a person can place one's life.

V. RELIGION AND SOCIAL NETWORK

The next level of social organization is what is now termed the "social network" (Pattison, 1977; Pattison *et al*, 1979). People are not linked amorphously to culture at large. Rather, each person is embedded in a finite number of social relations of about 1500 to 2000 persons. I shall briefly describe the nature of social network structure, and then proceed to illustrate some issues of religion at this level, particularly in religious cults.

People are linked to each other in a variety of patterns, termed "networks". Depending upon the specific social action, we can trace these networks throughout this finite number of people. Thus, there are rumor networks, political networks, informational networks, work networks, friendships networks, etc. Not all people are involved in all the networks, and many people in a network, which is an invisible social construct after all, do not know one another, nor are they aware that they belong to the same social network. Yet their social actions influence one another, and through appropriate social action the invisible social links can be made visible to all – as, for example, a community response to a disaster or political action campaign.

I shall discuss only personal networks here. That is, the networks of social relations identified with one person, who is consciously related to a finite number of persons. Even though all these persons do not know one another, they are all socially related to the identified subject. This is called an "ego-centric" network. And, even more limited, I shall discuss only the persons deemed most "important' to the individuals who comprise the "intimate psychosocial network" of the individual. This limited group of people, about 25 persons in normal networks, we find to be a basic social unit of function.

In order to study the personal psychosocial network, we have devised the Pattison Psychosocial Inventory. This consists of three major elements. First, we ask subjects to simply list all the people who are important to them, regardless of whether they like the persons or not, arranged in four subgroups of family, relatives, friends/neighbors, and social/work associates. Second, the subject specifies which people have ongoing relationships between them, apart from their relation to the subject – these are the links or "connections" in the network. Third, the subject rates the nature and quality of interaction between the subject and each person on five variables that have been shown to be critical elements of significant interpersonal relationships. The first variable is contact; there is a high degree of *interaction*, whether face-to-face, by telephone, or by letter. In other words, the normal person invests in those with whom he has frequent contact. Second, the relationship has a strong *emotional intensity*. The degree of valued investment is reflected in the intensity of feeling toward the other. Third, the emotion is *positive*. Negative important relationships are maintained only in the face of constraint (e.g., a boss or spouse). Fourth, the relationship has an *instrumental base*, i.e., the other person is not only positively valued but can be counted on to provide concrete assistance. Fifth, the relationship is *symmetrically reciprocal*. The other person returns a strong positive emotional feeling and may count on you to, in turn, provide instrumental assistance. So there is an affective and instrumental quid pro quo and mutual exchange of both positive feelings and instrumental assistance between the subject and the others in his personal network.

With this method we have studied a national sample of normal populations and a wide variety of persons with different types of psychopathology. We have discovered three main types of personal social networks. First is a highly replicable social network for normal persons. Second is a "neurotic-type" network common to persons with neurotic disorders, alcoholics, and suicide attempters. Third is a "psychotic-type" network common to acute and chronic schizophrenics and manic-depressive, sociopaths, and heroin addicts.

The normal network has about 25 persons. There are five or six persons in each subgroup of family, relatives, friend/neighbors, social/work associates. In a normal network, each person relates to about six other persons apart from the subject. The relationships are rated highly on each of the five variables of interaction. That is, the relationships have frequent contact, positive and intense emotional investment, provide instrumental assistance, and are symmentrically reciprocal.

What does this normal social network provide the subject? First, it provides a relatively consistent set of norms and social expectations for the management of intercurrent stress. Second, individuals and groups can be readily mobilized in the network to respond to the subject when under stress. Third, there is a rather continuous flow of positive emotional support to the subject. Fourth, the network provides ready and available instrumental assistance to the subject. Fifth, the network is relatively conflict-free and tends to be stress-reducing, rather than stress-inducing or stress-maintaining. Sixth, the network is semipermeable across multiple areas of life interaction, so that the subject is consistently reinforced in function throughout his life-space, yet not subject to a single group of people who might impose a closed "group tyranny". Seventh, the network consists of selected persons drawn from a larger pool of other relatives, friends/neighbors, social/work associates, so that the loss or addition of important persons in the network can be readily accommodated. In sum, the normal social network is a flexible and responsive social resource in which the person is embedded.

Our data revealed that effective personal function is intimately linked to one's intimate psychosocial network. It is noteworthy that healthy networks have a moderate degree of compliance built into their structure. Neurotic networks are characterized by low compliance and psychotic networks by excessive and coercive compliance. The significance of these variations in compliance is highlighted in the following excerpts from my study of religious youth cults (Pattison, 1980).

Religious youth cults offer a religious healing system in opposition to standard mental health norms and methods. These religious youth cults proclaim a superior route to insight, understanding, satisfying relationships with others, and peace with self and the world. They do not offer "psychotherapy", but growth and learning. They do not offer "mental health", but health of the whole person. They do not intend to help one cope with reality but, rather, offer a new sense of reality. They are "alternative healing systems" that share many of the goals of the mental health system, but differ radically in method, content, and context. Many young people deliberately turn away from traditional psychotherapies and look toward a religious cult as the answer for what we might consider mental health problems of anxiety, depression, apathy, disinterest, meaninglessness, isolation, and confusion.

Religious cults are not new phenomena. There is a circular pattern in which religious protest movements arise out of social alienation as socially isolated cults, move into partial social accomodation as sects, achieve social respectability as denominations, and lose social relevance as homogenized "civil religion". This in turn creates an existential vacuum within which the new cultic movements are spawned. What may seem an exotic cult may be a religious movement in one of several stages of social accommodation. Similarly, there is a spectrum of religious youth movements in the United States today. Our concern here is with one end of the spectrum that I shall define as "cult", as follows: they are primarily composed of young adults, with an explicit religious orientation, offering a radical world view in distinction from the common culture, with a strong emphasis on separatism from the "world at large" which is reflected in some degree of small group communality – ranging from total community living to frequent communal gatherings.

Although strikingly different in theological content, they demonstrate similar sociological characteristics. There are cults derived from eastern mysticism, such as the Hare Krishna, the Divine Light Mission, the lovers of Meher Baba; syncretistic derivations from main line Protestantism such as the Moonies; and extentions of fundamentalism as in the Jesus People. All are derivative forms of major cultural religions but without participation in the larger culture, for the devotees live in a "separtate reality'.

Although our data are sparse, the scattered studies reveal that those attracted to religious youth cults are not the ethnic poor from out urban ghettos or rural backwaters. Rather, these are middle-class, affluent, educated, and sophisticated youth. Indeed, part of the popular uproar about such religious youth cults comes from bewildered parents, educators, and mental health professionals, who cannot comprehend why these youth who have been socialized into the mainstream of society with many seeming advantages should turn their backs on their cultural heritage to enter such a "separate reality".

Studies of youth cult members reveal relatively similar psychological patterns. Devotees show increased anxiety, decreased personal integration, and increased impulse expression. However, after conversion and participation in the life style of the cult, these youth demonstrate a reduction in anxiety and of life. One could interpret such data to indicate that the participants are "neurotic", and that these cults provide "psychotherapy". An equally tenable interpretation is that these young people exhibit emotional responses to the "existential dyslocation" in life which is ameliorated through an "existential resolution" provided by the religious cult.

The youth who turn from psychotherapy toward religious cults are the harbingers of the shift in western cosmologies now under way. These youth no longer "buy into" the western scientific rationalism of their parents. They face an existential angst that the western modes of psychotherapy do not address. It is not surprising to see new supernaturalistic social organizations form which address the existential situation of these youth. These youth cults arise out of conventional cultural religions but depart from the cosmological moorings of the conventional religions, whether eastern or western.

The sociological distinction of these youth cults, then, is the "separate reality" of a new cosmology, where the devotees come from the bourgeousie. In contrast, the poor and ethnic minorities form religious cults which protest the conventional cosmology of the culture, while the socially marginal and inept join cults which are merely off-beat transformations of popular culture such as Scientology, Theosophy, astrology, or the Church of Satan.

A second major theme is the radical change in family structure. The religious youth cults are an alternative family structure for youth who find themselves lacking a viable family structure.

As the religious framework of family structure lost much of its strength due to secularization, family, filial, and parental ties were considerably weakened. At the same time, the extended family kinship system was being eroded by industrialization and urbanization. As a result, there was increasing "nuclearization" of family structure, such that, in the middle class, the nuclear family became the conventional model of family life. There was great concern that the isolated nuclear family would not long exist without the instrumental and affective supports of the extended kinship system.

It is not that the youth lost their nuclear families. In fact, many of the youthful devotees proclaim that they love and respect their parents – but that is not enough for them. The problem lies in the fact that the nuclear family alone is separated from the ongoing processes of society. The nuclear family may provide affective ties, but it appears irrelevant to the instrumental nature of modern bureaucratic society. As Kenneth Keniston (1960) has stated:

> . . . there is a loss of a sense of historical relatedness, the loss of traditional community, and the intact task, and perhaps most important, the loss of a compelling positive vision of the individual and collective future. (p. 475)

It is noteworthy that the religious youth cults have not recruited membership from the working classes and ethnic classes where the extended family kinship system, often with strong religious ideologies, still remains a modal family structure.

The extended family kinship system is a social institution which integrates the young into the culture. The extended family kinship system provided continuity of values, continuity of capital and property, continuity of technical skills, and continuity of life styles across generations.

But, though the extended family system provided for integration in the culture, it was a system that was essentially conservative in nature and changed only slowly over time. Not only did the extended family system disintegrate with the rapid expansion of technology and social movement, but its inflexibility made it non-adaptive to periods of rapid social change.

It is striking that so many young people look with nostalgia back toward the old extended family kinship system and attempt to recreate that family structure in communes. However, the communes as reconstituted extended kinship structures do not servive for long because, like the extended kinship system, they represent an anachronistic social structure that is not malleable and adaptive to rapid shifts in social roles, skills, economics, etc.

Among the religious youth cults, those which are most communal in structure (such as the Moonies) tend to hold their devotees for relatively short periods of time, from a few months to a few years. However, those youth cults which are more culturally integrative (like Meher Baba and the Jesus People) are likely to develop longer term participants who also live and work in the dominant culture.

Those religious youth cults which replicate the extended kinship system are less viable institutions, whereas the cults which approximate the normal social network systems I described are likely to attain longer term viability.

Recent studies of the new wave of consciousness among the youth who are joining religious cults reveals both a set of deprivations which these youth experience and a search for new social structures which will promote integration into the culture. Sociologist Charles Glock (1964) defines four major deprivations of these youth: social, organismic, ethical, and psychic.

It is striking that the traditional extended family kinship system provided for social, organismic, ethical, and psychic well-being, whereas many of the middle-class youth of today have experienced loss of the social supports of the kinship system, organismic loss often associated with drug use, ethic losses due to secularization, and, finally, many psychic symptoms as noted earlier. We have been that the normal social network provides social support, promotes organismic health, probably will generate ethical norms, and provides for psychic well-being.

Let us focus our analysis now on the youth cults. Here we find a social system that begins to look curiously much like our normal social network systems. Many of the youth cults are organized into small, functional units of around 30 people. They emphasize both affective and instrumental ties between the members. There is strong social support with opportunities for frequent interaction. There are usually strong interdictions against drug use and the active promotion of healthful life styles. They generate strong ethic norms, built on explicit religious ideologies. And, as we have seen before, there are indications of salutary psychic improvement in the psychological adaptation of the devotes.

It is no wonder that the names used by these youth cults indicate the nature of their social structure: the Family of God, the Children of God the Holy Family, etc.

There has been a loss of symbols in western psychotherapy. The mystery, awe, and sense of transcendence in the process of healing have been demystified as psychotherapy is promoted as a science. In contrast, we see a rich symbolization of healing in the altered states of consciousness and rites of mysticism and meditation so central to the religious youth cults. Such experiences may not be pathological regressive states but rather 'transformational' symbolic experiences of the new cosmology of the youth, which may be ego-integrative.

Finally, how do we interpret psychic symptoms? Where the social network is not adequate, a person is likely to experience inability to cope with life stress, hence generating symptoms of psychic distress and behavioral dysfunction. The problem is not just personal neurosis but rather an ineffective social network for adaptation. The data on devotees of religious youth cults reveal psychic distress among these youth. This is not surprising where the social network of an extended family system has proven inadequate. However, when they affiliate with an adequate social network – a religious youth cult, we observe a decrease in psychic symptoms and improvement in life adaptation.

The above interpretations are supported by a new comprehensive study of religious sects and cults sponsored by the Province of Ontario (Hill, 1980). That report finds that there are indeed casulalties, particularly among the highly coercive "total community' groups. But importantly, such casualities were already emotionally "high-risk" subjects. Further, recruitment into such groups is not just through bald coercion – but a series of differential decision points to deepen one's affiliation.

In sum, we may suggest that a moderate degree of participant compliance is characteristic of the healthy and normal social network. Obviously some people seek even stronger social affiliation where the compliance is more total. To many observers, such willingness to submit to rigid norms of total compliance seem onerous at best – and frightening to some. Yet the Hill report found the casualty reports highly exaggerated. Even more striking was the finding that ex-commune members, drop-outs, and the disenchanged were *not* universally negative in their judgments of sect participation. Rather they reported personal benefits and substantial elements of satisfaction, even though they did not choose to remain within the "religious-culture".

VI. RELIGION AND THE FAMILY

Religious beliefs, values, attitudes, and practices are an integral part of family life in some manner for most American families. In fact, social scientists assert an interdependent link between family and religion. For example, family sociologist C. C. Zimmerman (1974) says:

> Religion is a collective and not an individual fact. Thus the family is only partly subservient to individual wishes. It is also a religious and legal-political institution. When a couple join in matrimony the biological mating has religious and political significance. The moral and political rights, obligations and duties of the couple and their children are also altered. Family, society, and civilization intertwine through religious beliefs. This system of interrelationships explains why times such as the present see a concurrent weakening of faiths, family relations, and public order. (p. 2)

Although there is an apparent diminution in the strength and vitality of family and religion in our culture, this may be more apparent than real. From a historical perspective, Zimmerman observes that during periods of rapid social change both families and religion tend to decline in strength and together reemerge with social re-consolidation. He predicted the emerging vitality of both family and religion which we now see.

I shall focus now on some of the major psychodynamic patterns involving religion in the family. I shall describe four major psychosocial aspects of religion, with clinical examples for each.

Sacralization

This refers to the patterning of family structure and function provided by a religious framework. The religious structure defines beliefs, attitudes, values, and interactions of family life. This may include the choice of a marital mate from a specific religious background; patterns of courtship; the nature of marital vows and marital expectations; the expected roles of mother, father, children, and kin; patterns of child-rearing; patterns of worship, recreation, and education; methods of resolving conflict and defining desirable mode of interpersonal interaction. In other words, there is a 'sacred order' that provides not only overarching beliefs and values, but also defines the social patterning of the family down to very specific details of behavior.

Thus, religion is not merely an epi-phenomenon of family belief, but also an intrinsic part of the structure, order, and dynamic of family life and function.

The advantage of sacralization is that it provides a high degree of consensual agreement among family members about roles, behaviors, and goals. Thus, we may expect high degrees of social cohesion and the capacity to mobilize the family unit to cope with stress and crisis in an effective manner.

Example: A young family was confronted with a major crisis when one of their children suffered severe brain damage in a car accident. Both parents and children immediately responded to this family trauma in terms of their religious belief that the event was within the province of God's will for their family. Each family member supported the other in emotional ways and immediately re-assigned family tasks so that the injured child could be cared for. In addition, other kin and friends who shared the same religious perspective reinforced the emotional coping style of the family and quickly provided concrete assistance in everyday family tasks.

In the above case there was no great emotional decompensation on the part of any family member, nor the family as a unit. Crisis intervention from mental health agencies was not needed, because adequate coping capacity was present within the family and their extended kin and friend support systems in the church.

The disadvantage of sacralization is that the specific 'sacred order' in the family may not be adaptive to the needs of the family or to the changing sociocultural milieu of the family. Thus, when change in family function is required, it may be seen as a threat to the established sacred order, and the family capacity to adapt and respond may be restricted or compromised.

Example: A middle-aged family with five children had centered their life in a small urban Mennonite church. Both parents were professionals who still maintained a strong allegiance to a rural conservative Mennonite life style. As a result, the young children were sent to urban schools dressed in rural Mennonite clothes, and required to act in accord with rural Mennonite social traditions. Although the parents were able to tolerate the social conflict of living in two different cultural worlds, the children could not. Soon the children began to exhibit school phobias, nighmares, and manifest neurotic symptoms.

In this case, individual psychotherapy with the children had been of little avail. Only when the family was able to address the implicit sacralization of family function was change effected in the family life style with resolution of the children's symptoms.

Family Coalitions With the Supernatural

In this situation religious figures, such as God, Christ, a saint, the Virgin Mary, angels or devils, may be invoked as personal beings who are drawn into the personal interactions between family members. Parents may comfort children by telling them that angels will watch over their bed at night, or threaten children by the punishment of the devil. Coalition with a supernatural figure may be made by a family member to gain additional strength in family arguments, to gain extra power, control, authority, or sanction.

The advantage to such a coalition when developed at a somewhat abstract and general level is that it provides a common source of overarching values that may command family member commitment beyond the immediate narcissiastic positions of each family member. Thus, parents are to be obeyed, children treated with respect, and marital partner treated justly, nor just on the basis of personal power, personal proclivity, or personal need, but because of Godly sanctions.

An eloquent statement of this view is provided by Regina W. Wieman (1941) in her book, *The Family Lives Its Religion*, where she says:

> The family that lives for the sake of great things itself becomes great. . . . Complete commitment to the Creativity of God is the great source of security, of freedom, of richness, and of meaning for the family.

Example: A middle-aged family was faced with a request to provide emergency shelter for two orphaned children. Each family member was faced with different personal problems in this situation. In a family conference, after consideration of the individual personal conflicts, the family sought a resolution on the basis of their shared religious commitments, rather than on personal need and conflict.

The disadvantages of coalitions lie in the opportunity for avoidance of personal responsibility and the projection of power and authority to an invisible family member with whom there cannot be joint family interaction. Instances of family myth and family mystification lead to implicit "curses" on family members due to such coalitions with the supernatural.

Example: A little girl came home from Sunday School and immediately began to brush her teeth. When her parents told her it was not necessary to brush her teeth she vigorously opposed them, saying that she had learned in Sunday School that Jesus would cry if she did not brush her teeth. And since she did not want Jesus to cry, she was going to brush her teeth regardless of what her parents said.

Example: A seven-year-old boy was consistently annoying his parents, teachers, and family friends. Whenever he was reproached, he would reply that he was an evil person inhabited by a devil who made him do all these annoying things. So he couldn't change.

Example: A young couple came for marital counseling. The wife stated that here first love was Jesus Christ, who was telling her how to treat her husband. Therefore she had no need to pay any attention to her husband's opinions.

In these examples, it is evident one cannot dismiss such coalitions out of hand as mere superstitions, but must appreciate the dynamic function of such coalitions.

Religious Conflict as a Projection of Family Conflict

It is not unusual to find religious issues used as a 'stalking horse' to present and represent an underlying family conflict. As Draper, et al. (1965) have shown, religious ideas, values, concepts, can be a rich and accurate reflection of psychodynamics. Especially in deeply devout or strongly religious families, religious metaphor may be a dominant mode of family communication. On the other hand, I have seen many ostensibly non-religious families who have employed religious metaphor and symbol as a convenient arena for projection of family conflict.

Example: A yough Jewish family with no ostensible religious commitments suddenly began to bring violent religious disagreements to family therapy sessions. On the surface the issue was whether to provide a BarMitzvah for the children. Soon the family was engaged in an intense and rather bitter exploration of what religion meant to each family member. In this process, a latent strong difference in religious orientation between two families of origin was uncovered, which in turn was embodied in a basic conflict between mother and father over patterns and responsibilities of child rearing. This in turn emanated from basic conflicts around marital trust, sharing, and reciprocity. Although this family subsequently developed a rather strong religious commitment, conflict over their religious commitment subsided when the underlying family conflict was uncovered.

This example is instructive in that there was genuine religious movement occuring in this family, which was being distorted by the spurious projection of family conflict into their religious exploration.

Family Conflict as a Projection of Religious Conflict

Not all religious conflict is a projection of other family conflict, however, for just the reverse can occur, in which religious conflict in its own right can produce disruption of effective family function. Perhaps the most striking example is the fact that marriages of mixed religious background have much higher probabilities for marital conflict, dissatisfaction, and divorce. Differing degrees of religious commitment and religious practice may serve as the nidus for conflict. For example, a husband may become jealous of a wide who spends time in religious work to the seeming neglect of her husband. Or there may be fundamental differences in religious frame of reference where husband and wife really have divergent views of life.

Example: A young couple sought marital counseling because of mutual dissatisfaction with the marriage. Both had experienced a religious conversion as "Jesus People", and both were engaged in similar religious vocations. Yet, in the six years of marriage, the wife had developed a profound religious commitment, whereas the husband maintained only a superficial allegiance to the allegedly shared religious viewpoint. Although they had shared a similar life style at the onset of marriage, it was clear that they had grown quite apart in religious life style. The marital conflict arose directly out of now fundamentally different religious commitments.

Example: A middle-aged couple had reared four children in a devout, pietistic conservative Brehteren church. As each child grew up through adolescence, they gave up any religious belief and refused any participation with the parents in the religious activities that had been the center of family life. Although the parents respected the autonomy of the children. strained and distant relationships resulted from the loss of shared religious commitments, for the parents maintained their intense religious life, which was now discontinuous with their children.

In sum, religion may play a major role in the structure and function of family life. As we have seen, religion can promote health and moral family function, or religion can be destructive.

VII. RELIGION AND THE INDIVIDUAL

The effects of religion in relation to personality development, psychodynamics, and behavior has been extensively studied (Pattison, 1969; Pruyser, 1968; Strommen, 1971). Although there is a wealth of empirical and clinical data, one can draw no simple conclusions. The patterns of "being religious", as noted earlier, are critical to our interpretation.

As important example of this problem is found in the research on the relationship between religion and prejudice. On the one hand was the pious assertion that devoutly religious persons should or would love everyone in the world, without prejudice. On the other hand, there was substantial data on the positive correlation between religiousity and prejudice. This paradox was considerably resolved by the work of Gordon Allport (1967) who found that some very religious people were much less prejudiced than agnostics, atheists, and irreligious, while other very religious people were much more prejudiced.

The least prejudiced religious held to what Allport terms "intrinsic religion" – a commitment to universal norms and values of high moral intention. While the most prejudiced religious held to "extrinsic religion" – a commitment to a particularistic and ideological group membership norm.

These two styles of being religious can be related to norming and valuing processes of psychodynamics. I have termed the broader ego dynamics of this process "ego morality" (Pattison, 1968), to contrast with the superego morality functions which are more primitive and narrow.

Most clinicians are well acquainted with the development of the superego, which is the internalized injunctions of parental figures. The internalized superego norms are subsequently experienced as "guilt feelings". This is often assumed to be the essence of "conscience" or "moral norms". Indeed, religious norms may be internalized as unconscious contents of the superego. As a result, we can observe religiously determined behavior, which is unconsciously determined. This represents a major source of "extrinsic religious compliance". However, it can hardly be called morality, except in the most primitive sense. Such moral behavior is not necessarily moral in consequence. In fact this type of religious psychodynamic often results in immoral behavior pursued in the name of religious morality, as in the religious zealot or the moral masochist. What we in fact have is not morality, but a private moral code of the unconscious, which is at best quasi-morality or moralism.

In contrast, 'intrinsic religious morality' is related to ego development and mature ego function. Edith Jacobson (1964) had described these functions thus:

> The mature self-critical ego, though participating in this moral evaluation, also judges our ego functions and our practical relations to reality . . . evaluates behavior not only in terms of correct or incorrect, true or false, appropriate of inappropriate, reasonable or unreasonable . . . and ego goals.

The achievement of mature moral ego functions is shown by Kohlberg (1964) to be related to the following moral capacities of ego development:

(1) The ability to withstand temptation and to behave honestly.
(2) The act in conformance with social norms that require impulse control.
(3) Capacity to defer immediate gratification in favour of more distant rewards.
(4) Maintain focused attention on one task.
(5) Ability to control unsocialized phantasies.

But formal moral capacity and actual moral behavior are not necessarily congruent. Moral performance is learned through the observance of older children and adults, leading to role imitation, role practice, and role learning. And most importantly, moral behavior is strongly determined by the social and situational context of significant others (Aronfreed, 1968).

Moral or 'pro-social' behavior is based upon social learning and social reinforcement, which catalyzes the translation of principle into action. Moral character is both an attribute of the person and a situational social response. Pro-social behavior results from affective and cognitive developmental integration of the self along with socially learned and reinforced role behaviors.

In terms of religion, we can see that, where a religious system is primarily assimilated into a primitive superego structure, we will find strong unconscious religious behavior – which may not necessarily be related to higher moral values or moral behavior. Whereas, a religious system that is assimilated into mature development or discriminative ego functions and provides social contexts supportive of actualization of high moral commitment may produce behavior in compliance with high ethical principles.

VIII. RELIGIOUS PHILOSOPHY

Up to this point in my demonstration, I have suggested that religion is perhaps the strongest force in human history that can be crystallized into human good or human evil. Religion can promote mental health or create mental illness. But let us consider the term "mental health" in a broader sense than merely the absence of manifest psychosis or neurosis. What do we mean by "mental health" and how do we relate religion to mental healthiness? Here I should like to entertain a consideration of religious philosophy – or simply our fundamental assumptions about the image of man or nature of man. In particular, I shall focus on psychoanalytic thought as it has influenced our mental health assumptions.

Perhaps because we are so deeply socialized into current conventional wisdom, it is easy to accept the assumption that the mental health enterprise is based on empirical science, in which the nature of man can be derived solely from experimental scientific data. I shall not belabor the point that this assumption itself implies a particular concept of man. At point is the issue that we interpret, value, and ascribe meaning to the data; assemble, organize, and cohere the data into constructs of man, based on philosophical and theological assumptions. Such basic assumptions about the nature of humanity thus guide the formulation of empirical questions, the methods of data collection, and the interpretations thereof.

Major works have been devoted to the analysis and critique of the various "images of man" that lie behind the various experimental "psychologies", including psychoanalysis as an experimental psychology (Cox, 1973; Galdston, 1963; Klausner, 1965; Rosenthal, 1971).

In brief, classic western thought through the medieval period envisioned a static universe, with man partaking of both good and evil, caught betwixt the tensions. The onset of the Enlightenment Period did not forsake the tension between good and evil, but foresaw the power of rational man to overcome evil and pursue good. Thus, each man possessed the potential for moral action with internal and social balances against evil as God endowed each man with unique personality characteristics (Curti, 1980).

The critical transition in western thought occured in the 19th century with the ascension of empirical science wedded to a philosophy of materialistic naturalism. The human enterprise was naturalized and secularized. Psychology became a "natural science". Good and evil, right and wrong, were expelled from psychological discourse. There was no longer any "ought", only "is".

Man was a natural animal, a biologic organism. Psychology in the end is a biology. Society became an epi-phenomenon of biological "herd instincts". Coupled with this image of man was both a biological and a social evolution of man. The evil man or bad man was the primitive man. Man was evolving into a good man, and *pari passu*, society was evolving into a good society. Empirical science was handmaiden to rational man, to hasten and refine this natural progression to "higher forms". It is noteworthy that the concept of "original sin" was jettisoned, for man is not a flawed creation, but merely an organism moving along a natural line of development. There is no sin or evil in the world – only more or less adaptive behavior. Maladaptive behavior is primitive, adaptive behavior is mature. Health is homeostatic adaptation that promotes survival (Wallace, 1981a, b).

Psychoanalysis, in general, has been a major legatee as well as promotor of this naturalistic image of man. It is no wonder then that we do not find evil and sin as concepts in psychoanalytic thought. This does not mean that psychoanalysis discarded value judgements. Rather psychoanalysis participated in a subtle but radical *re-definition* of evil and sin. Evil, if there be evil, was the distortion of the natural nature of man by oppressive forces of society.

It is beyond our scope to fully elucidate the antimonies of thought reflected in the entire corpus of Freud. Certainly he was more complex than his subsequent redactors. Yet, the basic thrust of his thoughts, which have influenced psychoanalysis as an intellectual movement, are clear, as shown in the exegesis by Roazen (1968). For Freud, the attributes of human existence to be highly valued were *rationality* and *independence*. Freud was a child of the Enlightenment. Yet, at the same time, he was a precursor of modern existential man – man, the individualist – modern man existing in ennui and anomie.

The ideal image of man that Freud portrays is man who can reckon with his own impulses, who can overcome himself. Where id was there, shall ego be, indeed. But, Freud was also an elitist who saw few who could achieve the Stoic ideal of toleration and control of the self. For the average man in the street, religion, "the opiate of society", would be necessary to assuage anxiety and control aggression.

In this view, man is not evil, but merely inadequate, immature, unsophisticated, irrational, or neurotic. Perhaps victimized by his own natural impulses, but not evil. We must acknowledge that Freud was both an idealist and a realistic pessimist; whereas, subsequent psychoanalytic theorists have been more wont to stress the idealist nature of man, and ignore the seeming ineluctable expressions of human destructiveness. This latter trend reached its apogee in the humanistic thinking of Abraham Maslow and Carl Rogers, for whom man has the natural ability to become good – obstructed only by the vicissitudes of constriction enforced by society (Pattison, 1965a).

If there is no evil in man, it cannot be said that there is no evil in society. But rather than to define evil social action, it is society or culture itself which is evil – in the sense that culture constricts, distorts, enmeshes the individual, and thereby reduces individual freedom. If maximization of individual choice and individual action is a value axiom of psychoanalytic thought, then evil is any social force interfering with individual freedom. As Roazen (1968) has demonstrated, Freud came periously close to social anarchy in his social and political perspectives. Society did not contribute anything positive to the human enterprise, except as a second assist to inadequate souls who could not cope effectively with just their own individualistic resources. Freud and his followers saw only negative coercive aspects of society, and failed to appreciate either the social nature of individual development and function or the constructive and critically necessary components of social coercsion.

Finally, without explicit values to be found in the individual or the society, Freud completed the naturalistic and materialistic transition by finding value and defining good and evil in terms of the abstract notion of health, Mental or psychological health became the summum bonum. Roazen (1968) comments:

> The notion of health inherent in Frued's concept of psychoanalytic treatment is of crucial importance .... his concept of psychological normality is one possible answer to the liberal quest for an elucidation of the value of self-fulfillment ... psychic health was for Freud in part a normative concept .... he was demonstrating in practice the importance of health as a goal. (p. 283)

Note that we have shifted subtly, but profoundly, from social goals to personal goals, from moral goals to biological goals. Health is good, ill-health is bad. The mature genital character is good, the neurotic character is evil. Good health is the goal of existence, and good actions are those which promote individual good health. With health as the fulcrum of good and evil, it is easy to see how such a conceptual framework fitted the western drift toward narcissistic culture, individualistic culture, a culture pre-occupied with individual self-satisfaction and self-gratification regardless of the cost. It is no accident that, in western culture, health services consume increasing portions of the national budget, with escalating personal and social costs. Goodness is healthiness. To be sick is evil.

In sum, a broad sketch of psychoanalytic thought presents us with a naturalistic and materialistic image of man, in which the values of existence are rationality, individuality, and freedom. As a natural organism there are no good or evil attributes of man, but merely degrees of effective survival or adaptation. Society, in turn, is the product of man. Social action is a necessary evil, to be tolerated and minimized, until such time in social evolution when natural man is no longer dependent upon culture, and the values of existence have been transformed into health values. Good health promotes individual survival and social evolution. Bad health is evil in that it interferes with individualization and promotes dependency.

As might be expected, Freud does not directly take up the topics of either sin or evil. The index to his collected works contains no entry for sin. The one entry for evil refers to his case analysis of obsessional neuroisis, in which Freud interprets possession by evil spirits as a symbolic representation of possession by forbidden impulses.

As Wallace (1981b, c) has noted, Freud's thinking was both vacillating and ambiguous about the exact nature of evil, but in all, evil was that part of natural human instinct that needed to be channelled and controlled by the good instincts. The exact good or bad instincts varied in Freud's analysis. In 1915, the egoist instincts were good and social instincts were bad. In 1920 and 1921, the aggressive drive was bad and libidinal drive was good. In 1930, uninhibited sensuality was bad and aim inhibited libido was good.

Now the valuation of human instincts as either neutral or intrinsically good or evil is a conceptual problem. Freud opted to assume that instincts were naturalistically neutral in the formal sense, yet he never altogether abandoned the sense of intrinsic evil drives or instincts. On the other hand, we can with equal logic assume good and evil drives (the assumption of Plato and western thought up through medievalism). Or we can assume that value neutrality of instincts and drives, and still assume an original sin, an implacable evil aspect of man: that is, the flawed incapacity of man to transcend his own nature. In sum, the description of drive and instinct psychodynamics do not imply any particular conceptual assumptions about the nature of evil. However, it was the *naturalistic assumption* of Freud and the psychoanalytic movement that arbitrarily removed the concept of evil from our consideration of human nature.

It is striking that Freud himself avoided a direct confrontation with the conceptual, philosophical, or theological implications of his own assumptive position. On occasion, he sought refuge in a reductionistic avoidance of the issue, as when in his letters he branded any asking of big questions as pathological (Freud, 1960):

> The moment a man questions the meaning and value of life, he is sick, since objectively, neither has any existence; by asking this question one is merely admitting to a store of unsatisfied libido to which something else must have happened, a kind of fermentation leading to sadness and depression. (p. 436)

Or he appealed directly to his naturalistic assumption as in his monograph on *Civilization and Its Discontents* (Freud, 1930), where he asserts one has:

> a right to dismiss the question of the meaning of life, for it seems to derive from human presumptuousness. . . . Nobody talks about the purpose of life of animals. (p. 64)

Yet despite such overt aversions to the "big questions", Freud persisted after morality as a central issue of his thought, as Reiff (1959) has shown. Freud lived and practiced a scrupulous conventional life, despite a libertarian, anarchic, intellectual stance. This paradox, says Kung (1980) reflects the fact that Freud knew evil and eschewed it, but did not know why. It is illuminating of Freud's own personal paradox to contrast his reductionistic dismissal of evil and morality in his official publications, with his personal statements as in the following letter to Oskar Pfister (Meng and Freud, 1963):

> . . . Moral demands may be the correct expression of the valid order of things analagous to the hygienic order. . . . Immoralism cannot possibly be the last word, otherwise hypocrisy

and lies would be as good and valuable as honesty and integrity, and battling with the drawn sword for truth would be folly. ... Your morality, my dear professor, has made a deep impact on me. ... I am oppressed by the lack of seriousness ... regarding confrontation with the highest ethical values ... I prefer to deal analytically with the moral imperative, which I regard as an inadequate expression of a system of imperatives intended for the good of mankind. If this highest biological and ethical principle is deprived of its moral impulse, the effect is oppressive and alarming, while the reestablishment of the higher meaning leads to release and healing ... I prefer complete moralisation. (pp. 136–137)

If the above quotation seems like a complete reversal of the more familiar Freudian quotations, it should be recalled that the personal words above are actually more consonant with his obdurate personal life and implicit admonitions about the goals of psychoanalysis. If should not be surprising, in fact, that there is such a wide divergence between Freud's theory and life. In fact, Karl Menninger (1963) has commented that Freud's moral and theological operations were the major unanalyzed segment of his own life.

In sum, Freud left an ambiguous and conflicted legacy of thought and action in regard to evil. As I read the record, Freud persisted in grappling with the problems of evil, throughout his work and life. But he was inconsistent. His formal and official positions were modified by his many asides. He never integrated what he knew of evil into his formal psychoanalytic concepts. Yet his awareness of evil remained.

As we pass from Freud to his followers, the record becomes more meager. The official Freudian assumptions became essentially the psychoanalytic frame of reference, without much attempt to examine either the philosophical assumptions of the psychoanalytic movement or to elucidate the psychological assumptions about the nature of man (Menninger, 1963).

A major classical contribution to moral thought was *Man, Morals, and Society* (Flugel, 1961). Here Flugel concentrates on the vicissitudes of superego development as the main moral agency of man. Like Freud, he locates the concept of evil in the instinctual drive of man:

In dealing with immorality and criminality ... we are all of us born criminals in the sense that we are extensively endowed with impulses which, if unchecked, lead to antisocial conduct. This is no doubt the element of truth in the doctrine of original sin. (p. 187)

Consistent with the naturalistic assumption, Flugel analyzes individual problems of superego malfunction. But Flugel does not look at the issue of social evil, nor question the limitation of moral function to solely superego operations.

Of the nature of evil, that issue is virutally ignored or dismissed by most of the major psychoanalytic theoreticians. The assumption that scientific man will rationally achieve health is the pervading theme. For example, H. S. Sullivan (1956) says:

I found myself defining evil as the unwarranted interference with life. (p. 329)

In similar vein, Franz Alexander (1961) defines social life as lived by biologically independent organisms, in which social problems are due to ignorance. Alexander questions and answers:

Can psychoanalysis contribute to the social problem by increasing the social conscience in the individual? Obviously sound education is the only possible course. (p. 406)

The traditional psychoanalytic view has pursued the theme of good and evil beyond just instincts, to include good and evil object relations. Thus Fairbairn (1954) observes:

It is to the realm of these bad objects . . . that the ultimate origin of all psychopathological developments is to be traced, for it may be said of all psychoneurosis and psychotic patients that, if a True Mass is being celebrated in the chancel, a Black Mass is being celebrated in the crypt. It becomes evident accordingly, that the psychotherapist is the true successor to the exorcist, and that he is concerned, not only with the "forgiveness of sins", but also with the "casting out of devils". (p. 70)

Note how consistently he has subjectivized evil here. The problem of evil is a therapeutic problem, not a moral issue. Human values are persistently defined as health values (Masserman, 1960).

In sum, we may conclude that traditional psychoanalytic thought treats evil not only in purely secular terms, but in personal and individual terms. There is not objective evil, there are only evil psychological processes. Sin has been thoroughly transformed into sickness. There is no justice for evil, nor forgiviness of sins; rather there is therapy for neurosis.

The consequences of this formulation for a psychoanalytic theory of morality has been significant. Morality is considered solely in terms of superego function. Morality as a conscious and personal aspect of ego function, interdigitated with social learning and social values is almost totally neglected in traditional psychoanalytic concepts of moral function (Pattison, 1980). If social values are merely epi-phenomena of individual values, if individual values maximize self-health and self-freedom, and if there is no social evil, but only descriptive natural process, then it is logical to focus solely upon intrapsychic processes as the center of moral inquiry – as indeed the classic psychoanalytic formulations still do (Lewis, 1971; Post, 1972). The consequence, as we shall later examine, is an extraordinary neglect of not only the empirical evidence on moral process in psychological function, but also a reduction of moral inquiry to individual psychopathology.

In contrast to the traditional psychoanalytic formulations that tend to fill the textbooks and standard journal articles, there have been some significant reformulations within the psychoanalytic tradition.

Heinz Hartmann (1960) addressed the moral dimensions of psychoanalysis in remarkably perceptive manner. He notes that psychoanalysis as a therapy may provide integration and unity of psychological processes, and thereby increase the capacity for moral thought and action. Yet Hartmann is careful to conclude that psychological healthiness by no means guarantees moral action or a moral persons. Thus, Hartmann does separate healthiness from goodness. Yet, Hartmann limits his discourse to the psychological processes of self-knowledge, and does not explore the larger normative issues of good and evil. To him thse are "beyond scientific discourse".

Attempts at practical definitions of good and evil within a psychoanalytic framework have focused on differences between 'creative ethics' and "defensive ethics" (Levine, 1972); on the separation of moral values as a social enterprise from the moral values within the conduct of psychoanalysis (Academy of Religion and Mental Health, 1965). The normative aspects of good and evil are explicated within an *adaptive* frame of reference, hence relativistic and not normative. This is clearly seen in the work of Erik Erikson (1964), who staunchly sets forth the Golden Rule and proclaims social virtues in the name of human dignity and social survival. Adaptation is the key concept in all this recent work, which rests on a latter day humanism – pessimistic about the human condition and pleading for mankind to save itself. In this case we have moved from naturalism (traditional psychoanalysis) to humanism (contemporary psychoanalysis).

But if contemporary psychoanalysis in its humanistic form acknowledges evil, it is sanguine; this position is philosophically naive in its underpinnings. For where is the ground of certainty for such a humanism or its rationalistic enterprise? Some perceptive psychoanalytic voices have begun to ask normative questions about evil. To mind come the assertions of Robert Coles about social inequity, or the existential anxieties of the atomic age and our moral turpitude about war examined by Robert Lifton. The soft underbelly of rationalism in the modern age is exposed by Allen Wheelis (1971) who finds that psychoanalysis as science has no answer for the problem of evil:

> Science and faith do not now contend for the same domain, and faith is undiminished by the growth of science . . . life proceeds on something dark and deep, and, however clothed in he garb of reason, ultimately arbitrary . . . .
>
> Certainty is the basis for attacking evil. Knowing absolutely what is right authorizes the assault on what is wrong. But certainty is hard to find . . . . we have lived a delusion, we cannot know the world. (pp. 108–114)

So we have come a far distance in psychoanalytic thought from a passionate attack by the rational materialists in the time of Freud, through the comfortable assurance of traditional scientific psychoanalysis, to a disquieted contemporary psychoanalytic humanism, to, finally, existential angst in which psychoanalysts proclaim normative evil and see no answer to that evil in the therapeusis of the individual.

Now, I should like to call attention to several strains of thought which challenge the basic psychoanalytic assumptions outlined.

First, let us consider the assumption of man as a natural organism and, particularly, the reduction of man to a homeostatic biologic organism.

For example, Chein (1962) argues that the key issue is the choice between two images of man: either as a helpless, powerless reagent or an active responsible agent. If we choose the latter, then evil is a viable option of man in action, and man is a conscious moral agent. Similarly, Henry Murray (1962) admonishes that the image of man as a computer, animal or infant is Satanic in its intent and end. Murray argues that such a psychological image is not only a *reduction psychologem*, but a *reduction ad absurdum*. To Murray, the existential age of the absurd is the product of a psychology which had reduced man to the absurd. Among many contemporary sources, it will do to cite Easterbrook (1978) who trenchantly recasts the human free will as the key element to moral choice and moral responsibility, which is always set within the social context. The biologic and naturalistic image of man is not humanness, asserts Eisenberg (1972), but rather the unique human trait is moral choice against the evil action of mankind. Nor is a successful psychoanalysis a preventive safeguard against evil action. As Marmor (1979) has observed:

> The plain fact is that graduated psychoanalysts, no less than other people, continue to exhibit a wide variety of characterological patterns that are not ideal. Some show an undue amount of narcissism, others are exploitative, others noticeably obsessive-compulsive, others abrasively aggressive or competitive, still others overly dedicated to the worship of money, and finally, some are even known to become erotically involved on occasion with their patients. (p. 488)

In sum, the image of man as simply a natural organism who *is*, is challenged by the notion of man who *ought*. This latter position perceives of man as capable of evil choice and action – of man who possesses moral responsibility – of man who chooses to sin.

The second line of criticism is voiced against the notion of society as simply an oppressive agent: the failure to grasp the *reality* of the social construction of evil. We must come to grips with objective reality of evil intent, evil action, and evil social organization asserts Doob (1978). Man is capable of immense evil, from which we try to escape, says Becker (1975). Elsewhere, Becker (1973) argues that it is the failure to confront his own evil and need for salvation that is the dilemma of modern man:

> Thus the plight of modern man: a sinner with no word for it, or worse, who looks for the word for it in a dictionary of psychology and thus only aggravates the problem of his separateness and hyperconsciousness. (p. 198)

If man has the potential for evil, then certainly society can be constructed to evil ends. But in contrast to traditional Freudian thought where society is the evil, the critique asserts the moral responsibility of man to create good or evil forces of society.

Implicit in the above critique is the notion that human moral capacity is an attribute not accounted for in traditional psychoanalytic formulations of superego operation. In her recent elegant summary, Jane Loevinger (1976) shows how empirical evidence of moral development and moral capacity must be framed in terms of the unconscious and conscious developments of ego function. In the end, moral function is found to be a specific attribute of ego function, not reducible to simple drive vicissitudes and superego operation. In turn, we can speak of moral anxiety and moral concern as uniquely human experiences in response to moral dilemma (Hiltner and Menninger, 1963).

The final step of the critique is to question the transformation of all issues of evil and sin into health issues. Hiltner (1962) puts the critical questions succinctly:

> Do you believe that virtually all of man's troubles and sufferings are of the nature of sickness and illness? . . . Do you imply that he, as a subject, has no kind of responsibility for confronting and dealing with his condition? . . . If man's actual condition involves more than deviation from health, however, what else do you include? (p. 260)

A similar critique is made by the European existentialist Ludwig Binswanger (1963):

> Psychology must take the place of theology, health of redemption, symptom of suffering, the physician of priest, and that instead of the meaning and substance of life, pleasure and unpleasure have become the major problems of life. (p. 179)

What we are left with then is the age-old problem of man's inhumanity to man. Whence comes social evil into the world and how might we promote the social good? In their recent analysis of the roots of evil, Sanford and Comstock (1971) find the social tree of evil rooted in personal maldevelopment, in family dysfunction, in community dysfunction, and in the social sanction of dehumanization.

Since we have already seen how religion can be a powerful force for either good or evil at each level of the tree of humanity, it seem plausible to consider how we might address the application of religious forces for human good – and thereby mental health. I suggest that religious philosophy profoundly influences how we define good and evil in each culture. And I propose that each religious philosophy implicity directs how we use the forces of the mental health enterprise toward good and evil. It remains our further task to more closely examine the mental health enterprises in our respective cultures to determine the following:

(a) What are the religious assumptions of the mental health enterprise in our culture?

(b) What are the implicit religious definitions of good and evil upon which our mental health enterprises operate?

(c) What are the actual consequences of these assumptions that mold the nature of our own particular mental health delivery systems?

Should we be so bold to address the questions in our respective cultures and mental health delivery systems. I would not be surprised to find that some parts of our mental health systems do indeed contribute to the social good, some parts are neglible in effect, and some parts no doubt contribute to personal and social evil.

IX. TOWARD A SUMMARY

In this address I have linked religion to profound influences on human affairs at the psychological, social, and cultural level. I have suggested that religion can be a force for good or evil. I have argued that our concern for mental health is ultimately rooted in our concern for good and evil. Therefore in a fundamental sense the religious quest for the "good" is a mental health quest at the same time. In turn, we must pursue the moral assumptions, meanings, and consequences of the religious assumptions built inevitably into every mental health delivery system of a specific culture.

Professor and Chairman,
Department of Psychiatry,
Medical College of Georgia,
Augusta, Georgia

REFERENCES

Academy of Religion and Mental Health
1965 Moral Values and Psychoanalysis. Academy of Religion and Mental Health, New York.

Alexander, F.
1961 The Scope of Psychoanalysis. Basic Books, New York.

Allport, G. W. and Ross, J. M.
1967 Personal Religious Orientation and Prejudice. Journal of Personality and Social Psychiatry 5: 432–433.

Aronfreed, J.
1968 Conduct and Conscience: The Socialization of Internalized Control Over Behavior. Academic Press, New York.

Baroja, J. C.
1964 The World of Witches. University of Chicago Press, Chicago.

Becker, E.
1973 The Denial of Death. Free Press, New York.
1975 Escape from Evil. Free Press, New York.

Bellah, R. N.
1975 The Broken Covenant: American Civil Religion in Time of Trial. Seabury Press, New York.

Binswanger, L.
1963 Being-in-the-World. Basic Books, New York.

Bourguignon, E.
1973 Religion, Altered States of Consciousness, and Social Change. Ohio State University Press, Columbus.

Chein, I.
1962 The Image of Man. Journal of Social Issues 18: 1–35.

Cox, R. H. (ed.)
1973 Religious Systems and Psychotherapy. C. C. Thomas, Springfield, Illinois.

Curti, M.
1980 Human Nature in American Thought: A History. University of Wisconsin Press, Madison.

Dillenberger, J.
1960 Protestant Thought and Natural Sciences. Doubleday, Garden City, New York.

Doob, L. E.
1978 Panorama of Evil. Greenwood Press, Westport, Connecticut.

Draper, E., Meyer, G. G., Parzen, Z., and Samuelson, G.
1965 On the Diagnostic Value of Religious Ideation. Archives of General Psychiatry 13: 202–207.

Easterbrook, J. A.
1978 The Determinants of Free Will. Academic Press, New York.

Eisenberg, L.
1972 The Human Nature of Human Nature. Science 176: 125–128.

Ellenberger, H. F.
1970 The Discovery of the Unconscious. The History and Evolution Dynamic Psychiatry. Basic Books, New York.

Erikson, E.
1964 Insight and Responsibility. W. W. Norton, New York.

Fairbairn, W. D. R.
1954 An Object-Relations Theory of Personality. Basic Books, New York.

Flugel, J. C.
1961 Man, Morals, and Society. Viking Press, New York.

Freud, E. (ed.)
1975 The Letters of Sigmund Freud. Basic Books.

Freud, S.
1923 The Ego and the Id. Standard Edition. Vol. 19, Hogarth, London.

Galdston, I. (ed.)
1963 Man's Image in Medicine and Anthropology. International University Press, New York.

Glock, C. Y.
1964 The Role of Deprivation in the Origin and Evolution of Religious Groups. In: Lee, R. and Marty, M. (eds.). Religion and Social Conflict. Oxford University Press, New York.

Glock, C. Y. and Stark, R.
1965 Religion and Society in Tension. Rand McNally, Chicago.

Hartmann, H.
1960 Psychoanalysis and Moral Values. International University Press, New York.

Hill, D. G.
1980 Study of Mind Development Groups, Sects and Cults in Ontario. Report to the Ontario Government, Toronto.

Hiltner, S.
1962 Man's Problems and Potentialities. In: Doniger, S. (ed.). The Nature of Man, Harper, New York.

Hiltner, S. and Menninger, K.
1963 Constructive Aspects of Anxiety. Abingdon, Nashville.

Jacobson, E.
1964 The Self and the Object World. International University Press, New York.

Keniston, K.
1960 The Uncommitted: Alienated Youth in American Society, Harcourt, Brace, and World, New York.

Klausner, S. Z. (ed.)
1965 The Quest for Self-Control: Classical Philosophies and Scientific Research. Free Press, New York.

Kluckhohn, C.
1966 Introduction: In: Less, W. A. and Vogt, E. Z. (eds.). Reader in: Comparative Religion: An Anthropological Approach. Harper and Row, New York.

Kohlberg, L.
1964 Development of Moral Character and Moral Ideology. In: Hoffman, M. L. and

Hoffman, L. W. (eds.). Review of Child Development Research. Vol. 1, Russell Sage Foundation, New York.

Kung. H.
1980 Freud and the Problem of God. Yale University Press, New York.

Levine, M.
1972 Psychiatry and Ethics. G. Braziller, New York.

Lewis, H. B.
1971 Shame and Guilt in Neurosis. International University Press, New York.

Lingeman, R.
1980 Small Town America. G. P. Putnam's Sons, New York.

Loevinger, J.
1976 Ego Development. Jossey-Bass, San Francisco.

Marmor, J.
1979 Psychoanalytic Training. Archives of General Psychiatry 36: 486–489.

Masserman, J. (ed.)
1960 Psychoanalysis and Human Values. Grune and Stratton, New York.

Marty, M. E.
1977 Science Versus Religion: An Old Squabble Simmers Down. Saturday Review. December 10, 29–35.

Murray, H. A.
1962 The Personality and Career of Satan. Journal of Social Issues 18: 36–54.

Neamans, J. S.
1975 Suggestions of the Devil: The Origin of Madness. Anchor Books, New York.

Needleman, J.
1970 The New Religions. Doubleday, Garden City, New York.

Needleman, J. and Baker, G. (eds.)
1978 Understanding the New Religions. Seabury Press, New York.

Pande, S. K.
1968 The Mystique of Western Psychotherapy: An Eastern Interpretation. Journal of Nervous and Menal Disease 146: 435–432.

Pattison, E. M.
1965 Contemporary Views of Man in Psychology. Pastoral Psychology 16: 21–26.
1968 Ego Morality: An Emerging Psychotherapeutic Concept. Psychoanalytic Review 55: 187–222.
1977 A Theoretical-Empirical Base for Social Systems Therapy. In: Foulkes, E. *et al.* (eds.). Current Perspectives in Cultural Psychiatry. Spectrum, New York.

Pattison, E. M. (ed.)
1969 Clinical Psychiatry and Religion. Little, Brown, Boston.
1980 Religious Youth Cults: Alternative Healing Social Networks. Journal of Religion and Health 19: 275–284 (4).
1980 Moral Awareness. Academic American Encyclopedia. Arete Publishing Co., Princeton, New Jersey.

Pattison, E. M., Llamas, R., and Hurd, G.
1979 Social Network Mediation of Anxiety. Psychiatric Annals 9: 56–67.

Post, S. C. (ed.)
1972 Moral Values and the Super Ego Concept in Psycholoanalysis. International University Press, New York.

Pruyser, P.
1968 A Dynamic Psychology of Religion. Harper and Row, New York.

Rieff, P.
1959 Freud: The Mind of the Moralist, Viking Press, New York.
1966 The Triumph of the Therapeutic: Uses of Faith after Freud. Harper and Row, New York.

Roazen, R.
1968 Freud: Social and Political Thought. A. A. Knopf, New York.
Rosenthal, B. G.
1971 The Images of Man. Basic Books, New York.
Sanford, N. and Comstock, C.
1971 Sanctions for Evil. Jossey-Bass, San Francisco.
Sartre, J.-P.
1947 Existentialism and Human Emotions. Philosophical Library, New York.
Strommen, M. P.
1971 Research on Religious Development: A Comprehensive Handbook. Hawthorn Books, New York.
Sullivan, H. S.
1956 The Fusion of Psychiatry and Social Sciences. The Collected Works of H. S. Sullivan. Basic Books, New York.
Wallace, E.
1981a Freud and Anthropology: A History and Re-Appraisal. International University Press, New York.
1981b Freud and Religion: A History and Appraisal. Psychoanalytic Study of Society. Vol. X, International University Press, New York.
1981c Notes on the Compatibility between Psychoanalysis and Religion. Unpublished manuscript.
Wheelis, A.
1971 The End of the Modern Age. Basic Books, New York.
Wieman, R. W.
1941 The Family Lives Its Religion. Harper, New York.
Wuthnow, R.
1976 The Consciousness Reformation. University of California Press, Berkeley.
Zaretsky, I. I. and Leone, M. P. (eds.)
1974 Religious Movements in Contemporary America. Univeristy of Princeton Press, Princeton, New Jersey.
Zimmerman, C. C.
1974 Family Influence upon Religion. Journal of Comparative Family Studies 5: 1–16.

SECTION TWO

WORKSHOP REPORTS

INTRODUCTION

Workshops provide the opportunity for a more intimate exchange of information and views among the Congress participants and, to a large extent, they reflect the essence of the conference. The 1981 World Congress featured a total of 23 *Topic Workshops* which met on two afternoons, with some of the meetings continuing into extra evening sessions.

A number of the workshops are continuations from the Vancouver (1977) and Salzburg (1979) Congresses, covering the following topics: Migration; The Mass Media; Leisure and Changing Values; Sex Roles; School Mental Health; Healing Arts, Religion and Mental Health; Alcohol and Drugs – A Continuing Concern; The Family in the Face of Crisis; Children In Stress; and Mental Health in Primary Health Care.

The *Teaching Workshops* are a new addition to the World Congress. Their purpose is to provide participants an opportunity to acquire new knowledge and to improve skills in one's own field of specialization. The teaching sessions were led by faculty who are prominent in their special fields of interest.

Richard C. Nann, Dorcas Susan Butt, and Lourdes Ladrido-Ignacio (eds.), Mental Health, Cultural Values and Social Development, 155.

ALAN STOLLER, M.D. (Australia)

MIGRATION

This workshop, the third of a current series on this topic, followed on workshops in Vancouver (1977) and Salzburg (1979). The latter had stimulated the production of a monograph, "Uprooting and Surviving" (D. Reidel Publ. Co., Holland and U.S.A., 1982), filling in the gap since 1960, when WFMH had published the volume "Uprooting and Resettlement".

Attention was drawn early on to aspects of migration such as the diverse reasons for migration and the consequences for outcome, especially the movement from agrarian to industrial environments.

At the national level, there was often a lack of coherent planning by "receiving" countries; policies were often tied to manpower needs and varied according to economic circumstances. There was a need to keep families together and provide supports during the period of resettlement – up to 3 to 5 years. Efforts needed to be made to provide cohesive ethnic programs with supportive networks, provision of information and preservation of cultural strengths; additionally, opportunities to integrate with the host culture through the acquisition of language was essential. Special attention needed to be given to unemployment in the young male and females in low-paid occupations. Discrimination was seen as a feature of most societies and this varied from one nation to another and differentially for specific ethnic groups. This was a current problem with foreign workers and a need was expressed for the sending country to screen and brief its nationals prior to departure and for the host country to orient immigrants to patterns of living therein and prepare them for return. The latter is especially noted in regard to returning students who will not infrequently have absorbed the host culture and become alienated from their own traditions. Within the host country, attention should be given to orientation programs for such students as well as those who fail and are too embarassed to return, a feature which is significant in Asian students because of "loss of face". It was suggested that exchange student programs between countries should be encouraged.

Successful adaptation of children was assisted by a bilingual approach, since they were able to learn the new social system through the security of their own culture; also, bilinguality helped diminish tensions at home. A special child-at-risk was the young immigrant who arrived at a late stage of schooling.

A new picture of family life was emerging in early post-war immigrants, as the second generation was ageing and family cohesiveness diminishing. A significant number of husbands were leaving their wives after the children had grown up. Women's issues were becoming more significant in the host country, and patterns of working wives were taken up. Married women with poor language

Richard C. Nann, Dorcas Susan Butt, and Lourdes Ladrido-Ignacio (eds.), Mental Health, Cultural Values and Social Development, 157–159.

facility who suffered lower rates of integration were isolated within the family and suffered accordingly. Asian outmarriages were reported to be increasing in USA, indicating a degree of successful integration.

Much attention was given to aspects of Asian immigration in developed countries. The Chinese population in Vancouver has developed their own elaborate service agencies, with advocacy inbuilt; and indigenous services were already beginning to appear for the Vietnamese intake into the United States. Traditional host country bureaucratic services did not tend to adequately cover the needs of immigrants because of language problems and cultural differences and planning needed to take this into account. It was stressed that modern psychiatric concepts are foreign to many of the Asian and rural immigrants and that access to native healers is essential, with a bridge between the latter and host country mental health practitioners. Attention was drawn to the Japanese method of dealing with specialist and diplomatic personnel in developing countries, with initial orientation, total family involvement, a maximal stay of two years, and language tuition for the children on return, being part of the general policy towards displacement.

Attention was drawn to the need of more personnel for refugee camps by Mrs. Teresita Silva, Social Services Officer with UNHCR in Manila. More orientation programs were needed, as well as an enlargement of quotas by receiving countries or, alternatively, the raising of funds to place refugees elsewhere. The question of the definition of a refugee is still very much a matter of debate and needs exist far beyond the strict definition used by UNHCR.

Mention was made of the need for research into successful adaptation and the factors involved. A multifactoral model involving such factors as social network, levels of expectation, language attainment, identity formation and degree of culture shock needed to be considered in comparing ethnic groups, but, above all, cultural differences needed to be taken into account in the adequate assessment of the variables involved in coping. A comparative lexicon of mental health concepts could well be a task undertaken as a preliminary. Longitudinal studies are needed, but this would require adequate attention to mobility aspects. A useful exercise would be the comparative adjustment of Vietnamese refugees in USA, Canada and Australia. The utilization of services and its relation to poverty could be a profitable avenue for study. Other areas include the effects of involvement in decision-making, placement in scattered as compared with close-knit ethnic groups, parent-child conflicts and, possibly, basic comparative biological researches into emotional maladjustment. Service and research needs could be served by the creation of multilingual consultants in host countries, regular seminars, integration with national preventive health services and the provision of sociocultural centres.

Mrs. Cynthia Freier presented her findings in regard to the assimilation of Asian-Americans in New York. These comprised 311,000 residents, mainly Chinese, Japanese, Filipinos, Koreans and Vietnamese, the numbers having increased 300% between the 1970 and 1980 censuses. Attention was drawn to the diversity of migration experiences and the under-utilization of mental health services by some ethnic groups.

Chairperson:	Dr. Alan Stoller (Australia)
Co-ordinator:	Dr. Richard Nann (Canada)
Facilitator:	Ms. Corazon Alma de Léon (Philippines)
Resource Person:	Ms. Cynthia Freier (U.S.A.)

PURI NAVARETTE and FLOR MALICAY

MASS MEDIA

This workshop examined both the positive and the negative effects of the mass media on mental health, particularly with respect to the social and psychological development of young children. Discussion focussed on questions and issues stimulated by a paper presented by Dr. Tsune Shirai, based on a study of television viewing by pre-school children in Japan. Some related experiences in other countries were reported by workshop participants.

The results of the Japanese study included the following findings: there is a high correlation between parents' and children's viewing time; children whose parents watch television regularly also watch as much, with both parents and children oftentimes viewing the same programs; more than 50% of the children view adult programs. The toddlers (18 to 24 months) view television more than the others in the 2–5 age grouping.

These findings would seem to complement those from another study in Japan which discovered that: more than 30% of children between the ages of 2–5 view adult programs with their parents; more mothers view children's programs than fathers do; and mothers unwittingly allow their children to share certain adult programs which the children would not otherwise be allowed to view on their own.

One general conclusion from the Shirai study is that television can be used on a limited basis for value formation, value reinforcement, habit formation, and motivation towards developing attitudes. This seems to be consistent with experiences in the United States where, for example, it was found that 80 percent of children who view a program such as "The Electric Company" find it as an entertainment and highly stimulating medium only in terms of form, such as colour, sound, voice, music.

There was no consensus among the workshop participants as to the kind of television program children should watch. However, it was agreed that television as a medium is in itself powerful as it can influence some people's behaviour and thought.

Workshop participants expressed the view that the mass media should be responsible to the needs of audiences, and that the media must be instructive and educational. There is a need for co-active listening and viewing, where parents and children make use of mass media together.

The point was made that the use of television for therapeutic purposes, such as treatment of phobics, is still in a very preliminary state. In Denmark, an experiment is being conducted involving mentally ill patients for the promotion of mental health. A film has been produced with the patients portraying themselves, and talking about the various aspects of their illness with very little

Richard C. Nann, Dorcas Susan Butt, and Lourdes Ladrido-Ignacio (eds.), Mental Health, Cultural Values and Social Development, 160–161.

comment from the narrator. This is considered more effective in the promotion of mental health as compared to more directive approaches. As a general conclusion, workshop participants felt strongly that the inculcation of values and the bringing up of mentally healthy individuals rest primarily with the parents of a family. While the use of media such as television may be useful in some aspects of child development, there is no substitute for the tender touch and warmth of parental love and care.

WORKSHIP RECOMMENDATIONS

(1) The teaching of attitudes, habits and values to children should essentially be done by parents within the family framework.
(2) Media must refrain from deciding what is good and not good for its audiences.
(3) Production of radio/TV programs should take into consideration their effects on the psychological developments of children and adults.
(4) Media could be used in facilitating and promoting mental health by concentrating on preventive aspects and guidance in attitudes towards various family members.
(5) Research with controlled variables should be conducted on children comparing TV viewers and non-viewers regarding their achievements in school.

Chairperson: Mrs. Lourdes G. Ibarreta-Huelgas (Philippines)
Co-ordinator: Haider Maghazaji (Iraq)
Facilitators: Ms. Puri Navarette (Philippines); Ms. Flor Malicay (Philippines)
Resource Person: Dr. Tsune Shirai (Japan)

WESLEY SHERA, Ph.D. (Canada) and FRANK A. JOHNSON, M.D. (U.S.A.)

LEISURE AND CHANGING VALUES

The ongoing workshop on leisure followed meetings in 1977 (Vancouver) and in 1979 (Salzburg). Discussion focused on the changing values which are implicated both in the acknowledgement of the need for leisure and in the search for methods to heighten the experience of creative leisure time.

Definitions were reviewed. Leisure experiences are those activities outside of work, or the tasks connected with management of the home or personal living situation (the provision of food, shelter, comfort, protection). Leisure experiences include several areas of activities, including recreational, religious, aesthetic. Such activity is distinguished by a degree of choice, as opposed to compulsion or imposed obligation. Most leisure activity is disconnected from subsistance activities such as gainful employment, homemaking, child rearing, and family-support activities. The dimension of time (specifically the use of time and the psychological perception of time) is critical to the nature of leisure.

The North American approach to leisure presented by John Nesbitt emphasized the historical, cultural and esthetic dimensions of recreational experience. He suggested some resistance in the U.S.A. to the idea of play and leisure. Programs have been designed to respond to a variety of needs for recreational and leisure activity, including a scheme for realizing continuing goals during various stages of life.

Mr. Matsuda and Mr. Wagatsuma described the serious problem of dealing with leisure time in the future. The ten-year existence of the Japanese Institute for Leisure testifies to that country's foresight concerning the problem. This problem affects all industrial societies since, as nations achieve a plateau of productivity in both their internal and world markets, gross national product indicies will level (aside from inflation), whereas the number of employable persons will increase. This will lead to lower (relative) per capita income, shorter working hours, job sharing, earlier retirement and higher unemployment or underemployment. All of these adjustments produce increased free time for individuals, and thus, the need for access to authentic, economical and socially productive leisure. Fortunately, such schedules for leisure are already part of the expectation of the Japanese workers' relationship to both industry and government. In the absence of constructive leisure activity, deteriorating morale, hostile dependence, apathy and clinical disability are all possibilities.

The second day of the workshop began with a brief review of the findings of an international comparative study of values and wellbeing. This study, co-ordinated by the Leisure Development Centre of Japan, sampled a population 18 years of age and older in 13 countries, both developed and developing. The sampling strategies were diverse but appropriate to each of the countries involved

Richard C. Nann, Dorcas Susan Butt, and Lourdes Ladrido-Ignacio (eds.), Mental Health, Cultural Values and Social Development, 162–163.

and was carried out by an in-home interview using a structured questionnaire. In analyses and a preliminary report by Morton Beiser and Susan Butt in Canada, four scales were used to assess value systems: religiosity, satisfaction with material needs, satisfaction with job relations, and satisfaction with human relations. The results were highlighted and then discussed using the theoretical formulations of Erikson and Jung.

The Japanese resource people cautioned the group about the difficulty of not only doing, but interpreting, this kind of cross-cultural research. They suggested that in many cultures there are implicit values which control interviewees' responses. Other issues mentioned included the importance of sub-cultural groupings, concrete versus abstract questions, appropriateness of the division of life cycles, and the cultural relevance of various explanatory frameworks. An illustration of the last issue included a description of how Maslow's Need Hierarchy is not appropriate to the Japanese society since material needs are stronger than needs for self-realization.

During the remainder of the workshop, conflicts in values were discussed. Illustrations included the distinction made by the Japanese between leisure and recreation, the inability of many Americans to deal with controlled leisure and the Filipino struggle for independence and self-identity. These examples illustrate, not only conflicts within cultures, but also differences across cultures. The Filipino participants described how their society was attempting to resist Americanization and to preserve their cultural heritage in order to develop a new, integrated cultural identity. This implied a moving toward some independence for the Filipino youth but within the context of the rich social networks. This was contrasted with the interdependence of the Japanese and individualism of the Americans. The American approach to leisure and recreation was described as competitive and consumerist. Although this situation is somewhat similar in Canada, there is an emerging emphasis on co-operative games and recreation for children. The Federal Government of Canada has also taken a major role in promoting, through the media, the importance of a healthy lifestyle. This includes anti-smoking and alcohol campaigns and the promotion of nutritious eating habits and physical exercise.

Chairperson:	Dr. Wesley Shera (Canada)
Co-ordinators:	Dr. Frank A. Johnson (U.S.A.); Hiroshi Wagatsuma (Japan)
Facilitators:	Ms. Josefina D. Pineda (Philippines); Ms. Lina B. Laigo (Philippines)
Resource Persons:	Dr. John Nesbitt (U.S.A.); Yoshiyuki Matsuda (Japan); Natshiko Yoshida (Japan)

CAROLINA VERA LLAMANZARES

SEX ROLES AND MENTAL HEALTH

Some questions addressed were (1) What are the major problems which arise in society during periods of change in sex role expectations? (2) What are some ways in which the mental health professional may help with the problems identified? (3) What are individual expectations? (4) How may various goals be achieved?

The following problems were identified:
Parenting Responsibilities. These include: family planning as an integral part of mental health care; need for mother/father role in parenting; need for both parents in child rearing; and fathers' role change.

Sexism in Work Roles. These include: women's presumed inability to handle top level executive positions; women's presumed role to provide a support system in administration; women's having to cope with a male hierarchy at work; women's achievement (leaving husband behind); labour laws discriminating against women; no maternity leave for fathers.

Conflicts Due to Socio-Economic-Cultural Pressures to Adhere to Traditional Sex Roles. These include: women must relinquish their personal goals to the role of wife and mother (in actuality, she is hidden power of the family); men are expected to earn more (if they don't, they lose masculine image as head of family); women who work sometimes seem punished by controlling husbands who turn to other women (by other families putting pressure to take care of their children and by defensive children who make mothers feel guilty); women lack the opportunity to decide what they want to do besides rearing children and caring for a husband.

Various national problems were proposed:
Japan: fathers are absent due to work demands; mothers turn to children for emotional needs; mothers act as both father and mother; and the mother's need to go to work has surfaced due to the need for economic self-sufficiency.

Indonesia: sex taboos hinder education, sex therapy and sex information, thus blocking sex education and the fulfillment of partners in marriage.

Canada: women are caught in a male-oriented society; there is a need to understand men's approaches to women's achievement; the professions are sex oriented (decision makers in most professions are men); women administrators do not follow socially accepted role expectations; the loneliness of high-achieving women leads to crises and confusion of goals.

Richard C. Nann, Dorcas Susan Butt, and Lourdes Ladrido-Ignacio (eds.), Mental Health, Cultural Values and Social Development, 164–165.

Some specific positive suggestions follow:

During child-rearing, are children given opportunities to be flexible in expressing feelings such as the tenderness and the assertion important for survival and for life in 21st century? Are males and females considered to be partners, supportive of each other, and co-equal in both their needs for responsibility and their needs for self-actualization? Are there definitive studies on planned parenthood to help adolescents in making decisions? Are women aware of their potential for full development as persons, professionals, mothers, and wives, and given an opportunity to allow this to surface? Does this awareness create conflict and confusion in women? Are children given opportunities outside the home, especially in the school system, to have masculine as well as female role models? Is human sexuality information, education, and therapy available for coping with stress in middle age?

Workshop conclusions and recommendations follow: (1) Many of the participants were interested in continuing the work begun in 1977 with the first workshop on sex-role attitudes. There was a commitment from several delegates from various countries to pursue this topic. (2) There is a need for dissemination of information on this topic at regional and local levels to increase awareness. There is a need for cross-cultural research results to be shared. (3) There is a need for mental health professionals and workers in all countries to examine their own attitudes toward male and female sexuality during times of sex-role change.

Chairperson:	Dr. Rama Pandey (U.S.A.)
Co-ordinator:	Dr. Selma Hughes (U.S.A.)
Facilitator:	Ms. Carolina V. Llamanzares (Philippines)
Resource Persons:	Dr. Leticia Lantican (Philippines); Dr. Pirkko Niemala (Finland); Mr. Roberto Mendoza (Philippines); Ms. Ruth Ann Brown (U.S.A.); Dr. Eleanor Nash (Republic of S.A.)

MEI-CHEN LIN, M.S.W. (Canada) and MINDA SUTARIA, Ph.D. (Philippines)

SCHOOL MENTAL HEALTH

School may have either a salutary or deleterious effect on the mental health of individuals. This underscores the need for effective school mental health intervention programs.

One critical issue is whether or not to send a child for psychiatric treatment. There is evidence to suggest that caution needs to be exercised in referring children to a therapist whom they do not know very well. In the United States, studies cite 90% failure in cases where teachers withdrew children from their classes and referred them to a therapist. About 50% of the children referred did not return for treatment. A more effective type of intervention can be inferred from a successful seven-year experiment in California which tried out a system of specialized individual rewards, both at home and in school, for children who had problems. In Vancouver, Canada, mental health service is integrated in the total health, education and social welfare services in the school system. The adoption of a life enrichment program for children, using youth as trained tutors, produced gratifying results. Home-school liaison work has been introduced to facilitate the adjustment of immigrant students in primary and secondary schools, stressing early prevention and intervention. Services are also provided to assist their families with psycho-social and cultural problems they face as immigrants. In the Philippines, a parallel approach in a peer-facilitator program introduced in some secondary schools helped upgrade achievement, and consequently reduced school mental health problems.

To be effective, a school mental health intervention program must adopt a "wiser and a wider" approach, which means that it must have a plan of development, involve the whole system, be accepted by students, teachers and parents, provide a system of rewards for success in school, have a clear and precise discipline program, and make counselling and discussion available to students, teachers and parents. Such an approach would increase awareness among all involved of mental health concerns and should aim, through education and training, at having teachers serve as mental health role models.

An intervention process which was tried out in a school in Malaysia approximates such a "wiser and wider" approach. This process, which used psychiatric consultation, was introduced in a school that had low academic achievement and high incidence of petty crimes. It involved individual assessment of referred students, group therapy sessions led by a psychiatrist with a student counsellor as co-therapist, and discussion with the teachers, the headmaster, school supervisor, student counsellor and parents concerned. One useful insight gained from this experiment is that the young prefer to be treated as friends rather than being "mothered" or "fathered".

Richard C. Nann, Dorcas Susan Butt, and Lourdes Ladrido-Ignacio (eds.), Mental Health, Cultural Values and Social Development, 166–168.

There is a growing concern today about the mental health of children who are not in school and of those who go to school but do not benefit from it, as well as those who strain very hard in order to get through the "narrow gates" which school and other institutions set up for them. It is not only the young whose mental health is eroded by this *narrow gate syndrome* but also that of teachers and whole families.

Among the three main ethnic groups in Malaysia, the value of education is heavily stressed. In Kuala Lampur, a majority of school children receive supplementary tutoring beyond school hours. A significant number of students indicate that too much of their time is spent with study and household chores leaving little or no time for recreation. Associated stresses and pressures hinder the total development of children affected.

In Japan there is an alarming increase in the incidence of school refusal due to factors such as: the emergence of the nuclear family and the demise of the extended family system; extremely high expectations of parents for their children; keen competition in school; and attendance in very large schools which have engendered feelings of insecurity among children. The need for intervention programs which develops a sense of security in school is evident.

In postwar Japan, especially after 1970, a system of higher education entrance examinations has created stressful competition among students with a significant impact on individuals, families and teachers. It is not the aspirations for social prestige, but rather a struggle for family pride and survival which motivates the competition for economic and social security. The *Hensa-chi system* has come into use among teachers as an index for a student's achievement deviation from the class mean and also from the national mean. The system is used to predict candidates' success on University entrance examinations, thus reducing the "narrow gate" ratio of applicants to university acceptances. The system, however, created problems for a segment of teenagers who dropped out, exhibiting aggression and anti-social behaviours and showing tendencies toward apathy. The *Hensa-chi system*, while attempting to reduce "narrow gate" pressures, has also resulted in students' loss of self-determination in educational choices and other mental health problems. Its effectiveness is being evaluated while the search for more appropriate ways of dealing with *narrow gate syndrome* continues.

In Hong Kong, the highly competitive educational structure has exacerbated the mental health problems not only of students but of teachers and parents as well. Undue emphasis in the curriculum of higher grades on passing the government examination to qualify for limited employment opportunities has led to certain behavioural aberrations among students. Alternatives that may help solve the mental health problems of students include multisectoral intervention, curriculum development, specifically the preparation of multi-level materials, and improved mental health education for teachers.

In Taiwan, enrolment in elementary and junior high schools is high, yet there have been disturbing reports of maladjusted youth in schools. To increase parents' and teachers' understanding of and empathy with junior high school students experiencing educational and "narrow gate" pressures, in Taipei, student's opinions and feelings expressed in peer group discussions and diaries regarding parents' and teachers' attitudes and expectations are carefully studied. These are in turn considered by teachers, parents and government authorities in developing and implementing preventive and positive mental health programs for students.

Narrow gate syndrome is especially severe among junior and high school students preparing for entrance examination to the next academic level. In a Taipei pilot project, an experimental mental health scale was used to identify students suffering from intense anxieties or examination phobia. Attempts were then made to desensitize and alleviate these symptoms through group counselling for both students and teachers on study habits and teaching and coaching methods, utilizing audio-visual resources wherever possible. Marked improvement was noted among students receiving this counselling.

RESOLUTION

Whereas, the progress of a nation depends largely upon the development of its human resources;

Whereas, health and education are basic to the development of human resources;

Whereas, one phenomenon which has affected the mental health of children and youth as well as of their teachers and parents is the "narrow gate syndrome", that is an unhealthy expenditure of physical and mental resources in severe competition for limited academic and employment opportunities;

Whereas, the pernicious effects of the narrow gate syndrome militate against human resource development;

Whereas, unless governments and citizens take concerted action to eliminate factors causing *narrow gate syndrome*, the mental health of a citizenry may be severely threatened, with detrimental result to human resource development;

Therefore, be it resolved, that the World Federation for Mental Health bring to the attention of governments and citizens the deleterious effects of the *narrow gate syndrome* so that effective action can be initiated to counteract it.

Chairpersons: Dr. Minda C. Sutaria (Philippines); Mrs. Mei-Chen Lin (Canada)
Facilitator: Dr. Erlinda G. Lolarga (philippines)
Resource Persons: Dr. Milton Miller (U.S.A.); Ms. Peggy C. Y. Chan (Hong Kong); Ms. Elsie Ho (Hong Kong); Dr. T. W. Woon (Malaysia); Dr. Osamu Osato (Japan); Dr. Sachio Okada (Japan); Dr. Atsutaka Hashimoto (Japan); Dr. Hisao Nakai (Japan); Shozo Shimada (Japan); Dr. Sadaaki Shirataki (Japan); Dr. Susan Ong (Malaysia); Mr. K. L. Yeoh (Malaysia); Mr. Munekazu Hatanaka (Japan); Mr. Seijun Toguchi (Japan); Mr. Yung-Ho Ko (Taiwan); Dr. Emily Miao (Taiwan); Dr. Tsung-Yi Lin (Canada)

MORTON BEISER, M.D. (Canada)

THE HEALING ARTS, RELIGION AND MENTAL HEALTH

One of the major interests in traditional healing has been the hope that, through this phenomenon, the processes common to all healing can be understood. Much traditional healing seems aimed towards facilitating a patient's re-acceptance by the human group. Thus, re-assimilation into a significant group could be one of the important processes which occurs in healing. Another possibility is that certain mental states can be stimulated during healing, which will in turn evoke physiological responses leading to health. Some work suggests that the physiological state associated with the mental state many have called "hope" leads to recovery from illness. Conversely, "despair" co-exists with a physiological state leading to disease and perhaps even death. In some instances, healing cannot occur unless the patient feels that cultural imperatives have been addressed. For example, physical illness may be treated, but the patient will not feel better if he feels the illness was the result of a transgression or a curse that has not been dealt with.

Such statements about healing, which have appeared in western scientific literature, share a common limitation. Since they originate in a western framework of thought, a pattern which stresses analytical thinking, the formulations will inevitably be culture-bound. Other models of thought are also relevant in trying to achieve understanding. Perhaps we should be as concerned with *whether* something works as *why* it works. The danger in being overly-analytical is that, if we do not understand why something works – or if our treasured scientific theories (western) suggest that traditional healing should not work, we may block practices that are benefitting needy people. Such phenomena and experiences deemed to be a part of esoteric healing seem unverifiable. Should they be labelled non-existent because they cannot be "scientifically" measured? Or should we reserve judgement, recognizing that some may not be measurable because we currently lack the tools for that purpose?

The practice of psychic surgery, of opening the body and removing diseased parts by a healer without any surgical tools, has become associated in many people's minds with the Philippines. Psychic surgeons, as well as healers who work with prayer, visualization and magnetic healing practice in the Philippines and their work deserves study.

We must not romanticize healing. Healing can be used for "good" or "evil" by both traditional and western healers. Its use for "evil", that is, for selfish gains, for the purpose of "taking" rather than for "faith", must continue to be a concern for health care workers. Because medical manpower is scarce and expensive, people are at risk of being exploited by those unscrupulous enough to do so. So great is the potential for abuse in healing that several workshop

Richard C. Nann, Dorcas Susan Butt, and Lourdes Ladrido-Ignacio (eds.), Mental Health, Cultural Values and Social Development, 169–170.

participants questioned if the WFMH should not concern itself with trying to formulate a set of principles by which the ethics and practice of healing, both western and traditional, could be assessed.

Chairperson:	Dr. Morton Beiser (Canada)
Co-ordinator:	Dr. Antonia P. Perlas (Philippines)
Resource Persons:	Dr. John Spiegel (U.S.A.); Dr. Carlos León (Colombia)

PHILLIP LORENZANA III

ALCOHOL AND DRUGS: A CONTINUING CONCERN

There can be no doubt that dependence on alcohol and other drugs has assumed major importance as a health problem throughout the world. The factors responsible for this are complex and multiple; it is a serious error to think that the same factors are operating equally in all cases, yet homogeneity may be the implied assumption when terms such as "alcoholic" or "addict" are used.

The workshop sets out to explore "the anatomy" of dependence – its political, social, psychological and biological roots; the rationale (and irrationalities of the community response); and the role of the health worker in its prevention, detection and treatment. A multi-national gathering offers unique opportunities, and emphasis will be given to national variations and to cultural influences in all the above factors.

The first paper read, "The Ex-Addict as a Therapist: A Mirror View" by Fernando B. Perfas of the Philippines, expounded on the merits of employing "ex-addicts" in rehabilitation work. Mr. Perfas conducted a study of 8 "ex-addicts", two of them females, who have since been fully rehabilitated and who are presently employed by DARE Foundation (of the Philippines) in its rehabilitation program.

The study took the cudgels on behalf of the "ex-addict" as a therapist in rehabilitation work, maintaining that the "ex" is in a better position to understand and be in empathy with the "addict" because he or she, the "ex", once was in the same plight. Further, the "addict" will more readily respond positively to the "ex" because identification will be easier. Finally, the "ex" is living proof that full rehabilitation is possible: it has been done, and it can be done again. Mr. Perfas added that DARE Foundation, Inc. employs ex-addicts in all aspects of the DARE program of treatment and rehabilitation and so doing, has achieved and continues to achieve a significant ratio of success to failure.

In reaction to the paper, Dr. Cooper of New Zealand commented that the term, "therapist", in his experience, referred to the medically trained personnel, including those in medically related fields, while others were referred to as "support personnel or staff". Dr. Theodore Abas of the Philippines, co-ordinator, explained that in the Philippines, the term was used to include anyone who has a direct bearing on the rehabilitation of the addict. Thus, even patients/residents in a therapeutic community centre may at times assume the role of a "therapist". In fact, it is one of the distinguishing elements of the therapeutic community approach to rehabilitation and one that differentiates it from other approaches.

Dr. Cooper wanted a clearer definition of the term "addict", and "addiction". Dr. Basil James of New Zealand, co-ordinator, replied that the term has the Latin root *ad dicta*, which means at someone's beck and call; literally, a slave.

Richard C. Nann, Dorcas Susan Butt, and Lourdes Ladrido-Ignacio (eds.), Mental Health, Cultural Values and Social Development, 171–177.

The term therefore has a wide range of meaning, a latitude broad enough to encompass many shades. Dr. Abas added that to him, a person who does not suffer withdrawal symptoms (should the substance abused be withheld) is not an "addict" but a mere "habitue". A general discussion followed on the pros and cons of employing "ex-addicts" in rehabilitation work.

Capt. Charles Reed of the United States Air Force disclosed that two government programs in the United States each tried a different approach in the employment of "ex-addicts" and "professionals", one employing solely "ex-addicts" and the other employing solely "professionals", in their rehabilitation work. Their statistics show that both approaches showed the same ratio of success to failure. Neither had the edge over the other. Mr. Phillip Lorenzana III of the Philippines, facilitator, commented that such statistics would tend to show that the "ex-addict", as therapist, is at least as good as the "professional". Capt. Reed agreed that the statistics from these two programs would tend to show just that.

Dr. Francy Mateus, psychiatrist from Hawaii, U.S.A., commented that whatever be the efficacy of the "ex" as a therapist, he reverted soon enough, in her experience, to the abuse of drugs once he leaves the rehabilitation centre. The "ex" remained "ex" only so long as he remained a "therapist" in the centre. Capt. Reed inquired into the motivation of "ex-addicts" in staying with the rehabilitation community: he questioned whether the over-riding factor was fear to return to "normal" society lest the "ex" revert to the abuse of alcohol and/or drugs. Mr. Perfas answered that in DARE Foundation, the problem was not of over-staying "ex-addicts" but rather of the swift turnover of "ex-addict" staff personnel because they, the "ex", preferred the outside community, recognizing that it represented the real challenge.

A question arose as to what determines demand for a particular substance abuse. Dr. Cooper wrote on the blackboard on equation with total demand *Qd* on one side, and the factors that affect demand on the other side. He postulated that *Qd* is a function of several factors or variables. Algebraically,

$$Qd = f(\text{price, income, tax, individual taste, prices of other goods, advertising, societal pressures, etc.})$$

or

$$Qd = f(P, Y, T, P1, P2, \ldots Pn, Fn).$$

Dr. Cooper explained that the equation as written on the board by no means exhausted the list of variables that affected total demand. The elements that constituted the function would make a very long list, indeed. For the sake of brevity and clarity, however, we could exclude most of the minor elements without sacrificing the relevance of the equation. For the most part anyhow, the elements excluded will be those which cannot be practically determined. Individual taste or preference, for instance, would be a value so difficult to determine that we would be forced to assign to it an arbitrary constant. All other minor elements could be lumped under one catch-all parameter which could assume a plus or minus value depending on its collective effect on total demand. This way, we could greatly simplify the model and with greater facility isolate and study the major variables that determine total demand for a substance of abuse.

Thus, the model becomes,

$$Qd = f(P, X)$$

where

= Qd represents total demand.
= P represents the major variables under close study,
= X represents the minor elements lumped under one parameter.

With this highly condensed model, we could now study the effect of one major variable, for instance, Price, on total demand Qd by assuming all other variables to be, ceteris paribus, parameters.

By isolating Price to be the major variable under study, the model now becomes,

$$Qd = f(\text{Price}, P\text{-price}, X).$$

Ignoring for the moment the determinants of Price (for Price is itself a function of a set of other variables), we may determine the effect of an increase or decrease in Price on the total quantity demanded Qd. Empirical studies have shown that, for the vast majority of consumer goods, an increase in price brings about an opposite movement in quantity demanded, and vice versa. We could therefore safely conclude that a decrease in price of the substance of abuse would bring about an increase in its quantity demanded. The cheaper the street cost of a substance of abuse, the greater would be its consumption. If our aim is to effect a decrease in the consumption of a particular substance of abuse, we could achieve such by manipulating a variable or a set of variables that determine its demand. In our particular model, we could, or should, manipulate Price.

But Price is itself a function of a set of other variables: availability, cartage, prices of other goods, tax, etc. By manipulating the variables that determine Price, we manipulate Price itself and indirectly, the total quantity demanded of the substance of abuse.

Dr. Cooper went on to elaborate that in his country, New Zealand, the price of some substances of abuse, tobacco and alcohol, for instance, actually went down in real terms as against the prices of other goods. The percentage price increase was lower than that of other goods, thus making tobacco and alcohol, in effect, cheaper than before.

Although price is probably not the single major cause of the continued abuse of tobacco and alcohol, its manipulation could bring about a decrease in the quantity demanded of the substances in question. Here, government could step in, in the form of policies and taxation, which are among the determinants of Price.

The participants voiced that such would be difficult in their countries for there, the tobacco and alcohol lobbies were both very active and influential. Even the advertising lobby, which has an effect on demand, would probably lend its weight in behalf of the tobacco and alcohol companies.

Dr. Cooper admitted that there would be difficulties, but he went on to say that here, at least, government had the power to manipulate demand through price whether or not it chose to do so. But in the case of other substances of abuse, government by legislating their illegality has done away with a potent tool at their command, that of the power to manipulate quantity demanded through price. Dr. Cooper advocated that certain substances of abuse that are readily available in the streets despite their illegality be legitimized so that government may exercise, through taxation, some measure of control in its demand.

The paper of Mrs. Leticia Generoso of the Philippines, "The Philippine Response to the Drug Problem", focussed on the current state of the drug problem in the Philippines and touched on the Anti-Drug Abuse law, the various rehabilitation and treatment centres and their approaches to the problem, and the governing body, the Dangerous Drugs Board.

For a start, Mrs. Generoso reported that the Philippines is one of the few Asian countries with a minimal heroin problem. The declaration of Martial Law in the Philippines in September of 1972 greatly curtailed the illicit sale of this drug, a declaration that was timely because heroin abuse then was at its highest in the Philippines. Prior to Martial Law, smuggled drugs coursed through 34 ports of entry in the Philippiness, including the two American military bases, Clark Air Base in Central Luzon and the Subic Naval Base in Northern Luzon.

In 1980, however, statistics showed a precipitate increase. While opium and its derivatives continue to be hard to come by, marijuana and restricted pharmaceutical drugs such as cough preparations are easily available and are widely abused. In this year alone, the total number of cannabis plants/seedlings seized by government operatives exceeded by 50% the total amount seized during the nine-year period 1971–1979. Further, the Philippines remains a transit country in the international traffic in illicit drugs. Drug contraband continues to be smuggled through the Philippines to the U.S.A., Canada, Japan, Australia and Hong Kong, with the last named figuring prominently as the country of destination in 6 cases of trans-shipment of heroin from Bangkok through Manila. Government operatives conducted 1,411 arrests, resulting in the apprehension of 2,587 persons. Of these, 72 were foreign nationals, 47 of them Americans. The courts resolved 176 cases involving violations of the dangerous drugs act, in the process disposing of 126 convictions.

The paper also enlarged on the service offered by the different treatment agencies and explained the different approaches each agency employed in their treatment of drug and/or alcohol dependents.

Participant reaction took the form of requests for elaboration on the various treatment agencies and their approaches to the problem. It was stressed that the different Philippine rehabilitation centres as a rule co-ordinated with one another. Most of the after-care work from cases treated by the private organizations were undertaken by government agencies, principally the Dangerous Drugs Board.

Dr. T. Hemmi of Japan, in his paper, "Are Alcohol and Drug Taking Political Issues?", focussed on the running controversy between mental health workers and politicians in Japan in the battle against alcohol and drug abuse. Japanese politicians do not want "open" treatment of patients with alcohol and/or drug taking problems and this frustrates mental health workers who claim that this attitude worsens the problem because patients who should or must receive treatment do not receive such due to the interference of politicians. Dr. Hemmi went on to cite several instances involving alcohol and/or drug abuse. He concluded by saying that this issue should be openly discussed in Japan so as to arrive at a working accommodation beneficial to all.

A participant reaction took the form of a question into the motives of Japanese politicians in not wanting "open" treatment: could it be that they do not want the real dimensions of the problem to be made known to the general public?

Dr. Hemmi said that in Japan advice is a matter of shame. He went on to add that the Japanese typically has a low tolerance to alcohol which appears to be biologically based and thus, refrains from abusing it. Since 1955, however, the incidence of alcohol intake in Japan has risen tremendously. This does not mean an increase in the number of cases of chronic alcoholism; rather, the statistics reflect an increase in the number of acute cases of intoxication, enough to warrant hospitalization.

A participant asked whether the typical Japanese would seek the help of a doctor should he have a drinking problem. Dr. Hemmi replied that the traditional Japanese would rather seek the help of his Buddhist or Shinto priest. Dr. Hemmi's reply, bringing in religion in the context of culture, sparked a lively discussion of society and its ills. Participant involvement was animated as others shared their own culturally defined responses to the problem of substance abuse. Asked whether, in the context of Japanese culture with its many restraints, alcohol is a coping mechanism for the expression of emotions normally restrained, Dr. Hemmi replied that in essence, no. As in all cultures, the Japanese have socially acceptable forms of outlets. Alcohol abuse is a phenomenon common to most, if not all, societies. It is true, however, that it is a social problem.

As to drug abuse, Dr. Hemmi said that although the Japanese have a low incidence of addiction, the problem is compounded by the Courts, which have an "either or" attitude when resolving drug cases. Thus, for a Japanese to undergo compulsory treatment for drug dependency, he first has to be found guilty of a drug crime. He will then be given compulsory treatment while in prison. Otherwise (if found not guilty), he is allowed to go home with no court provision for treatment. In Japan, courts do not order compulsory treatment, even when the patient-accused is obviously addicted to drugs. This "either or" attitude (either one is guilty, in which case one receives compulsory treatment in prison; or one is not guilty, in which case one goes home) is lamented by Japanese mental health workers.

Dr. Hemmi was asked to elaborate on aspects of Japanese society/culture which act to depress the rise of substance addiction in his country. He attributed the low incidence of substance abuse in Japan to four major cultural/societal factors: (1) The Japanese, as a people, do not like sedatives. Their drugs of choice are amphetamines. But since Japanese are typically hard-working, most do not need chemicals to spur them on; consequently, only a few use them. (2) Drug Laws are strictly enforced in Japan. This is because the police have the wholehearted support of the people. Also, Japan has a tradition of strict law enforcement, not only in drugs, and the people have traditionally supported the government and its laws. (3) The attitudes of the people regulated substance abuse. The community looks with intense severity on the addict, whether on alcohol or drugs. (4) The high sense of personal dignity of the individual Japanese, and close identification with the family mitigates against substance abuse.

Often, the community's condemnation (which also reflects on the addict's family) added to the deep shame felt by the Japanese addict, brings about an unbearable situation. Many Japanese addicts have committed suicide rather than go on living a life of humiliation.

Dr. Datu Mahadevan's paper, "Alcohol and Drugs: A Continuing Concern", was an overview of the state of the drug and alcohol problem in his native Malaysia and in many countries of the world. The paper touched on the studies and approaches made by different countries and the conclusions and recommendations derived therefrom. Finland, for instance, in a study of 9,000 families found that parents with a history of alcohol abuse tended to have children with congenital deformities.

The paper, covering as it did several countries and planning a multitude of approaches to the drug and alcohol problem, stimulated diverse participant reaction. Among subjects discussed were: the case of countries whose economics benefitted from illicit drug production and supply to other countries; the case of preventive education being a double-edged sword; the case for the legitimization of certain substances of abuse so as government can better control its abuse; the case for international sanctions against countries or governments which allow trans-shipment of illicit drugs, etc.

What stimulated participant reaction most, however, were discussions on society. The phenomenon is a social problem. The root cause is in society. The participants agreed that, "We live in a contradictory society. Society, with one face, says, 'Do not take it', but with another face, it says, 'Take it, for it is acceptable – and profitable'."

The participants, however, also agreed that while the root cause may be in society, the root "cure" is also in society. Dr. Cooper moved that we study the dynamic aspects in society that minimizes substance drug abuse among its members. "Start with society," he urged.

Workshop conclusions and recommendations were as follows: (1) Substance abuse, though common to most societies, is a social problem. Its cure must be found in society. (2) Preventive education is a double-edged sword and one that must be used with great care. (3) The worth of the ex-addict, or a rehabilitated addict, as a therapist is at least equal to that of a professional. The ex-addict should be given every chance to prove his worth in other aspects of employment. (4) A country should seek endemic solutions to this social problem. The conclusions or recommendations of other cultures lifted in toto will not be sufficient to deal with the problem. (5) Addiction is not criminal; it is a disease, and the addict is a victim.

Chairperson:	Dr. Datu Adnan Bin Haji Abdullah (Malaysia)
Co-ordinators:	Dr. Theodore B. R. Abas (Philippines); Dr. Basil James (New Zealand)
Facilitator:	Mr. Phillip Lorenzana III (Philippines)
Resource Persons:	Mr. Fernando B. Perfas (Philippines); Mrs. Leticia Generoso (Philippines); Dr. Datu Mahalingan Mahadevan (Malaysia); Dr. T. Hemmi (Japan)

OLGA RUIZ DE ARANA and ELEANOR ELEQUIN

REHABILITATION OF THE DISABLED

This workshop followed a pre-Congress seminar aimed at maximizing interaction and including attitudinal and behavioural changes among service providers. Disabled persons, his/her family and practitioners in mental health attended. Paper presentations focus on the context of disability, intervention programs and research findings for particular categories of disability.

"Disabled persons have the right to participate fully in the life and development of the society in which they live. It is our duty to enable them to exercise that right." With this frame of reference, the importance of understanding attitudes toward disability was a priority issue. The paper by Asai *et al.* underscored the significance of the family's concept to mental disorder and the attitudes to the mentally ill member. Another paper, in view of the increasing number of chronic psychiatric patients, presented sports therapy as a rehabilitative approach. Indicators of its effectiveness in the motor and behaviour areas were presented. An alternative strategy came from behaviour modification techniques. Its use in Guam on mentally retarded and chronically ill patients hospitalized for an extended period of time was reported.

The differences in attitudes toward disability between control groups and different categories of the disabled in Denmark and Japan were reported by Shibata. Another study compared the attitudes of Chinese (Taiwan) with Americans in terms of degree of positiveness towards the disabled. Knowledge of the handicapping conditions was suggested as a variable which would help to explain the range of differences. The need for cross-cultural studies was also underscored.

The culture accommodation model (New Zealand) was presented as a framework for translating into practise what already exists in the community. Such programs may feature concern with accessibility, administrative openness, acceptability, continuity with cultural beliefs and satisfaction by the user.

The importance of culture was discussed on the policy level. Despite differences in the scope of target groups, education is recognized being universally important on a social level. The need to identify strengths as a focus for policy development was suggested.

The group emphasized concern with global problems, such as hunger, energy, unemployment, and poverty. Education is needed to enable people to respond to these issues and problems in terms of new structures, academic programs and research. Education in relation to the needs of the disabled should be a priority concern. Social awareness and social conscience are necessary if we are to instill values supporting concern for the disabled in our world citizens.

The psychology of the disabled and the handicapped emphasizes the strengths rather than the weaknesses of those conditions. In-country intervention

Richard C. Nann, Dorcas Susan Butt, and Lourdes Ladrido-Ignacio (eds.), Mental Health, Cultural Values and Social Development, 178–179.

approaches show the multi-disciplinary and multi-national insights of the providers of services. A frequent question was: How can society, the specialist-professional and the research specialist serve the cause of the handicapped and the disabled?

Three recommendations were: provide more sensitization and information about the disabled and the handicapped; carry out cross-cultural studies of intervention programs; and emphasize innovative social action programs for the covertly disabled.

Chairperson:	Prof. Charlotte A. Floro (Philippines)
Facilitators:	Dr. Olga de Arana (Philippines); Dr. Eleanor Elequin (Philippines)
Resource Persons:	Dr. Michael Caldwell (Guam); Fr. Robert Ronald (Taiwan); Mr. Ryochi Shibata (Japan); Dr. Nick Higginbotham (New Zeland); Dr. George Kallingal (Guam); Dr. Philip Crunk (U.S.A.); Dr. Nobuo Namikoshi (Japan)

SOLEDAD DUTERTE

LINKAGES VITAL BETWEEN POLITICS AND MENTAL HEALTH

This workshop was concerned with three general subjects. These were: mental health principles and issues inherent in politics; the politics of mental health work; and political skills that a mental health worker must learn.

With the need for an integrated total development program for sound mental health, the establishment of vital linkages with other agencies involved in the promotion of good mental health has become a necessity. The linkages which must be established with agencies, both public and private, need the political acumen of mental health leaders.

Prof. Carlos pointed out that mental health should be the main concern of the political scientist because it is the political system that determines policies. In this aspect of society, mental health and politics are partners in achieving the same goal.

The workshop hoped to determine specific definitions of who is mentally ill and of the value system inherent in political factors. The group defined politics as a mental process by which one changes the systems of which one is a part. Dr. Ayo Binitie introduced an effective definition of mental health taken from the Nigerian constitution as that which is for the welfare of individual citizens. He also deliberated that the most important points so far as economics and politics are concerned is that the distribution of human resources touches both individuals and families.

Gomez drew the attention of the workshop to a young society, coping with problems such as disturbed, irrational and anti-social groups, in addition to political difficulties.

Dick Hunter addressed the question of how to *cope* with problems in face of political realities. He cited several pragmatic approaches: (1) How to *agree* specifically on the problem area. What solutions are available, such as legislation, coalitions of groups, etc. (2) One has to know how to influence the people who will determine changes in legislation.

Jim Ricks stressed ways to use the political system. In this regard, he raised three questions: (1) If one can only do a little, what should one do? (2) How can one sell one's idea? (3) How does one keep it from being unworkable?

Question (1) elicited the *mental illness model*. All one can do is: (a) treat the patients; (b) apply social controls; (c) clean up neighbourhood. Second is the *network model*. Here, efforts are grouped together to produce harmonious and successful results.

Reactions from delegates: (1) Reactions of delegates from developed countries were quite different from those of delegates from the developing countries. (2) No generalization could be made because each country has different social

Richard C. Nann, Dorcas Susan Butt, and Lourdes Ladrido-Ignacio (eds.), Mental Health, Cultural Values and Social Development, 180–182.

systems, as well as different forms of government. (3) Forms of government influence mental health policies. (4) Developing countries find it hard to influence their systems of government. (5) Individuals, families and communities are instruments of change, but they differ in developed and developing countries. (6) Funding for institutions such as mental hospitals is at the mercy of politicians. (7) Government should not be the only agency for funding purposes. (8) How can there be mental health in the troubled countries? (9) Mental health depends on the economic, social, cultural status of the individual. (10) Each system of government, democratic and communist, has its own merits and demerits.

Propositions: by Brenda Wattie

(1) Culture and societies vary greatly. The developing countries should not simply adopt western technologies of mental health care, but respect and use their own natural resources. They should not make the mistakes of western countries, such as putting major resources into building psychiatric hospitals. Instead, they should use their own community resources, which in many respects, especially in terms of family stability, are strong. Western societies have had to construct artificial self-help groups and networks to support mental health programs.

(2) It is necessary to broaden the base of decision-making and participation beyond a small number of people, who are often the people close to "government" in the Third World countries. In order to do this, we must broaden literacy, information and participation in decision-making throughout society.

(3) There is no conflict between therapeutic "membranous systems" and confrontation in the cause of gaining mental health resources. The two activities strengthen each other.

Propositions: by Rodolfo Escosa, M.D.

(1) People should be mobilized to think and act on problems of increasing crime, armed conflicts between and within countries, violence, terrorisms, riots, labour unrest. Persons unable to support themselves should be helped and all people should have meaningful participation in community activities.

(2) Through communication and technology, a greater number of people are becoming more acutely aware, not only of the variety of crises that confront individuals and cultures, but also of the reasons why they occur.

(3) Lay people, scientists, technocrats and politicians are increasingly knowledgeable about how our many human problems and crises are brought about by inability of our existing institutions to provide services to people that would enable them to live in harmony with each other. At present, the socio-political systems and structures are unable to satisfy the basic needs of 20% in developed areas and of 66 to 75% in less fortunate places.

(4) The politicians and their advisers who determine how people and available resources shall be managed and disposed are becoming less arbitrary in their decision-making procedures as more people are becoming enlightened, politicized and vocal about their demands for a bigger share in the enjoyment of human rights to satisfy basic needs.

(5) Mental health leaders would like the politicians who manage the community's means and resources to increase the small share that has so far been granted to their projects. This is an immediate need. Those who have must be more receptive to rapid changes in the basic structure and operations of the economic system so that those who are deprived may have a chance to contribute more to the fulfillment of themselves and others.

(6) This long-range objective of affecting changes in socio-political relationships would entail changes in the values and attitudes not only among rich nations, but also among the masses of deprived people who should be better organized in their demands for a more dignified existence.

In conclusion the World Federation for Mental Health has much work to do in promoting mental health. We hope that someday, socialist and communistic countries and Christians and non-Christians can come together and prove that to be able to survive in this world, we have to understand, to abide, and to value human life.

Chairperson: Ms. Brenda Wattie (Canada)
Co-ordinator: Dr. Benjamin Marte (Philippines)
Facilitator: Mrs. Soledad R. Duterte (Philippines)
Speakers: Prof. Clarita Carlos (Philippines); Prof. Lourdes Gomez (Philippines); Dr. Ayo Binitie (Nigeria); Mr. Dick Hunter (U.S.A.); Mr. Jim Ricks (Canada)

MANUEL BONIFACIO and ESTER GAJO

MENTAL HEALTH AND RURAL COMMUNITIES

A number of subjects were discussed in this workshop relating to mental health and rural communities. These included: problems in organizing and developing a mental health service program in a rural setting; the effects of rapid development and modernization on the mental health of rural communities; preventive mental health in a rural village; and the effects of urban and rural life styles on the fertility patterns of women.

There are many issues and factors to be considered in the provision of mental health services in a rural setting. Community support services are usually not well developed or are completely absent. A study of rural after-care services for discharged mental hospital patients in the Philippines found one of the greatest problems to be the non-acceptance of the patients by their families and by others in a rural community.

Rapid development, urbanization, modernization, and industrialization carry through to the mental health of rural communities with the erosion and disruption of tradition, values, culture, beliefs and family solidarity. A study of community development in rural Malaysia found that pressures and frustrations are often created by the mass media accelerating desires and wants of modern products – wares, clothes, radio and other electronic gadgets – without cognizance of the usually low purchasing power and more simple and complacent lifestyle found in rural communities. Rural communities usually have problems adjusting to the rapid conversion and development of inherited farmlands into housing subdivisions, wide cemented roads, factories or country clubs. There can also be unrealistic expectations if a rural development program requiring resources and trained personnel is implemented in a depressed community with very limited resources, materials and trained manpower.

In the face of large scale change, there is need to strengthen the idea of a therapeutic community as a mental health strategy for rehabilitative and preventive services. What is required is the creation of a new culture which has continuity with the past.

Traditional spiritual values and human support systems have important roles in the prevention and rehabilitation of mental health problems. Three basic ingredients have been identified as essential for good mental health. These are: (a) FAITH, the ability to put aside our day to day routines of life and to see that there is meaning beyond ourselves; (b) honest BELIEF that our work is important, be it at home or outside, and satisfying, fulfilling and relatively enjoyable; (c) the ABILITY to share our hopes and joy with each other, instead of just releasing our sorrow and anger and frustrations. These three ingredients are intricately interwoven in the traditions, religion and way of life of the rural community.

Richard C. Nann, Dorcas Susan Butt, and Lourdes Ladrido-Ignacio (eds.), Mental Health, Cultural Values and Social Development, 183–184.

Conscious attention to the longitudinal development process of a child and the complex interaction of biological and social aspect of child development are important elements in preventive psychiatry in the 1980s. This conscious attention and care to the child's bio-social development may effectively and positively improve the neurological and psychological development of the child as shown in a current study on preventive psychiatry in a rural village in Japan.

According to an initial report on a study of women living in Mexico City who come from urban and rural backgrounds, changes in lifestyle affect fertility patterns and mental and behavioural attitudes. Other consequences of change include: tendencies to be less tolerant, more easily frustrated, and more likely to develop tension and depression. These findings seem to have major implications related to the migration of rural families to urban communities.

WORKSHOP RECOMMENDATION

(a) To recognize traditional belief and value systems in the development of mental health programs.
(b) To strengthen the notion of therapeutic communities.
(c) To involve behavioural scientists in the planning process of national mental health programs and formulation of policies.
(d) Maximize community participation in the development of human resources and health services for preventive purposes.
(e) Emphasize the total health of the community in development plans.
(f) Collaborative regional studies on mental health problems of rural communities with the support of mental health regional office.

Chairperson: Dr. Manuel Bonifacio (Philippines)
Co-ordinator: Ms. Ester B. Gajo (Philippines)
Resource Persons: Dr. Flocerfina B. de Jesus (Philippines); Prof. Deva Dass (Malaysia); Dr. Sadaaki Shirataki (Japan); Dr. Federico Puente (Mexico)

ESTER DE JESUS-AMOR

CRIMINAL JUSTICE SYSTEM: ITS FUNCTIONS IN CONTEMPORARY SOCIETY

INTRODUCTION

The workshop speakers and participants discussed human rights and criminal justice in the light of events in contemporary society and within the framework of philosophy, concepts and practices in various countries. Values intrinsic in the planning and implementation of criminal justice were considered, as well as the central role of education in the home and in the school to inculcate a set of values to prevent the onset of delinquency, or to intercept the further entry of the offender into the formal penal system. Laws, traditions, culture, and development were reviewed and analyzed in the light of incidence of crime and the relationship of mental health to behaviour which society finds disruptive of peace and order.

Decriminalization and alternatives to prison as punishment were discussed. There was agreement that, even if it was difficult to achieve, countries must continually strive to strike a balance among protecting the rights of offenders; seeking redress for the unlawful act committed against the offended; and the protection of society itself from behaviour which is harmful to other persons and which disturbs the community's peace and order. There was concern that the enforcers of law could be just as harmful as the criminals.

COURSE OF THIS WORKSHOP

A total of six papers were presented during the course of this workshop. Two speakers from the Philippines used the Philippine experience to point out generic concepts in criminal justice and human rights.

The first speaker described justice as giving the person, particularly the child (both as offended and offender) what is due to him and to make opportunities for a better quality of life available. He pointed out that Criminal Justice in the Philippines is law tempered by compassion and concern for the offended, for the offender, and for the society which must be protected from the harmful effects of the crime. The International Year of the Child and the Philippines' Decade of the Filipino Child have provided impetus to a more humane approach to youth offenders.

Human rights are transformed into basic services which have been improved through the following measures: the integration and professionalization of the police; circuitization of municipal courts and filling of vacancies for speedy trial of cases; the establishment of a probation system, and the Board of Pardons and Parole; and the decentralization of prison. Community participation has been

Richard C. Nann, Dorcas Susan Butt, and Lourdes Ladrido-Ignacio (eds.), Mental Health, Cultural Values and Social Development, 185–188.

activated with government and non-governmental organizations extending services especially to the youth. There are also services geared towards child advocacy and crisis intervention outside of the formal judicial system.

The second speaker spoke on the implications of human rights and criminal justice for mental health. She discussed the substantive rights of a person which are the accepted standards of justice and human dignity and values. Recent trends in the Philippines include:

(1) The right to treatment and rehabilitation to enable the offender to become sufficiently responsible to assume his place in society;

(2) The right to a public trial but the need to protect persons from excessive publicity through television, which would cause the public to equate the trial process with forms of entertainment; and

(3) The need to seek help from mental health associations for evaluation and management of cases.

Discussion in the workshop focused on the attitude of law enforcers and the need for a psychiatric team to assist the courts in the evaluation and/or management of cases. The complementary role of the professionals – medical psychiatrist, psychologist, social workers, lawyers, and others in the helping process – was underscored in the prevention and management of disorders.

Particular attention was given by the workshop to the subject of juvenile offenders. A Philippine study shows that delinquency is influenced by the quality of family relations, the content of the mass media, and the state of economic and social security which are fundamentally determined by the social and economic system. In turn, there are variables which correlate with poverty and a lack of education, namely, unhappy and broken homes, death or separation of parents, parental overstrictness or inconsistency in disciplinary methods, idleness, inadequate recreational facilities and religious and moral training.

Discussion of causative factors and preventive measures brought up the following points:

(1) It is not only poverty that causes delinquent behaviour because delinquent behaviour is found among affluent persons. Delinquent behaviour may also be due to not having direction in life and to the values of such persons.

(2) A Philippine delegate described the program for youthful offenders in Bacolod, and reported the lack of proper guidance as a contributory factor to delinquency. The majority of the offenders who are released return to the courts and this is attributed to the inability of offenders to make a decent living.

(3) There is the possibility of temporal lobe epilepsy and other behaviour disorders as contributing to the incidence of delinquent behaviour.

(4) Emphasis on value development is needed as a preventive measure with the home being reinforced by the school in the inculcation of desirable values to prevent/deter delinquent behaviour.

The workshop also heard a presentation based on observations of criminal justice systems in various countries. Emphasis was made on the importance of decriminalization of some crimes that do not pose danger or disequilibrium to society. Police harassment is an example of the hunter being just as feared as the hunted. In some countries, an offense may be punishable according to one statute, and again punished in a special law. Imprisonment is not a reliable means of reformation as attested by the incidence of recidivism, quasi-recidivism, and habitual delinquency. An "ideal criminal justice system" requires strict and faithful implementation of criminal laws, a fearless judiciary, measures for rehabilitation and reformation of the offender, but without sacrificing other important human values of society.

The speaker from Canada briefly traced the historical background of the Centracare Saint John Incorporated with a slide presentation. He described the services and facilities of a forensic unit and the psychiatric facility located in New Brunswick, Canada. The forensic unit offers court assessment, treatment, long term planning for offenders by a multidisciplinary team composed of a psychiatrist, psychologist, criminologist, social worker, occupational therapist and head nurse. Security arrangements on the unit have been designed to integrate containment with responsibility. All professionals interact with patients within the context of a modified therapeutic community where patients participate in various activities. Emphasis was made on the intensive training given to the multidisciplinary staff on forensic work for the unit to be a highly specialized clinical entity.

The forensic unit collaborates with the Department of Justice. The referrals are from the courts which can be for fitness to determine the level of functioning and their understanding of courtroom proceedings, or for sentencing recommendation for which the team assesses the patient's cognitive and perceptual abilities, their personality characteristics and their suitability for therapy, if treatment is indicated.

Discussion focused on the need for a Human Rights Commission, the need for members of the law enforcement agencies to successfully pass a course on Human Rights and the need for more alternatives to imprisonment.

RECOMMENDATIONS

(1) There is a need for procedures and guidelines in criminal justice harmonious with human rights to fully protect the fundamental rights of all persons in addition to the general rights embodied in a Bill of Rights and the specific provisions in the penal code and statutes.

(2) There is a need for co-ordinated planning of services and implementation of laws.

(3) Officers and officials within the criminal justice system entrusted with the implementation of laws and regulations should be required to complete courses on human rights.

(4) The services of a forensic psychiatric team should be made available to

the courts within a given geographical area or jurisdiction to assist in the evaluation and/or management of cases.

(5) A Human Rights Commission may be established to safeguard the rights of the offended and the offender, and to maintain a balance between individual rights and the rights of society to be protected against violent, disruptive acts.

Chairperson:	Justice Roberto R. Concepcion (Philippines)
Co-ordinators:	Ms. Ester de Jesus-Amor (Philippines); Dr. Roger Guzman (Canada)
Facilitator:	Dr. Araceli N. Maravilla (Philippines)
Speakers/Reactors:	Hon. Jesus N. Borromeo (Philippines); Judge Leonor Ines Luciano (Philippines); Fiscal Fe Gutierrez (Philippines); Mr. Merlin Magallona (Philippines); Judge Alicia Sempio-Dy (Philippines); Dean Antonio Gregorio (Philippines); Justice Jose B. L. Reyes (Philippines)

BEN CHUD, M.S.W. (Canada)

THE FAMILY IN THE FACE OF CRISIS

There were more than 40 participants in this workshop. Four formal papers were presented. The remainder of the time was given to discussion.

Ben Chud, co-ordinator of the workshop, presented an introductory paper. In his remarks, Mr. Chud pointed out that much of the literature on the topic of the family originates in North America and the industrialized world. Yet the concept of the family and the role that it plays is variously understood around the world. Similarly, the notion and the theoretical formulation of crisis and crisis intervention originated in North America, the pioneer work being done by Gerald Caplan and his associates. Jacobson Parad Rapaport and others elaborated on the theme.

The paper gave a brief formulation of the concept of crisis and the methodology involved in crisis intervention. He challenged the members of the workshop to discuss the applicability of the work done in the industrialized countries to the developing nations of the world. He concluded his paper by posing a number of questions for discussion.

The second presentation, "Responses of Japanese Families to Mental Disorders", was the result of a research project at Asai Mental Hospital in Japan conducted by a team that included Kunihiko Asai, Toshio Asai, Yoshihiro Asai, Sanji Bunai, Tadao Ryuchi and Yoshitomo Takahashi. This study included 49 case histories first seen between March 30th and June 30th, 1980. Information in this paper was derived from interviews with the patients and their families, and mainly concerned the interpersonal process that took place from the beginning of deviant or morbid behaviour to the decision to take the ill member of the family to a psychiatrist. Interviewees included parents, spouses, siblings, children, grandparents and other family members.

Areas studied were: the family's interpretation of psychotic problems and its relation to the time interval from onset to referral to a psychiatrist; the family's attitude to the neighbours' reactions; the changing relationships in the family following the onset of psychiatric problems; the family response to psychiatric attention; the patient's attitudes to consulting a psychiatrist; the family's understanding of the purpose of the hospital visit; the family's expectation for the level of recovery after hospitalization.

The study concluded that Japanese families responded to the onset of mental illness, psychotic manifestations in particular, in characteristic ways. They tend to minimize the onset either through denial, rationalization or somatization. The stigma of mental illness, traditionally prevalent in Japanese society, is still very pervasive but seems to have diminished in the last decade. Mental illness in a family seems to negatively affect family relations in about half of the sample.

Richard C. Nann, Dorcas Susan Butt, and Lourdes Ladrido-Ignacio (eds.), Mental Health, Cultural Values and Social Development, 189–191.

The family assumes major responsibility in the choice of modes of intervention, often disregarding the wishes of the ill member. The families who minimize mental illness tend to keep the ill member at home longer and consult a psychiatrist, with reluctance, as a last resort. This they do only after the family resources and tolerance are exhausted. Families have a fairly realistic expectation about the recovery of the mentally ill or the outcome of psychiatric treatment.

Kunio Hishihara of the National Institute of Mental Health in Japan presented "The Japanese Family and Social Care for the Mentally Ill". The paper indicated that, unlike the West, almost 90% of Japanese patients in mental hospitals are involuntary admissions. Twenty percent are admitted by two government appointed psychiatrists on grounds that the patient may be injurious to themselves or to others: seventy percent are admitted involuntarily by members of the family who take on the role of legal protector.

Historically, the roots for such a system began when the family was the ultimate source of welfare for each individual. Whereas this has changed considerably since World War II, the Mental Health Act still reflects a strong traditional pattern, as indicated by the pattern of hospitalization.

In 1959, there were approximately 30,000 mental hospital beds in Japan. In 1979, this number had increased to approximately 300,000. There is a remarkable difference among districts in Japan. Whereas the national average is 25 per 10,000 population, some districts have a rate of about 40 beds, while others are below the national average. For this study, the investigator chose two districts: one in Kumamoto prefecture (Southwest Japan) and the other in Miyagi (Northeast District). One of the distinctive features of these districts is that Miyagi has a more traditional family structure, whereas Kumamoto has a less extended family ideology.

Based on questionnaires from 2,952 families (65% return), two hypotheses were tested: that the differences in family relations accounts for the differing attitudes towards the care of the patient; and that family attitudes towards patients in Kumamoto where the extended family ties are looser would be more negative than in Miyagi where traditional family ideology still prevails.

The study concluded that the different family structures and ideologies in these two districts were reflected in the medical service systems. In Miyagi, where the traditional family ideology prevails, there were fewer in-patients. The families in Miyagi showed a lower level of sympathy for the patients. Thus, local background and extended family ideology are not necessarily related to good human relations between patients and their families.

The final paper, presented by Fe Maddela Valdez, dealt with "Prevention Approaches to Family Crises in a Community Outreach Program". A description was given of a non-governmental, church-associated program for distressed families in the lower socio-economic group in Manila. The interdisciplinary team comprises social workers, nurses, a physician, a dentist, a clergyman and a group of volunteers. The self-help program emphasizes self-reliance and consciousness-raising, and cooperation and mutual aid between neighbours is stressed. The educational aspect of the program includes hygiene, first aid, health care and household management. Participants also learn to deal with behavioural problems and psycho-social ills within the family, and income-generating skills are also taught. Recreational, social and spiritual activities round out the program.

A survey conducted by the agency and based upon 64 returns revealed the following:

Respondents rated poverty as by far the most important stress factor in producing a crisis. The second and third most frequent causes were quarrels between parents and serious illness in the family. The loss of job by the breadwinner, death in the family, childhood delinquency, separation of parents, cruelty of father and religious differences were additional stress factors.

When questioned about crisis situations, the parents' responses indicated that most felt that they were part of daily living. The same high percentage (91%) felt that crises were an avenue for growth. Approximately 25% felt that "maybe they are a part of God's plan", and 3% felt they were a form of punishment. When asked what they would do in the face of crisis, these respondents said that they would seek God's help. All respondents also said that they would strive to solve the problem; 95% felt that they would seek help from others; and 3% felt that they would keep the problem to themselves.

When asked about the team, 38% of the mothers said that the members displayed kindness and understanding. A similar percentage felt that the behaviour of the team members was warm and friendly and that the team members "seemed interested in my family". Twenty percent of the respondents felt that the team members were approachable and handled problems skillfully. Ninety percent felt that the team was well liked by the community and 18% felt that the team member was "a good teacher".

In summary and discussion, there was general agreement as follows: (1) Mental health knowledge, skills and attitudes can help prevent deep-rooted family crises arising out of socio-economic and psychological strains and thus improve the quality of life. (2) Family and community self-help and mutual support is an important factor in dealing with crisis situations. (3) Those who are of assistance to families in crises can themselves grow in the process of helping. (4) While professionals are most helpful at every level of providing service to families in crisis, non-professionals also can and should play an important role. This is particularly true in the developing countries where there is such a dearth of professionals. Here, the role of professionals should be to train para-professionals and educate the public at large.

Chairperson: Mr. Antonio Ulgado (Philippines)
Co-ordinator: Mr. Ben Chud (Canada)

DANILO PONCE, M.D. (U.S.A.), EMILY MIAO, Ph.D. (Taiwan) and
EVA GONZALES, Ph.D. (Philippines)

CHILDREN IN STRESS

Growing up in today's world is a complicated, demanding and, consequently, highly stressful process. Dr. Ponce's paper, "Today's Children: Tomorrow's Casualties or Tomorrow's Leaders?", set the tone for the discussion that followed. He outlined various contemporary psycho-social stressors that impinge on the growing child and his or her family. These included: (1) advances in technology, particularly in transportation and communication; (2) dwindling energy and fuel resources; (3) deteriorating world-wide economic conditions, brought about primarily by soaring energy and fuel costs; (4) geo-political instabilities and power shifts, particularly in fossil-fuel rich and poor countries; (5) escalation of military capabilities in these countries because of these instabilities; (6) advances in medical technology resulting in longer average life expectancies; (7) increase in world population, severely straining available food supplies and the capacity of countries to provide optimum nutrition to their populace; (8) urbanization and industrialization of less-developed countries; (9) exponential increase of indices of social disorganization.

These stressors may appear to be unconnected and tangential to the child developmental process as we know of it today, from the works of Erikson, Piaget, Freud, Kohlberg, and other developmental theorists. However, the stressors are in fact not only interrelated; they reinforce each other. The effects of these stressors are borne by the child and his or her significant others. One can trace world-wide economic deterioration to soaring energy and fuel costs; which is fed in part by the need for fossil fuel as a result of technological advances in transportation, communication, health care services, need for fertilizers for crops to feed the masses, and so on. The rise in cost of living is most concretely felt by the nuclear family. It forces a realignment of roles and rules in the traditional family system. Mother, father and every available adult are forced to work to earn a living and, hence, caretaking of the young is often left to strangers. The impact of this on the continuation of traditions, customs, belief and value systems on the growing child is obvious.

The impact of these stressors on the growing process are most visible in three areas: (1) drastic changes in the nature and the evolution of the developmental process; (2) demand for novel and more adaptive coping mechanisms and strategies to deal with the stressors; (3) redefinition of the context in which the growing process takes place.

Inability to deal adequately with these stressors by the child and his or her significant others could lead to: (1) developmental discontinuities; (2) developmental gaps and fixations; (3) diminishing sense of personal, familial and social history; (4) difficulties in the bonding, attachment and loss processes, processes

Richard C. Nann, Dorcas Susan Butt, and Lourdes Ladrido-Ignacio (eds.), Mental Health, Cultural Values and Social Development, 192–194.

that are so vital in the growing process; (5) increasing dependence by the child on gadgetry and mechanical objects as adults spend less time with him or her; (6) increasing dependence on mind-altering substances to substitute for decreased contacts.

Various coping strategies that are assumed to be adaptive to the demands imposed by the stressors were discussed: (1) ability to cope with ambiguities and uncertainties; (2) ability to cope with a discontinuous developmental process; (3) ability to cope with transitory relationships; (4) ability to cope with and create personal meaning and history; (5) meta-learning (i.e., "learning how to learn" skills); (6) ability to determine what is relevant to the present situation from the wealth of competing and conflicting information; (7) ability to synthesize conflicting data; (8) ability to use play and leisure time in a personally meaningful way and as tools for age/stage task mastery; (9) ability to master mechanical gadgetry.

The paper concluded by posing a potentially disquieting philosophical and moral question to the participants. The coping strategies required for a child to survive the exigencies of living in today's world would seem to indicate the next generation of adults will be self-centred, socially isolated, detached, individualistic – albeit competent and efficient. The question then is: Is it possible to encourage the development of these coping strategies without compromising humanity, compassion, and social conscience in the developing child?

Following this paper, Dr. Miao, co-ordinator of the workshop, presented "A Multi-Media Approach to Alleviating the Narrow-Gate Syndrome". She focused on the "Narrow-Gate Syndrome" as an explanation for stressful responses in school children in Taiwan. In Asian countries like Taiwan, Hong Kong, Japan, Korea, Philippines, Singapore, children and parents are preoccupied with one educational goal: to pass entrance examinations for progressively higher educational levels and better schools. Stressful responses range from dysfunctional parental attitudes, maladjusted behaviours, truancy, school phobia, school drop-outs, substance abuse (e.g., glue-sniffing) and delinquent behaviours. Extreme forms are withdrawal, apathy, lack of motivation, lack of direction and sense of purpose, and clinical depression. Ironically, one finds this cluster of responses even in those who have successfully completed and hurdled the "Narrow Gate" to higher education.

Following this, Dr. Miao enumerated several multi-media approaches designed to deal with this syndrome, such as encouraging students to write journals and diaries, and publishing them.

The ensuing discussion included the following: (1) need for a more precise definition of "stress"; (2) more specific discussion on the impact of stressors on the child and his or her family (e.g., how does one recognize a child undergoing a lot of stress); (3) clearer exposition of specific methods and strategies to diminish stress at the individual, family and community level.

Dr. Ponce offered the classic definition of stress by Hans Selye, that is, "a non-specific response of the body to any demands made upon it". Most participants in the workshop were connected with school systems and the discussions centred on stress as experienced by students. The questions and comments focused on the plight of today's youngsters with reference to the "Narrow-Gate Syndrome". It was suggested that stress created by the syndrome is differential and class-related (that is, upper-income groups have more options available and, hence, are able to deal with it more effectively. Lower-income groups have little or no options at all.). The group criticized educational systems that allow children to move through without necessarily learning anything.

Of particular interest to the participants were the practical methods described by Dr. Miao. There was discussion on the need to sensitize and train teachers to become more attuned to the "affective" components of teaching to complement the "cognitive", as she so touchingly described. Dr. Ponce shared some information on this from Hawaii, where the Department of Education trains teachers in "Affective Education". In the final analysis, coming to grips with casualties of the "Narrow-Gate Syndrome" is such a difficult undertaking that it takes governmental priority to deal with it.

Suggestions and recommendations from the workshop were: (1) more in-service training of teachers in the "affective" aspects of education to complement the "cognitive" aspects; (2) more availability of simple diagnostic tools to spot learning disabled children sooner; (3) generate "volunteerism" among professionals (psychiatrists, psychologists, social workers, etc.) to help in schools to combat the stresses of "Narrow-Gate Syndrome"; (4) applied research on the developmental needs of children so that appropriate interventions can be made; (5) implementation of interdisciplinary programs (e.g., parent-education in well-baby clinics); (6) service deliverers (e.g., teachers, mental health workers) must recognize the limitations of their professions and feel frustrated by them.

Chairperson: Dr. Danilo Ponce (U.S.A.)
Co-ordinator: Dr. Emily Miao (Taiwan)
Facilitator: Dr. Eva Gonzales (Philippines)

CELIA YANGCO

SOME CRITICAL POINTS IN THE HUMAN LIFE CYCLE: ADOLESCENCE

The objectives of this workshop were: (1) to discuss developmental and clinical issues related to adolescence as a critical point in the human life cycle; (2) to share experiences in youth programs; and (3) to identify possible national and regional programs of action for youth.

A recently concluded three-year research project on Philippine adolescents conducted in a rural and an urban community produced the following findings: The family is the main transmitter of culture of which values are an important component. Family solidarity is an outstanding value. Relationships with mother and father are marked by respect and affection, harmony and understanding. Sibling jealousy is minimized because children are trained to be close to one another and to share their possessions. In addition to their parents, children have access to other siblings and close kin. The eldest sibling acts as a parent surrogate.

Adolescent expectations and aspirations reveal that they expect to surpass their parents in such areas as education, travel, health, income, friends and prestige. Perceived avenues for upward mobility are education, business, hard work and social skills.

Philippine adolescents seem content with their identity, expressing the attitude that God made them who they are and they do not wish to be anyone else. This attitude of self-acceptance, however, was expressed more often by girls than by boys. Career aspirations reveal that medicine, engineering, law and commerce are rated highly, while teaching is not considered a desirable career.

While the double standard of morality (different moral norms for men and women) still prevails, Filipino wives nowadays show less patience with erring husbands, and more women resort to separation, divorce and annulment. Adolescent offspring seem more willing to admit that their parents are separated or divorced. Despite these changes, however, the family remains the source of moral, emotional and financial support.

There seems to be no "youth culture" in the Philippines. The *barkada* or peer group does not supplant the family except in deviant cases. The family still stands as the strong but flexible link that binds all stages in the life cycle.

In Finland, a recent study examined the relationship between occupational choice of students and parental attitudes. Occupation selection was viewed as a successful resolution of personal identity crisis. The study included three groups of students who belonged to religious organizations studying in: theology, political science and various other disciplines. The three groups of students were compared on various background variables such as school achievement, social affiliation, leisure time and other activities. Special attention was given to the

Richard C. Nann, Dorcas Susan Butt, and Lourdes Ladrido-Ignacio (eds.), Mental Health, Cultural Values and Social Development, 195–197.

students' parents – their religious life, social relations, and characteristics such as the use of power and control in parent-child relations and demonstration of love and warmth. The main findings of the study were: (a) religiosity of parents was positively related to religious activities of students and the choice of a religious-oriented career (i.e. theology); and (b) students who identified with their parents described their parents' relationship as closer and happier than did students who did not identify with their parents; the former also reported relations to their mothers during early years as being significantly close.

Young people in Japan today encounter a number of special problems which include: school phobia, violence against teachers, violence in the family, and suicide. These problems seem to stem from the need to participate in a highly competitive society – a need that is not really internalized by the adolescent but rather represents an external expectancy from society.

The cry of the adolescence for independence, while true for all cultures, seems to vary in degree and manifestation from country to country. In the Western culture being independent means almost totally free from parental supervision socially, economically and emotionally. In Finland and in the U.S.A., for example, independence of the young from parents would include the provision by the youth for his own needs and, therefore, in his indulging in work or occupation at an early age.

This is not the case, however, in most of the developing countries like Malaysia and the Philippines, where the youth, though wanting to be independent, are generally dependent on their families for emotional and economic support. This case is also true, to a certain extent, in Japan.

What value an adolescent places upon his schooling, and eventually his choice of his career, are influenced by his aspirations and by a number of other factors. What are the aspirations of the young? The answer to this question again varies in different cultures. In the developing and the less developed countries, youth aspirations are linked by their desire to reach a higher economic level. Thus, choices of careers are geared towards those professions that they think would give better income return for them and their families. This was observed to be happening in countries such as Malaysia and the Philippines. Conversely, this is not the case in developed countries like Japan, Finland and the U.S.A. In these countries, the youth aspirations seem to be more geared towards more self-esteem as, for example, serving one's country and fellowman.

There is a relationship between the career choices of youth and their countries' economic development level. Career choices, however, are also directly related to a country's educational system. The discrepancy between the educational facilities and the aspirations of the young is an area which requires further research. Likewise, the discrepancy between opportunity structure and the amount of labour available also needs to be better understood if the youth are to be helped in their career choices. One other area urgently requiring further attention is school-related problems. This phenomenon is not limited to Japan but in fact occurs in most countries. Also, the needs of the out-of-school youth cannot be ignored. The availability of recreational/leisure and other facilities serving the young are essential for their healthy development. There are generally not enough facilities providing recreation and other opportunities for the young.

RECOMMENDATIONS

In view of the identified areas of concern, the following recommendations are made:

(1) That more developmental and preventive programs should be developed for the adolescents; both for those in-school and out-of-school, including: facilities which provide wholesome activities along with recreation and programs for improving economic productivity, skills and job opportunities.

(2) That educators must take greater responsibility for addressing problems in school and school-related problems of the adolescents.

(3) That governments should take into account the link between the educational system and manpower needs in order to prepare the young to be contributing members of their community.

(4) That traditional institutions (family, school, church) should be strengthened to provide better mental health for the adolescents in the 1980s.

Chairperson:	Dr. Cornelio Banaag (Philippines)
Co-ordinator:	Dr. Patricia B. Licuanan (Philippines)
Facilitator:	Ms. Celia Yangco (Philippines)
Resource Persons:	Prof. Akira Hoshino (Japan); Ms. Anja Riita Lahikainen (Finland); Dr. Paz P. Mendez (Philippines)

LOURDES A. CARANDANG, M.D. and GRACE A. CABANOS (Philippines)

SOME CRITICAL POINTS IN THE HUMAN LIFE CYCLE: YOUNG ADULTHOOD

Although much has been said and written about various stages of human development, there seems to be very little attention given to the young adult years. Literature on the young adult tends to be scattered among articles concerning specific areas of concern such as sex roles and career expectations. Little is written about a member of the young adult age group as a total person incorporating intellectual, emotional, moral, physical and economic aspects.

The young adult comprises the vital work force of any nation, people who are at the peak of their productivity. What are the issues and stresses confronting this age group? What are their concerns? And, how are they coping with these stresses in life? What really distinguishes and characterizes the needs and conflicts confronting the young adult? All of these questions, of course, cannot be adequately addressed in one brief workshop. Instead, two or three specific issues formed the foci of discussion.

The developmental theory of Erik Erikson identifying the 8 Stages of Man refers specifically to the young adults' conflict of intimacy and isolation. This notion seems very useful in interpreting research findings from a study of Nigerian women whose husbands' work called for their absence from their homes. In many of these cases, the psychiatric symptoms disappeared after arrangements were made for the husbands to work within the locality in order to be with their families. Similarly, a Philippine study found that "talking to a friend" is a highly-ranked coping strategy among working young adults who encounter problems.

It is a well-known fact that identity crisis is characteristic of the adolescent stage of development. Perhaps more intense identity issues confront the young adult because of the need to come face to face with the realities of life in areas such as occupation, parenthood and conflicting roles. Stresses experienced in performing multiple roles, among females include those of wife, mother and career women; among males are those of husband, father, and provider. For both females and males, there is resulting difficulty in integrating the social, moral, emotional, physical and economic components of one's personality.

In the area of occupation, special problems are encountered when young adults shift from one occupation to another. Moreover, there are some young adults who seem unable to commit themselves to a particular job or career.

Inadequate decision-making skills among young adults seem to relate to conflict between personal needs and values versus social, emotional pressures; and to family economic needs versus relative economic status that must be considered in making decisions in life.

Richard C. Nann, Dorcas Susan Butt, and Lourdes Ladrido-Ignacio (eds.), Mental Health, Cultural Values and Social Development, 198–199.

RECOMMENDATIONS AND SOLUTIONS

(1) Schools can provide better preparation in areas such as:
   (a) Family Life Education, tackling topics such as: love, courtship and marriage; parenthood; budgeting; etc.
   (b) Decision-making skills focusing on the PROCESS, or the HOW of decision-making, relative to the choices one makes in life. This can be related to value systems and should be geared to the age levels of the students.

(2) *Support groups* for the young adult presently coping with stresses be made available; for example: seminars on relationships, communication, decision-making, parenthood. These support groups could be incorporated in existing structures such as church groups, community sharing groups.

(3) In the work environment, provisions for counselling be made available, and a mechanism for more dialogues between employer and employees be made available.

(4) The use of mass media in terms of informational dissemination on the Nos. 1, 2, 3 items mentioned above.

(5) That we continue to be passionate ADVOCATES of the "ignored" age group: the young adult – realizing the fact that this is a "make-or-break" period in the human life cycle.

Chairperson: Dr. Lourdes A. Carandang (Philippines)
Co-ordinator: Ms. Grace A. Cabanos (Philippines)
Resource Persons: Dr. R. Olukayode Jegeda (Nigeria); Dr. Lourdes K. Ledesna (Philippines)

MARIA PAZ DE GUZMAN, M.A. (Philippines)

SOME CRITICAL POINTS IN THE HUMAN LIFE CYCLE: MID-LIFE

There is a stage in human development distinctly identifiable, occurring between 40 and 60 years of age. Similar to adolescence, it appears to be a crisis-prone stage. About a third of the groups studied in the works of Levinson, Vaillant and Neugarten go through a stage where specific behaviours and feelings create distress, confusion and ill-will.

Unlike adolescence, however, the mid-life transition is more linked to anxiety and depression than to hostility and rebellion. The person in mid-life transition is likened to someone reaching that point in the tunnel of his/her existence, and suddenly realizing that much of what illumines his/her passage or pathway is the light coming from behind rather than in front. Unlike the adolescent who can see many choices and possibilities before him or her, the person in mid-life sees that there is little left ahead. This phenomenon may underlie the psychological component of depression and anxiety in mid-life. While it is agreed that there are identifiable physical and cognitive changes associated with the aging process, there is also a consensus that the quality of one's mid-life transition is determined by factors other than biological ones. These factors can be identified as follows:

(a) There is continuing pressure to excel than what one already has achieved. The person in mid-life who fails to determine when he or she has reached limits may be unconsciously responding to these implicit pressures. For those who have reached the top, and find that there is no more room beyond this, there is a need for a quick shifting-of-gears if one's equilibrium is to be maintained. For those who have not yet reached the top, they are faced with competition from younger colleagues as they try to accelerate.

(b) There is the disintegration and/or weakening of earlier ties, or relationships that coincide with middle age. Examples of this are:
   (i) the empty-nest syndrome when all of the children go their separate ways;
   (ii) the relocation of one's family to a new place or a foreign culture, or finding one's old neighbours, chums and associates all slowly moving away. This hyper-mobility of people can renew or heighten feelings of separation or of being left alone;

(c) There is the premium and value placed on youth and physical attractiveness by society. The increasing difficulty of maintaining one's ideal weight, stamina, and attractiveness to the opposite sex creates stress to the already beleaguered person in mid-life. Added to these are some culture-specific values which differentially affect the male and the female.

Richard C. Nann, Dorcas Susan Butt, and Lourdes Ladrido-Ignacio (eds.), Mental Health, Cultural Values and Social Development, 200–202.

In the Philippines, for example, a man in mid-life can openly have a mistress or two without getting much censure from their families, church or society in general. The Filipino woman is hardly able to "get away" with the stigma of reparation, let alone living openly, with someone who is not her legal spouse. How does one conceptualize the mental health status of the so-called "happily suffering" Filipino wife or the sociopathic Filipino husband? Is her "masochism" "culture-syntonic", and is his "sociopathy" a defect in the society's collective superego, rather than that of the individual's?

WORKSHOP CONCLUSIONS/RECOMMENDATIONS

Mid-life is a transition in human development. It is thus a stepping-stone to the next higher stage. The quality of one's mid-life will depend upon the quality of one's early adult life, inner resources for coping, and the options still available for him at the "tunnel" of life. If society continues to view mid-life as the peak after which everything else is downhill, it is no wonder then that mid-life is fraught with anxiety, self-doubts and depression. There is need to re-examine generally accepted notions about late maturity and the provisions that individuals and societies can promote in order to ensure mental health for those leaving mid-life and entering late maturity.

The following action plans or strategies are recommended:

(1) A re-examination of the retirement laws in each country in the light of research findings that arbitrary cut-off points for retirement age may be promoting mental illness rather than mental health.

(2) A provision of meaningful programs and activities which will continue to affirm the importance and usefulness of a person past mid-life.

(3) An encouragement of family interdependence in order to promote continuing bonds among family members so that one is able to count on other members in moments of crisis.

(4) A provision of community education, disseminating information that mid-life can be a crisis-laden stage so that "warning signs" can be identified and thus support and understanding can be delivered.

(5) A toning down of the over-glorification of being young, and a stressing of the values and virtues of late maturity.

(6) An understanding of basic research on the 60% to 70% of those in mid-life who "breeze through" without leaving in their wake emotional distress.

(7) A designing of exercises for the developing skills for coping with transition into mid-life.

(8) A promotion of nation-wide/worldwide awareness of the importance of physical and mental fitness that will prepare one for coping with crises that tend to coincide with mid-life.

Chairperson:	Dr. Juliana Seneriches (Philippines)
Co-ordinator:	Mrs. Maria Paz de Guzman (Philippines)
Facilitator:	Dr. Antonio Guazon (Philippines)
Resource Persons:	Dr. Norma C. Panahon (U.S.A.); Rev. William Morrissey (Philippines)

Mrs. BERT KRUGER-SMITH (U.S.A.)

SELF-HELP FOR THE AGED (OLD AGE AND MENTAL HEALTH)

Because concepts of aging and independence vary widely in developing and developed countries, the group decided to give broad definitions to the terms "aged" and "self-help".

The workshop participants shared the belief that many "advantages" touted by developed countries may work to the disadvantage of specific elements of the population. For example, reverence for the aged, family care of old people, and the extended family decline in urban, "developed" societies where more than 50 percent of women are in the work force and where mobility and urbanization result in nuclear family patterns.

The papers presented indicated the need to sensitize society and governments to "future" planning and to consider a "Council for the Third Age" devoted to the fundamental interests of aged persons. Stimuli for creativity, initiated in North America to help keep older people community-bound and alert were discussed. These included a program of day-activity centres, a puppetry program, a drama group, and a discussion program to help the children of parents who are growing old.

The changing quality of life for the old in Hong Kong was described. Here, congested living environments often lead to family conflict. Self-help programs are geared toward helping the elderly be independent and givers as well as receivers. Volunteers among the elderly play an important part in self-help programs.

In Malaysia, public expectations for help, coupled with an increasing number of aged people, create difficulties at all levels. The government provides homes for the aged, but "begging" is a common phenomenon as a means of self-help for this group.

Workshop conclusions and recommendations follow.

Self-help, ranging from government intervention to aid private foundations to "begging" by the elderly, demonstrate the range of possibilities in adaptation to old age. Workshop participants felt that an initial step towards self-help programs might be to discuss and revise the resolutions prepared by the World Health Organization during the Helsinki Symposium in May 1981. These resolutions grew out of a meeting on "Old Age and Mental Health" organized by the Finnish Association for Mental Health.

The revised resolution follows:

HELSINKI SYMPOSIUM RESOLUTION

Participants from 10 countries in Europe: Austria, Belgium, Denmark, Finland,

Richard C. Nann, Dorcas Susan Butt, and Lourdes Ladrido-Ignacio (eds.), Mental Health, Cultural Values and Social Development, 203–205.

Greece, Italy, Norway, United Kingdom and West Germany, and also from Canada, and the European office of WHO attending the Helsinki Symposium in May 1981, on "Old Age and Mental Health", organized by the Finnish Association for Mental Health, under the auspices of the European Region of the World Federation for Mental Health, agreed upon a resolution for presentation to the World Health Organization, the World Federation for Mental Health, and the National Government of all the countries represented. The following is the basic resolution but includes (in capital letters) changes made after discussion at the Manila Congress:

"WE RESOLVE THAT in order to meet the challenge of the social and medical requirements for the mental and physical health of the elderly people, AND TO IMPROVE THEIR QUALITY OF LIFE, we urgently request that emphasis is placed upon the following:

(1) development of national policies for aging people which must be formulated and carried out within the context of social and economic development WITH PARTICULAR EMPHASIS ON FINANCIAL SECURITY, HOUSING, HEALTH, AND TRANSPORTATION POLICIES;
(2) PROVISION OF RECOGNITION OF THE ELDERLY'S CONTRIBUTION TO SOCIETY, ACKNOWLEDGED OR NOT;
(3) (a) effective education and training program AT ALL LEVELS with full involvement of institutions of higher education and teaching hospitals for those involved in care,
    (b) for the general public, basic knowledge and skills TRAINING, and
    (c) pursue the research into the NEEDS OF older people, with particular emphasis on prevention, HEALTH SERVICES DELIVERY, COMMUNITY ATTITUDES, URBANIZATION AND MIGRATION.
(4) acceptance of the concept of choice and, when necessary, risk, for elderly people;
(5) provision of a range of services INCLUDING RESIDENTIAL to meet different degrees of need and the establishment of criteria for the inclusion or exclusion in institutional care of all kinds;
(6) redefinition of the role of primary health care multidisciplinary teams in work with elderly people;
(7) COMMUNITY SUPPORT SYSTEM – a key element of normal living and housing elderly people in the community, whether in care or in their homes;
(8) the full involvement of the whole community, and especially old people themselves in identifying their needs and in finding SOLUTIONS FOR THE PROBLEMS IDENTIFIED;
(9) STIMULATION OF THE SELF HELP POTENTIAL OF ELDER PEOPLE WHENEVER POSSIBLE.

All participants, in approving this resolution, added their own personal commitment to strive to secure implementation of these principles in their own country and in the organization with which they are associated.

Following formation of the resolutions, the group decided to propose to the World Federation for Mental Health that a "World Inventory of Community Support Systems and Self-Help for the Elderly" be undertaken. Such an inventory, carried out broadly and analyzed carefully, could help to develop a positive and manageable thrust for such self-help models possible in both the developed and developing worlds.

Chairperson:	Dr. Alex Kwan (Malaysia)
Co-ordinator:	Dr. Gaston Harnois (Canada)
Facilitator:	Mrs. Luvimin A. Custodio (Philippines)
Resource Persons:	Mr. William W. L. Wong (Hong Kong); Mrs. Bert Kruger-Smith (U.S.A.)

LOURDES LADRIDO-IGNACIO, M.D., MARILOU LEGASPI, M.S.W., and ZENAIDA NISCE (Philippines)

MENTAL HEALTH IN PRIMARY HEALTH CARE

"Health for All by the Year 2000" is a worldwide goal and many countries have initiated and developed health care programs in order to achieve this goal. The primary health care concept underlies these programs. The International Conference in Primary Health Care, held in 1978, provided that primary health care should include the promotion of mental health. The workshop, therefore, sought to confront the following key issues, which are central to the understanding of mental health in primary health care. (1) Clarification of the primary health care concept. (2) Clarification of the inter-relationship between primary health care and mental health in terms of: how does primary health care influence the mental health of the community; what mental health knowledge and skill can be applied in developing and providing primary health care; is it feasible to provide mental health care in general health care. (3) Discussion and adaption of strategies of action by participants relevant to specific conditions in their respective countries. Such strategies should focus on programs for mental health in primary health care.

The chairman, Dr. Amparo Banzon, presented a paper on Mental Health in Primary Health Care, which defined mental health as the condition which promotes the optimal development of the individual – physical, intellectual and emotional. This definition highlighted the individual and societal aspects of mental health – that the individual must be first psychologically capable and have access to resources and opportunities to realize his other aspirations within society. The implications of such definition can be seen on two levels. On the individual level, there is a need to re-examine norms and values of a particular culture as they relate to mental health, including a recognition of the contribution of traditional cultural patterns in the promotion of mental health. On the institutional level, government policies should be reformulated to include a broader definition of mental health in order to encourage and support the re-orientation of various institutions to be more responsive to community mental health needs. Within this context, an efficient and effective primary health care program is most important since its ultimate objective is to increase community access to resources and opportunities.

Dr. Sergio Gasmen reiterated the importance of the involvement of the community in his paper. He pointed out that the participation of the community in primary health care promotes mental health since it allows those who are most deprived to be involved in shaping and designing their own lives.

Dr. Kunihiko Asai centred on the patterns of help-seeking behaviour of Japanese psychiatric patients. He noted the important role the family plays

Richard C. Nann, Dorcas Susan Butt, and Lourdes Ladrido-Ignacio (eds.), Mental Health, Cultural Values and Social Development, 206–208.

in assisting the patient to seek treatment and services. Discussion followed on the ethics involved in the concept of community participation. An underlying assumption was that communities need the help of a health team, in meeting their needs.

Who are the primary health care workers and how can they be trained? Dr. Evangeline Suva shared her experiences in training workers at the health centre level. Given proper training, and the necessary government support and guidance, workers at the health centre can provide mental health care, specifically early detection of mental disorders; can carry out simple and circumscribed tasks in the care of psychiatric emergencies, the psychotic patient and anxiety and depressions; and can be sensitive to the social and psychological aspects of health and illness. The main focus of the training program is to make the health worker comfortable in providing mental health care among the members of the community.

The group agreed that it is not only feasible to provide mental health care in general health care but it is, in fact, necessary since there is a very close relationship between the provision of basic health care and the promotion of mental health. The mental health knowledge and skills needed in the implementation of primary health care were identified. These centred on the importance of having an understanding of the community, its cultural patterns and other socio-economic dimensions of community life. This means recognizing and using the indigenous structure, values and patterns that promote the mental health of the community. Health workers must be sensitive and responsive to the socio-psychological dimensions of the lives of the patients and the communities they serve. Additional knowledge and skills are required in the diagnosis and treatment of patients with mental health problems, and in helping people carry out their life tasks, for example, guidance for mothers about their children.

To help ensure that these suggestions are acted upon, the following strategies were suggested: (1) The creation of a wider awareness about mental health among members of the community through education, focussing on primary concerns in specific countries, including the stigma of mental illness. (2) A reorientation of the health care system to encompass the total health care process from in-patient to out-patient, from hospital to the community, and from urban to rural. (3) The enhancement of health workers through training in mental health, as well as maximizing their use in the mental health field. (4) Ensuring that mental health considerations are central to any government national health plan. (5) The organization of supportive associations, such as mental health clubs. (6) The participants decided to communicate with each other regarding the progress of their efforts in promoting mental health in primary health care during the next three months, using the office of Dr. Banzon, Chairman of the workshop, and the National Co-ordinator of primary health care in the Philippines, as the clearing house.

Chairperson:	Dr. Amparo Banzon (Philippines)
Co-ordinator:	Dr. Lourdes Ladrido-Ignacio (Philippines)
Facilitators:	Ms. Marilou Legaspi (Philippines); Mrs. Zenaida Nisce (Philippines)
Resource Persons:	Dr. Kunihiko Asai (Japan); Dr. Sergio Gasmen (Philippines); Dr. Evangeline Suva (Philippines)

HERIBERTA CAGNIOA

ORGANIZATION AND ROLES OF MENTAL HEALTH ORGANIZATIONS

This workshop examined the experiences of mental health associations in the several countries represented by the participants in attendance.

MALAYSIA

There are three mental health associations in this country, whose objectives are: (1) to educate the public on mental health; and (2) to urge government to provide and support mental health programs. However, the government is very reluctant to spend money on a disease or disorder which does not kill. One of the main activities of the mental health associations is the provision of a counselling program for secondary students and some primary pupils in schools where most of the teachers are not trained to handle emotional problems. The main function of the mental health organizations in this country is not in a hospital setting but in the community.

PHILIPPINES

The Philippines Mental Health Association has fourteen local chapters. The Oriental Negros Chapter is one of these. In serving twenty-four towns, this local Chapter has the following objectives, which are consistent with those of the parent national organization: (1) promotion of mental health; (2) prevention of mental illness; and (3) rehabilitation. With the support of other agencies and civic-minded citizens, the local Chapter was able to raise sufficient funds to construct a mini-hospital and a rehabilitation centre. The Chapter has a close linkage with the University of the Philippines College of Medicine. A lack of funding for ongoing programs is one of the main problems experienced by the local organization. A new local Chapter in Dipolog was just recently started last year with a small grant from the National PHMA.

THAILAND

The development of mental health services and organizations in this country has taken place in the private sector. Despite the existence of major social problems such as crime and drug addiction, the government has not actively been involved in mental health programs. There is a lack of effective co-operation between

Richard C. Nann, Dorcas Susan Butt, and Lourdes Ladrido-Ignacio (eds.), Mental Health, Cultural Values and Social Development, 209–211.

government and psychiatrists, and even among psychiatrists themselves. Mental health workers do not work as a team, and this tends to result in confusion. There has been some success in providing information and education on mental health through the use of the mass media. In some respects, mental health organizations are seen as a threat to the government.

ZAMBIA

The workshop Chairman had prepared a paper on "The Organization and Roles of Mental Health Associations", which was circulated at the meetings. The objectives of the Zambia Mental Health Association are directed to the promotion and sustenance of good mental health for all the people at both the national and international levels. The organization is a non-governmental, non-professional body. It brings together people of different backgrounds who share a common interest in mental health. It is managed and administered by an Executive Committee elected every two years. Its day to day work is co-ordinated by an Executive Secretary, who is the only non-volunteer. There are three sub-committees: (a) Research, Conferences and Publicity; (b) Management, Finance and Fundraising; and (c) Projects Development. At present, the Association has three district branches, but hopes eventually to establish a branch in each of the nine provinces in Zambia.

One of the major differences between experiences in developing and developed countries is that the former has had to assume responsibility for the provision of clinical and professional services because governments are not doing it. Unfortunately, the provision of direct services by mental health associations very quickly exhausts all resources and energies. There are many other tasks and programs to be done by a non-governmental organization.

During the workshop discussions, participants exchanged views on ways to make mental health associations more effective. Some suggestions which emerged from this discussion are:

(1) Public information programs must be dramatic enough to ensure impact. A problem in public information service is how to make the program compelling and appealing.

(2) There is the mistaken notion that mental health associations deal only with those who are mentally ill. There is need to communicate a better understanding of the role of these associations, and to dispel the stigma attached to mental illness.

(3) Time, effort and concentration are necessary to establish linkages with other civic groups. There is need to improve collaboration and encourage co-operation of other interested agencies and civic clubs.

(4) It is the responsibility of national associations of mental health to provide support and help to local chapters. Very often, the problem is communication.

(5) There should be an international exchange program. This should include an information centre and a program where persons can visit other countries and observe and learn from other countries. The WFMH should be playing this role.

Chairperson: Hon Isaac K. Mwendapole (Zambia)
Co-ordinator: Mr. George Rohn (Canada)
Facilitators: Ms. Elvie Sabado (Philippines); Mrs. Heriberta Cagnioa (Philippines)

Ms. JOSEFINA G. FERNANDEZ (Philippines)

TRAINING OF MENTAL HEALTH PROFESSIONALS AND VOLUNTEERS

A highlight of this workshop was the presentation of a paper entitled, "Professional Training of Psychiatric Nurses", by the main resource speaker, Yoshiyasu Yamaguchi. The paper was read in English, but copies, written both in English and Nipponggo, were furnished to the participants beforehand. Nenita Honda provided simultaneous translation to the large number of Japanese participants in this workshop. The language barrier slowed down the proceedings but the group's interest surmounted this problem.

Mr. Yamaguchi's paper gave a background on the role of the Japanese Psychiatric Nurses Education and Training Association, which evolved in response to changing needs and practices in the field of psychiatry in Japan. The highlights of psychiatric practice considered to be the basis for training are:

(1) Mental patients in Japan are considered to need treatment in specialized hospitals under secluded and intense care.

(2) Psychiatry in Japan is something left entirely in the hands of the private sector. Almost 82% of mental hospitals or facilities now existing in Japan are private operations.

(3) Psychiatry falls far short of demand in rural areas.

(4) There is now a greater awareness of the importance of psychiatry than at any other time, and at no other time have psychiatrists in Japan achieved today's visibility.

In the light of the foregoing phenomena, which called for the improvement of psychiatry and the care of mental patients in Japan, the Association has tried to contribute its share through the nurse education programs of its member organizations. The basic objectives of these programs are to develop a larger number of capable psychiatric nurses; to encourage psychiatric nurses to take pride in their vocation; and to improve themselves as professionals through enrichment of knowledge and technology.

The understanding of the morals and ethics of a professional psychiatric nurse is basic in the training. The nurse educational programs include courses in psychiatry, general and psychiatric nursing, clinical psychology, counselling, social welfare, laws and regulations, regional medical well-being, rehabilitation, recreational activities, nursing techniques, and case studies.

There are, in addition, a number of national and regional forums and symposia provided by the Association and its member organizations. These include: (1) National academic forums which consist of symposium and panel discussions which are all recorded and re-arranged for publication in the "Studies of Nursing", a documentary of the practice of psychiatry in Japan as it developed over the years. A regional academic forum is held every fall and the themes follow the

Richard C. Nann, Dorcas Susan Butt, and Lourdes Ladrido-Ignacio (eds.), Mental Health, Cultural Values and Social Development, 212–214.

ones discussed at the National Academic Forum for that season. (2) A second approach makes use of seminars addressed to different subjects like nurse management, leadership, nurses and trainees. (3) A third approach deals with seminars under different themes which are conducted for the training of potential managers of branch headquarters, lecturers of psychotherapy and clinical experts.

Mr. Yamaguchi closed his presentation with an invitation to all those engaged in psychotherapeutic nursing to attend the next academic study meeting which will be held in Sapporo in May 1982.

After the paper presentation, the following points were brought up in response to questions from the group:

(1) The Japanese Psychiatric Nursing Association was established to train nurses for hospital work without obtaining a Master's degree in a university. The job training is approved by the Minister of Health.

(2) Since it is difficult to induce psychiatrists to work in rural areas, a solution is to give seminars and to educate government doctors in those areas.

(3) In the United States, in just 18 years, 1,000 community mental health centres were established in the rural areas to treat people closer to where they live. However, due to some socio-economic issues, service and training budget have been reduced by 25 percent.

(4) Primary prevention should be concerned with identifying high risk groups such as people who survived major traumatic experiences, etc.

Another highlight of this workshop was the presentation of Angelita Vega-Cruz, on the contents of training programs for psychiatric nurses and nursing attendants in The Philippines. These programs include: the hospital psychiatric course, mental health and psychiatric nursing course, and the basic psychiatric nursing course for attendants. The topics included in the training programs for nurses are: psychological disorders, symptoms, causes, treatment modalities, nursing approaches, legal aspects of nursing, principles and concepts of mental health, communication skills, group dynamics, community mental health nursing, and the new performance evaluation. The training program for nursing attendants covers almost the same topics with the addition of anatomy and physiology, and remotivation techniques.

The existing shortage of personnel, particularly psychiatrists, necessitates expanded roles and duties of nurses, which includes making the regular rounds at the wards. By reason of their exposure, they have become skilled in helping and caring for the mental patients. They are trained in interaction and group therapy. The student nurses are also trained to have a one-to-one relationship with the mental patients. The shortage of nursing personnel would have been abated if the hospital has been allowed to use nursing students as volunteers. However, the Philippine Civil Service rules prohibit this.

Interdisciplinary training programs are also conducted in the Philippines, and are aimed at organizational development. For example, at the Ministry of Social Services and Development, team training is emphasized. Integrated training programs which incorporate common and specific knowledge to suit the need of the different staff are conducted.

A brief comment was made on the training of community psychologists in New Zealand, where an expanded role for such professionals has developed because of limited employment opportunities for clinical psychologists. The training is aimed at preparing the psychologist for alternative roles in the community which take on a preventive nature, for example acting as collaborator consultant for people with special needs; as a facilitator for groups; or as agents for social change. A six-year course, similar to the course for clinical psychologists, was developed to meet this particular need.

The question of how volunteers may be encouraged, trained, and effectively used was discussed in the light of varying socio-economic factors. In conclusion, the participants searchingly asked the question: Are we living in a dream world to expect volunteerism in developing countries?

RECOMMENDATIONS

(1) That the World Federation for Mental Health, through its member associations, provide those in the mental health professions with copies of training programs for mental health professionals and volunteers conducted in different countries. This can serve as a guide in preparing training programs where these may apply, taking into consideration the needs and resources and the socio-cultural background of the country concerned.

(2) That there be a mutual sharing of experience on motivating, training and effective usage of volunteers in the field of mental health among the different countries through newsletters, publications, and other media of communication.

Chairperson: Dr. Melvin Sabshin (U.S.A.)
Facilitator: Ms. Josefina G. Fernandez (Philippines)
Resource Person: Mr. Yoshiyasu Yamaguchi (Japan)

ALLAN BEIGEL and LORETO F. ROJA

RELATIONS BETWEEN LAY AND PROFESSIONALS

The topic, "Relations Between Lay and Professionals", was discussed within the context of guidance and counselling and the medical profession, and also within social work experience in the Philippines. Problems and issues were identified, and strategies for intervention were explored.

Among the problems and issues identified in the discussion are the following:

(1) Guidance counsellors and former classroom teachers, who leave their work temporarily to obtain a doctoral degree in the field of guidance and counselling, seem to meet with difficulties in re-adjusting to their former environments. One observation is that expectations from the community are too great for them to cope with.

(2) Medical students, especially from affluent families in urban areas, encounter adjustment difficulty in a rural setting.

(3) There is often a conflict in situations where a guidance counsellor wants parents and students to express their own needs, but the latter want to be told what to do, or expect direct solutions to existing problems.

(4) Relations between lay persons and professionals can be greatly influenced by the environment where the relationship exists or where the persons are working.

In considering strategies for improving the relationship between lay persons and professionals, the following suggestions are proposed:

(1) Have knowledge of the cultural backdrop of the population being served;

(2) Expose medical students to enable them to identify with the population being served, and to establish rapport with them;

(3) Develop a group of people (volunteers) who can serve as bridges or communication links between the lay and the professionals in the community;

(4) Be clear as to the kinds of decisions to be made by the lay person on the one hand and by the professional on the other;

(5) Encourage professionals to undertake activities and experiences which can sensitize them to what it is like to be a lay person;

(6) Find a neutral ground for communication between lay persons and professionals;

(7) Translate rhetorics of support to policy statements and action.

Workshop participants identified what they believe to be some critical elements in the relations between lay volunteer workers and professionals. These include: (a) a clear definition of the appropriate tasks of volunteers and the professional; (b) assurance that an activity is within the capacity of volunteers to perform; and (c) a mechanism must be set up for the training of volunteers who need it.

Richard C. Nann, Dorcas Susan Butt, and Lourdes Ladrido-Ignacio (eds.), Mental Health, Cultural Values and Social Development, 215–216.

Volunteers stay on when they feel they are able to contribute and, thus, develop a sense of worth and a sense of fulfillment. When there is extreme conflict between lay and professionals, two things may happen. Either the volunteer resigns, or if volunteers comprise the decision-making body, the professional resigns.

Chairperson: Dr. Allan Beigel (U.S.A.)
Co-ordinator: Mrs. Edita Martillano (Philippines)
Facilitator: Ms. Loreto F. Roja (Philippines)

Mrs. CARMEN ALCUAZ-REYES (Philippines)

MENTAL HEALTH SCREENING OF INDUSTRIAL WORKERS

Dr. Meltzer elaborated on the development of personality and the meaning of mental health. He emphasized the necessity for an "I-thou" relationship in fostering mental health. "Mental health would imply that in your head and in your heart you are relatively worthwhile." The person has sufficient self-regard and emotional acceptance. Some people are very ambivalent, their head and heart are not attuned to each other. This sometimes takes the form of neurotic thinking or thinking with a worry which can be exemplified by "If only . . . " statements. One who thinks with a worry "can tend to brood or develop physical symptoms which may give him a sense of failure and a pervading fear of failure." People can be taught to be healthy-minded, "To use their eyes and know what they are seeing", to "use their ears and know what they are hearing". After setting this broad framework, he dwelt on several topics: communication in industry, attempts to humanize organizations, the screening process, and the shocks of mankind.

Communication in industry is "not very human" and is often characterized by hierarchal communications. In particular, the appraisal interview which should be a constructive experience usually turns into an experience that tends to deflate the interviewee. He mentioned three styles of appraisal: "tell and sell", "listen and tell", and "problem-solving". The most desirable is the last because it provides an opportunity for mutual acceptance. Before moving on to the screening process, he talked briefly about efforts to make the organization more humane "The Industrial Revolution," he said, "advanced technology but dehumanized people."

Turning to the screening process, there is dissatisfaction with the word "screening" because it implies that the interviewer is the authority and does not allow mutuality. The most important tool in screening is the interview which should provide the framework for understanding the dynamics of the person. A battery of tests may be used as aids but this is secondary to the interview.

The history of testing was traced back to World War I and World War II when IQ tests were developed and given to enlisted men to help place them. In relation to IQ tests, the speaker warned against putting too much emphasis on the IQ because it is not constant and may often have very little relevance to the job. Other tests which are used in the screening process are special ability tests, interest tests, and personality tests including the projective tests such as the Rorschach and the TAT. Personality tests may help to answer questions such as "How energetic is he? How emotionally stable? How well can he get in touch with people?" Perhaps more important are instruments such as the Sense of Values Test and Projective Interviewing.

Richard C. Nann, Dorcas Susan Butt, and Lourdes Ladrido-Ignacio (eds.), Mental Health, Cultural Values and Social Development, 217–221.

Some of the principles Dr. Meltzer follows in trying to understand the person are:

(1) We all belong to the same human race.
(2) We are more like some people than others – more like those raised more similarly.
(3) In some respects, every single individual is unique.
(4) Personality may be organized rigidly, loosely, firmly.
(5) It is possible in the same person for some dimensions of his personality to be loose, while others are rigid and others firm.
(6) Rarely does a single personality grow up evenly.
(7) In the average personality, there are present unassimilated, undigested habit residues of growth.
(8) Every personality hangs on to some habits, to some feelings, some attitudes which are irrelevant to present circumstances and finds himself in need for a new perspective for further growth.
(9) Every personality passes through stages of development where the best habit he can have is the habit of changing habits.
(10) Personality growth is a continuing process. Using resources most effectively calls for periodic reconstruction or restructuring for greater effectiveness.
(11) There is no such thing as a developed personality. An alive person is developing.

Mr. Medina discussed the mental health screening of workers in an organization from the point of view of a user, a line manager. As a line manager what is of more interest to him is the state of mental health of people during employment. While screening procedures might ensure that people were in a good state of mental health at entry point, once in the organization their mental health could deteriorate.

A mental health check is needed at the entry level, when one moves into the supervisory level, and again at the managerial level because job demands and job structures change dramatically. The organization has not always recognized this nor has it prepared the person for the change. When one finds him or herself faced with a situation for which s/he is unprepared, s/he retrenches to old behaviour, which may not be appropriate to the situation. This neglect of the organization to prepare a person for a new job is an eroder of mental health. At the supervisory and managerial level some eroders are: the unmanageable desire for a taste of success, the need for recognition which is unrecognized by people of significance, the ambiguities of the job and the fear of failure because failure is treated as failure rather than as a learning experience. At the executive level the eroders are: power and the misuse of power, acquisition of power *per se* rather than power seen as a tool to get work done, success unless this is managed within the context of Christian values.

Mr. Medina noted that many managers within organizations do care about the mental health of their people and make an effort to improve the situation. He cited a research study that attempted to determine whether Herzberg's hygiene model really works in the Philippines. The subjects for the study were 250 marketing people, all college graduates. The findings showed that the desire for self-fulfillment on the job seemed to have been lost. More highly correlated with productivity was the satisfaction of social needs. But even this varied and correlated with age. In summary, the "new-hires" ranging in ages from 18–23 had very high social needs; those from 28–35 years of age had high economic and security needs. This was also the age at which many of them married and begot two children, thus the family demands for economics increased. At age 50–60, social needs rose once again. The implications of findings such as these, within the context of mental hygiene, indicate the importance of a company's ability to suit the fringe benefits, the recreation and socialization activities to the employees' needs to help them maintain their sanity.

He believes that within the context of the business organization it is important for managers to look at their environment and to manage it. And he noted that Joan Margolis stated at a conference of the IFTDO that they in the US are learning and picking up some things from developing countries on "humanizing the environment".

As a consultant to a number of industrial operations, one of Mrs. Diy's main concerns is how to help people become more productive and satisfied in work using a macro-approach. She is currently involved in research work with the Meralco Foundation spearheaded by Dr. Harry Oshima. Dr. Oshima has raised a number of questions regarding the varying degrees of productivity of the countries of East, Southeast and South Asia and the possible relationship of this to the work ethic, culture and religion. Some of the preliminary studies found, for instance, that it is the parents who curtail the child's curiosity and desire to work. When the children are young they tell them they don't have to work but should concentrate on playing and unwittingly create a dichotomy between work and play for their children.

Ms. Leonora Vasquez de Jesus presented a paper on "Mental Health Screening Practices for Overseas Workers to the Middle East: Issues and Problems" that focused on the present screening practices and problems and issues related to mental health. The employment of Filipino workers in the Middle East has grown from 2,000 in 1969–1971, to 14,100 in 1972, and 25,000 in 1977. Of this, 11,500 are in Saudi Arabia. Furthermore, 40 percent of these workers are rank-and-file craftsmen, construction or production process workers. The applicants are age 25–48; 73 percent are married; 42 percent are high school graduates, while 38 percent have some elementary schooling, 5 percent finished college, and 19 percent have vocational training. Work experience is varied. Many have been working in the Middle East and are re-applying. There are also those who would not find any employment in the Philippines. The returning workers' complaints regarding work conditions in the Middle East include: lack of water, physical discomfort, and lack of social life. Loneliness came next to biological needs. Despite all the difficulties encountered, workers still want to go to the Middle East, sometimes paying prohibitive recruitment fees to recruiters. The primary purpose is economic.

As the number of recruitment firms and workers leaving for the Middle East increased, so did reports of the number of workers showing signs of maladaptation and inability to stay in the job. This prompted several recruitment firms to consider mental health screening, although it appears that the main purpose was economic rather than a real concern for the workers' welfare. Because of this, the recruiters see to it that the cost of mental health screening is minimal, often choosing the lowest bidder among those offering professional services.

The screening process is "to determine the individual's capacity to adjust and to cope with a stressful situation". While standard instruments may be used as in other pre-employment screening structures, here not much weight is given to the applicant's mental abilities or aptitude for the job. Neither are the positive aspects of personality emphasized. The main concern is with the person's "ability to survive". Most of the practising psychologists use the same battery of tests: some administer one or two, others as many as five. Most also conduct an interview. The most frequently mentioned tests used are the MMPI, the Draw-a-Person Test, the Sentence Completion Test, the Hand Test, and the Luscher Colour Test.

The problems of screening include: (1) The relationship between the recruitment firm and the psychologists, e.g. while the recruiters are able to give very little information regarding the situation into which the workers will be placed, they want the psychologists to take full responsibility for the worker's behaviour once he is recommended. Sometimes the client firm has even requested a change in the recommendation since the applicant has important connections. (2) The instruments and test materials available, e.g. many of the tests are in English (which presents a difficulty for those who do not understand English), lack of alternative firms, no predictive validity studies because of poor-coordination between testing firm and recruitment agency. (3) There is a lack of co-operation between different testing firms, making it difficult to standardize screening practices and allowing for the practice of unqualified psychologists. (4) Problems of day-to-day administration, e.g. the question of re-testing an applicant in the hope of getting a better profile, the possibility of another person taking the test for someone.

The following questions were raised regarding ethical considerations: (1) Should other firms or other psychologists re-test an applicant who has already been tested before and rejected? (2) Should a psychologist service an illegally operating recruitment firm? (3) How do we safeguard the confidentiality of reports? (4) Who are psychologists responsible to – the client firm or the individual examiner? The following recommendations were offered: (1) Psychologists in this country must launch an education campaign to enlighten the public, especially client firms. (2) Practising psychologists in this line of work must organize to protect their own interests and to upgrade the quality of their services by setting minimum standards and qualifications for psychologists. (3) Research in the area must be encouraged and supported by the government.

Faculty:	Dr. Frank Johnson (U.S.A.)
Chairperson:	Dr. Hy Meltzer (U.S.A.)
Co-ordinator:	Mrs. Carmen Alcuaz-Reyes (Philippines)
Facilitators:	Comm. Rachel Fidelino (Philippines); Ms. Consolacion Cazenas (Philippines)
Resource Persons:	Mrs. Concepcion Diy (Philippines); Mr. Ramon Medina (Philippines); Ms. Leonora Vasquez de Jesus (Philippines)

ALICE AGPOON

CREATION AND USE OF COMMUNITY RESOURCES: GOOD PRACTICES IN MENTAL HEALTH

Participants from various countries presented a brief commentary of existing mental health resources in their own countries.

In the Philippines, hospitals are congested. There is a lack of awareness on the part of the community of mental health. There is the need to establish psychiatric departments in general hospitals all over the Philippines; to promote mental health concepts to the people and involve community participation; to implement a connection between the MSSD (Ministry of Social Services and Developments) and National Mental Hospital regarding establishment of the special care service of recovered mental patients in Southern Tagalog; and the need for MSSD to assist patients and families towards self-reliance.

In Hong Kong, institutions are available to care for mental patients. In Japan, there is an existing health services scheme. There are more hospital beds than psychiatric cases; mental health care is just beginning. Most psychiatric cases live with their own families. In Malaysia, foster homes are available for mental patients instead of long hospitalization.

From the ensuing discussion, workshop participants came to the following conclusions: (1) Mental health concepts should be available to the community; (2) There is need to establish welfare associations for patients similar to that in Malaysia; (3) Involve the community in mental health activities; (4) Patients should be helped in their re-integration into the community, as well as their families.

A paper presented by Mrs. Dulce Saguisag discussed a project to test the applicability of an operational model of community development in four barrios in Cavite, Philippines. Strategies tested in relation to identification, mobilization and utilization of community resources were: (1) establishing a community core group to plan, design and implement a community survey; (2) increasing community awareness to raise consciousness and to involve its citizens; (3) setting up task groups or committees to undertake a community planning course; (4) organizing workshops to identify needs, problems and solutions; (5) developing mechanisms to allow people to participate in development.

Recommendations emerging from this project were: (1) Agencies should initiate people slowly and gradually into roles in planning and implementation of a development program; (2) Define interfaces between agencies; (3) Concentrate on developing concepts of self-reliance, partnership and participation; (4) Establish workable mechanisms to allow people not only to benefit, but also to participate in development efforts by exercising their rights to determine what they need, how their needs can be met, and allowing them opportunities to deal with their problems.

Richard C. Nann, Dorcas Susan Butt, and Lourdes Ladrido-Ignacio (eds.), Mental Health, Cultural Values and Social Development, 222–223.

"Community Mental Health Services in Japan: A Study on Activity of Psychiatric Social Workers and Public Health Nurses" was presented by Tadaharu Nakao, which outlined attempts to study effective community mental health services by analyzing the influence of activities by psychiatric social workers (PSWs) and public health nurses (PHNs) on clients. This study discovered that the activities of PSWs and PHNs, and the development of available social resources benefitted their clients; that this correlated with the development of occupational training resources; and that the goals of the program should be social participation by the clients.

A proposal on the Special Community After Care Service For Recovered Mental Patients in Southern Tagalog (MSSD tie-up with the National Mental Hospital) was presented to the workshop. Due to time pressures, discussion on this proposal was limited, but the participants endorsed the aims of the project to de-congest the National Mental Hospital.

Faculty: Dr. Jan Praesetyo (Indonesia)
Chairperson: Dr. Datu Mahadevan (Malaysia)
Co-ordinator: Ms. Corazon G. de Leon (Philippines)
Facilitators: Ms. Alice Agpoon (Philippines); Dr. Flocerfina de Jesus (Philippines)
Resource Persons: Mrs. Dulce Saguisag (Philippines); Mr. Tadaharu Nakao (Japan)

Dr. ODITA D. YATCO (Philippines) and Dr. JAN PRAESETYO (Indonesia)

MENTAL HEALTH SCREENING OF CHILDREN

Following a presentation by Dr. Yoshihiro Asai, "Mental Health Screening of Children in Japan", discussion centred on questions of methodology, the instrument used, the cost funding and manpower requirement of the screening process. The screening was done by a team of psychiatrists, psychologists and psychiatric social workers and nurses. After the second paper, "Developmental Screening of Pre-School Children – Standardization of the Denver Developmental Screening Test (DDST) on Japanese Children and Its Implications for the Developmental Screening" by Dr. Reiko Ueda, questions posed were on modifications to the DDST, the variances in results, the elements of the test that were culture free and culture bound. The items modified were on language and the materials used. Also, the author commented on how climate influenced child-rearing, way of life, clothing and motor activity of the children.

The instrument takes about 20 minutes to administer, and it is readily used by other health personnel. The DDST has been tested in Japan and in the Philippines as well. Other comments focussed on the following: (1) In Japan the police force has devised a questionnaire purporting to detect future juvenile delinquents. (2) The need to periodically screen children at various ages: before 5 and every 2–3 years up until age 20 as well as the need to use different devices, the DDST being applicable only up until 6 years of age. (3) Screening would be integrated in the general health delivery, schools and mass media. (4) More and more the need of psychiatrists to team up with other disciplines.

At this point Dr. Praesetyo gave his reactions:

The first paper, which is based on a recent survey in Japan, attempts to show the importance of screening children at an early stage for early detection and early intervention of mental health problems. The examination done in this survey, I assume, was based on a clinical observational method examination procedure (physical and psychiatric). The important findings are revealed in the following points: (1) Those diagnosed as having physically and or psychiatric disturbances, showed a different outcome markedly by the end of the follow-up period. There was a marked decrease of physical disorders, whereas a striking increase of psychiatric disorders (its prevalence rate) was noted. (2) 75% of children with physical disturbance were discovered under the age of three, in contrast to only 20% of children with mental disturbance or mental retardation who were discovered within that age range. (3) It was mostly the mothers who took the lead in finding physical or psychiatric disturbances in their children, whereas the fathers accounted for only 5%. (4) The Japanese families tended to have difficulties in recognizing the signs of psychiatric disturbances or mental retardation in their children. This was in contrast to their attitudes towards their

Richard C. Nann, Dorcas Susan Butt, and Lourdes Ladrido-Ignacio (eds.), Mental Health, Cultural Values and Social Development, 224–226.

children's physical disturbances, in which case they consulted their doctors faster. Thus, physical needs better taken care of when compared to the psychiatric disturbances.

Besides examining the stigma towards psychiatric illness or mental retardation, the nature of these disorders were considered. Psychiatric illness and mental retardation, especially the mild types, are difficult to recognize in the earlier ages.

It is therefore necessary to establish a service, a screening method, that can be used practically to screen young children physically as well as mentally. The authors stressed the advantages of a combined physical and psychiatric approach to the study of child development.

The second paper attempts to describe the adaptation of the Denver Developmental screening test to the Japanese situation. There are indeed some differences in the developmental norms of children in various countries. However, the DDST has been found quite useful. It is practical, less time consuming compared to other psychological tests, it can be done by any health worker since it is not complex to interpret and does not need too specialized skill to administer the test. This achievement in Japan, may stimulate other Asian countries as well, to modify the DDST. In Indonesia for example, this test is used by pediatricians, but has not yet been standardized according to the Indonesian situation.

Now, going back to some basic issues regarding Mental Health Screening of Children. The definition of what is mental health, has been a hot issue, discussed during plenary sessions. What are we going to screen? If mental health is not only the absence of mental disorders, etc., are we able to screen it?

Mental health screening in this context is the screening of whether or not the child has overt or covert mental disorders and his or her abilities to adapt to his environment including his intellectual abilities.

If we want to screen something, we must have a comparative model.

What is the model used in this screening? Child psychiatrists, for example, especially in Indonesia and in the Philippines were not so familiar with this kind of test like the DDST. What use for screening is the clinical method, using models such as the developmental lines of Anna Freud, the Eriksonian stages of development, and the Piagetian model of intellectual development? Using these models, one can come to a profile of the child's developmental level and at the same time the personality profile of the child. What is really needed, is a general method, relatively easy to use by medical as well as non-medical professionals. The DDST seemed to be one with a promising potential.

RECOMMENDATIONS

(1) A clearing house for research be established in the various Regions of the WFMH for the purpose of: (a) identification of problems to be studied; (b) acting as a library of various research done in mental health; (c) offering aid to research that have been approved by the clearing house; (d) conducting seminars and training in research.

(2) There should be regular health screening of children from 0–20.
(3) Health screening of children be a part of parents' class.
(4) The DDST as modified and validated in Japan and the Philippines be disseminated to other countries in the Western Pacific Region for the establishment of in-country workers.
(5) A manual of instruction be composed which will be a basis of training with administration and interpretation of DDST and be disseminated to the countries of the Pacific Region.

Faculty: Dr. Jan Praesetyo (Indonesia)
Chairperson: Prof. Akira Hoshino (Japan)
Facilitator: Dr. Odita D. Yatco (Philippines)
Presentators: Dr. Yoshihiro Asai (Japan); Dr. Reiko Ueda (Japan)

Dr. CARMEN SENA (Philippines)

STRATEGIES IN MENTAL HEALTH CRISES

Two papers provided the focal points for this workshop. The first paper gave an account of an unique program of crisis intervention by telephone in Japan (the practice of Inochi-no-Denwa); the second reported on experiences in a Philippine refugee centre for displaced Vietnamese. An additional presentation was given by the Philippine Minister of Social Services and Development on crisis intervention practice.

The first Inochi-no-Denwa, or Life Line Centre, was opened in Tokyo ten years ago in 1971. Last year alone, 30,000 calls were received by this centre. At present, there are some ten telephone centres using the Japanese language, and one centre using English. In actual operation now is an *overseas* centre connecting Japan and Canada, which was opened in 1979. These centres render services 24 hours a day.

Inochi-no-Denwa aims to become a network for crisis intervention through telephone counselling. Psychiatrists and psychologists consider this as a very unique approach which has succeeded in opening a new field contributing to the psychotherapeutic process.

Inochi-no-Denwa has helped people in crisis, such as those who are lonely, frustrated and confused. It has helped prevent suicides in Japan as well as in other Western countries. Inochi-no-Denwa is not just a service centre but has become a sort of *social movement*. Lay volunteers have offered their services to work in the centres and have given their own unique contributions which could not be replaced by the professionals.

The characteristics of crisis intervention by telephone is the presentation of *confidentiality and anonymity*. Consequently, people who may feel ill at ease to disclose their problems in a face to face situation with another person find these centres not threatening. However, telephone counselling cannot be considered as a substitute for the traditional face to face counselling.

Telephone workers who are recruited as volunteers from the community undergo a structured training program conducted by mental health professionals. After a personal interview, the volunteer has to undergo group training in basic human relations including lectures on such topics as counselling, youth problems, family problems, marital and sex problems, community resources, etc. Their training may further proceed to an advanced training course or to an intern training. Continuing training while in service is provided by means of informal workshops.

Out of 31,925 callers recorded during a recent one year period, about 40 percent were men and 60 percent were women. The main problems presented ranged from "philosophy of life", to sex, marital, male-female relationships,

Richard C. Nann, Dorcas Susan Butt, and Lourdes Ladrido-Ignacio (eds.), Mental Health, Cultural Values and Social Development, 227–229.

personal mental health, to medical problems and mental illness. It is difficult to evaluate the effectiveness of the telephone life line centres. However, during the past 10 years that the telephone centres have been in operation, there has been a decline in the incidence of suicides in Japan. The statistics also show that about 10 to 20 percent of the callers belong to those who ages are less than 20.

The centre for Vietnamese refugees in the province of Palawan, Philippines received both refugees as well as repatriates returning to the Philippines. Since 1975 the total number of refugees taken in is around 19,000. About 10 percent of the group have been referred to general hospitals and to the psychiatric hospital for treatment. There have been 3 suicides recorded, two of these happened at sea on the way to the Philippines, and one occurred at the camp. There were 128 cases of excessive drunkenness and these were given counselling in the camp. The incidence of mental illness, however, can be considered small.

Vietnamese who were on board ship on their way to the Philippines suffered extreme physical hardships like hunger and thirst. It has been reported that such deprivation of basic needs forced them to extreme unorthodox practices like cannibalism. However, one cannot be certain. Leaving the home country for any Vietnamese is an experience of deep and extreme loss. Some say the Vietnamese places the love of country over and above that of family; leaving one's country serves to strip one of identity.

In spite of the hardships suffered by the refugees, very few of them openly complained of psychological problems. Perhaps this could be attributed to the basic attitude of Vietnamese people to "bow in resignation". Being together in a camp also offers some form of protection and emotional support.

Some form of community organization has been established in the camp, which is divided into zones. These are further sub-divided into sub-groups or units. These units are responsible for the organization of religious groups, athletic groups, vocational groups, embroidery groups, knitting groups, etc.

The camp has a program of counselling service which is usually provided by the leader of a zone. A bilingual staff is trained and given orientation and educational information concerning the host country as a means of averting "culture shock". The refugees are advised to cultivate a new identity once they are established in the host country.

In the area of interpersonal relationships, the refugees emit an attitude of suspiciousness toward foreigners. This could have been fostered and reinforced by the communist government in Vietnam which encouraged the family members to spy on one another. Another observation with regards to the attitude of the refugees is their expectation to be treated or received as "heroes" in their port of disembarkation.

The Palawan camp receives housing and food aid from UNHCR. The staff and other camp personnel are furnished by the Philippine government, and contributions from private citizens provide the refugees for their personal necessities. The refugees have built their own houses made out of native materials that are easily available in the nearby forests. Compared to the slum areas in some parts of the Philippines, the camp sites in Palawan and Bataan are far better off. This condition has apparently generated some feeling of enmity among the slum dwellers.

Crisis intervention, as practiced in the Philippines, is essentially eclectic in its approach. It is based on the following assumptions: an individual is subjected to stressful event throughout one's lifetime. During a crisis situation the individual encounters a state where equilibrium is endangered. The state of crisis itself *is not an illness* but represents the struggle of the individual within the crisis situation. When, during the stage of active crisis, help is made available, then one can successfully emerge out of the situation with better and new ways of adaptation which can serve to cope with future crises. Crisis intervention is a unique form of treatment adopted to the *critical period only* and not on a long term basis.

The Mental Health Program being pursued by the Philippine government embraces both the therapeutic and the preventive areas. The preventive field consists of education for public information, early detection of stress situations, problem identification and problem solving. For delinquent youths, facilities include rehabilitation centres in the 13 regions of the Philippines. For the elderly, there exist community centres as well as foster homes for the infirm.

Faculty: Dr. Carmen Sena (Philippines)
Chairperson: Min. Sylvia P. Montes (Philippines)
Facilitator: Ms. Erlinda Cordero (Philippines)
Resource Persons: Dr. Koichi Hasegawa (Japan); Sr. Pascal Le Phi Trui (Vietnam)

Dr. FRANCES RICKS (Canada) and
Dr. PILAR MAURICIO-FABIAN (Philippines)

PROGRAM EVALUATION IN MENTAL HEALTH

Frances Ricks presented a teaching workshop on evaluation in human service organizations. The workshop was based on three premises: (a) programs are delivered through organizations, therefore the appropriate framework for evaluation is a systems framework; (b) managers are responsible for organizations, therefore evaluation is a management function; (c) evaluation is the systematic collection of information about any or all parts of the system/ organization.

In view of the above a model (see Figure 1) for generic evaluation questions was presented. This model specifies what conditions need to exist in order to optimize case, program, agency, network and government (policy) evaluation.

The workshop responded to individual questions with regard to evaluation and how to do it "on a shoestring".

QUESTION(S)	CLAIMS	CASE
What do you do?	This is what we do This is whom we serve This is how we spend our time This is what we hope will happen This is what happened These are our resources	1. Standardized Case Files specify (a) demographic data (b) service received by type of service (c) treatment goals and service plans specified in behavioural terms. 2. Objective measures for case outcome have been developed, follow-up regarding outcome is systematic, and feedback to clinicians is provided. 3. A system exists to bring forward case(s) for review and/or follow-up. 4. Standardized Inventory of Resources.
What does it costs?	This is what our service(s) costs This is what it would cost if the service(s) were terminated This is what it costs for each increment in outcome level These are the benefit/ cost figures – for our program	1. Standardized Record Keeping System for Services Delivered is systematic and centralized providing the number of service hours by type of service per case. 2. Financial accounting system is centralized. 3. Community cost factor is determined.

Richard C. Nann, Dorcas Susan, Butt, and Lourdes Ladrido-Ignacio (eds.), Mental Health, Cultural Values and Social Development, 230–233.

How do you compare to others?	This is how we are doing compared to our previous performance This is how we are doing compared to objective/ normative standards This is how we are doing compared with alternative programs similar in intent	1. Standards for case management and planning have been developed, are in writing and monitored across time periods. 2. Standardized measures and change norms are available to measure outcome across cases. 3. Cases are matched on demographics, planned program and projected outcome.
Did your service cause outcome?	Our service(s) caused the observed changes	1. Matched sample or random assignment of cases is possible without jeopardizing standards and ethics of professional practices.

PROGRAM	AGENCY	NETWORK	GOVERNMENT
1. Program Objectives are identified in writing and specify target population, costs and volume. 2. Case file system for documenting case volume, case contacts and case outcome exists. 3. Objective measures for program outcome have been developed, follow-up is systematic. 4. Standardized reporting format of program data exists, and is used regularly to review program, fed back to staff and feeds agency level planning. 5. Standardized Inventory of Resources	1. A system for identifying, monitoring and reviewing programs (in terms of staff, costs, facilities, supplies, equipment, activities and outcome) exists and is utilized. 2. The agency has written statement of purpose, short and long term goals and specifies functions to reach goals. 3. Agency monitors short and long term goal achievement. 4. Standardized Inventory of Resources.	1. Each agency can furnish, upon request, a detailed classification of each of its program, the major activities within each, at least two indicators of program effort, two indicators of program effectiveness and two indicators of community needs, to which their programs are addressed. 2. Each agency in the network has a clear statement of purpose, goals and objectives. 3. Each agency can produce detailed information on clients seen, problems "treated", characteristics of clients, and staff time and activities in relation to client needs. 4. Each agency in the network maintains a list of unmet community needs/demands.	1. Sub-units within the Ministry are organized functionally in relation to programs. 2. Each functional sub-area has its own budget with flexibility to shift resources within that budget in response to changing needs. 3. Each sub-unit has a set of goals and objectives which are derived from a similar set of overall goals and objectives for the Ministry, derived from Government objectives. 4. Each group in the Ministry can provide a detailed analysis of *major programs*, activities, data on two indicators of effort and two indicators of efficiency. 5. Engages in community need identification, policy research and development, and long range planning.

1. Standardized Record Keeping System for services delivered is systematic, centralized and coded by program. 2. Financial accounting system is centralized and program based. 3. Community cost factor is determined.	1. Standardized Record Keeping System for services delivered is systematic, providing number of service hours by type of service per case per program. 2. Financial Accounting System is centralized and program based. 3. Community cost factor is determined.	1. Standardized record keeping for services is systematic across agencies. 2. Management has standardized reporting format to be used by all agencies and report cost/benefit data to network. 3. Community cost factor is determined.	1. Each group in the Ministry can provide a detailed cost analysis of *major programs*.
1. Standards for program(s) have been developed, are in writing, and monitored across time. 2. Standardized measures and change norms are available to measure outcome across programs. 3. Programs are matched in terms of program objectives and target population.	1. Agency standards have been developed and are in writing. 2. Standardized measures are available to measure agency outcome. 3. Agencies are matched in terms of agency objectives and target population.	1. Comparisons across agency/ time periods made based on standardized format, using standardized indicators or instruments. 2. Networks are matched in terms of objectives and target population.	1. Government uses cost/benefit/ effectiveness data on comparable agencies to allocate re-allocate existing resoucrces. 2. Government uses cost/benefit/ effectiveness data in the context of identified need. 3. Government provides need identification data and planning priorities information in advance of financial allocations/ re-allocations.
1. Matched sample or random assignment of cases to programs is possible without jeopardizing standards and ethics of professional practices.	1. Matched sample or random assignment of agencies/programs is possible without jeopardizing standards and ethics of professional practices.	1. Matched sample or random assignment of networks is possible without jeopardizing standards and ethics of practice.	1. Government uses control study data to allocate/re-allocate resources.

Figure 1
Program Evaluation Model Developed by M. Weinstein and F. Ricks

Dr. BASIL JAMES (New Zealand)

FUNDS FOR MENTAL HEALTH PROGRAMS: WHERE AND HOW

Mental health workers, professionals and volunteers alike are acutely aware of the need for more funds to be channelled into their various fields. Yet, few among them seem to be able to generate these funds directly or indirectly. A major failure is that attention and effort are not directed to the particular task. This failure is the result of several factors, including the assumption of value systems which appear at variance with those necessary for the mobilization of money; a neglect of the dynamics of the funding sources; a tendency to take for granted that virtue alone would triumph (in spite of countless experiences to the contrary); and an inability to find a common language with those whom one wished to influence. Yet, the challenge is real and must be addressed. Furthermore, there are good reasons why mental health workers should be adept at influencing behaviour; this ability, after all, would figure highly in their "raison d'etre".

There is a variety of perceived needs for which additional funding is required. These vary from country to country, but include funding for training and education, salaries, the evaluation of community centres and more substantial buildings. There is also the need for funds to implement nascent projects – both research and service.

Health as such is relatively low on the list of most government priorities (as opposed to illness), and within the field of health itself, mental health is particularly low. There exists a particular problem in articulating mental health concepts in terms which have clear meaning and relevance for legislators and funding bodies. Different "languages" must be used for different organizations. For example, research granting bodies require precision and a clearly worked out methodology and measurable end point. In this regard, the tasks of mental health personnel are clearly more difficult to define than those involving the more physically based sciences. Figures are available to show that this is the case. In terms of both total amounts funded and the percentage of requests approved psychologists tend to do rather better than psychiatrists, but both groups fare badly compared to such disciplines as physiology and biochemistry. In the formulation of research protocols, the likelihood of biological scientists being on adjudicating committees has to be borne in mind. Granting bodies may each have different priorities, and intending applicants are advised strongly to ascertain the composition of such groups so that the applications can be formulated with appropriate emphasis and in appropriate language. Ascertaining the kind of projects recently supported by funding bodies is also important. Personal discussions with individual members of funding bodies often help to clarify these issues, and such individual discussions often provide the opportunity for the intentions of the applicant to be made clearer to key persons.

Richard C. Nann, Dorcas Susan, Butt, and Lourdes Ladrido-Ignacio (eds.), Mental Health, Cultural Values and Social Development, 234–235.

Apart from specific Trusts and Research funds, the community at large is frequently a potential source of financial support. Several preliminary strategies may be articulated. There exist within most communities individuals and organizational networks (Jaycees, Rotary, etc.) who have a proven capacity for public involvement and, directly or indirectly, assistance for fundraising. Such individuals require identification: it is particularly helpful to identify individuals who have had direct experience in mental health matters such as someone being ill in their family. To such people, it is no longer a nebulous matter, but a matter of real and powerful concern. Recruiting such understanding and potentially influential individuals often facilitates amazing results.

Clearly, the mass media – newspapers, periodicals and television – are under-exploited in the field of mental health. Again, the search for individuals in key positions who have experience of, and sympathy with, mental health issues is an important preliminary step. Subsequent strategies can then be evolved using the "entreé" and knowledge that such persons have. The aims of any community project could be formulated as the "three I's" – Interest, Inform and Involve.

A similar strategy can be successful in penetrating policy-making and legislative machineries. It is important to be clear about goals, to understand how the "system" works, and where the points of sympathy and influence are. For example, major impetus in the United States for promulgation of mental health issues came from involved leaders, notably the late President, J. F. Kennedy and Mrs. Rosalynn Carter.

Perhaps these tactics seem obvious. What may be lacking is the commitment of mental health workers to be as active in, and as skillful about, such politicking in fundraising as they are in their individual clinical work. If the task were truly viewed as important, and allocated a sufficiently high priority, time would be given to them and one could earn one's success.

The workshop closed with a description of a community project in New Zealand via a "telethon" in which two million dollars were raised to inaugurate a Mental Health Foundation, and of a second project "Have Crisis Can Cope" – directed at community education and preventive strategies – involved 60,000 people in a population of three million, accomplished through the collaboration of the Mental Health Foundation, the New Zealand Jaycees, national networks of helping persons such as Marriage Guidance and Lifeline organizations, and finally, the community at large. Dr. James also showed a film, *Family of Ours*, produced as part of the "Have Crisis Can Cope" program, bringing home to the community at large the widely penetrating nature of mental health issues.

Faculty and Chairperson: Dr. Basil James (New Zealand)
Facilitator: Mrs. Cecilia Magalona (Philippines)

K. PATRICK OKURA (U.S.A.) and Dr. KNUD JENSEN (Denmark)

CONSUMER'S ROLE IN PLANNING MENTAL HEALTH SERVICES

In the past decade, a change has been taking place in countries having well-developed institutions for treatment of the mentally ill. After years of progress, development of psychiatric treatment has been stagnating. This has led to a more open debate on the suitability of established institutions, a debate in which patients and relatives increasingly take part. It is typical in developed countries that about half of all admissions to mental hospitals are re-admissions. This fact reveals the inadequacy of a treatment approach wherein patients are unable to copy with the demands of the environment on discharge. Consequently a new attitude towards care of the mentally ill is obviously needed.

Studies in many countries report that treatment of the mentally ill outside the environs of the mental hospital is fundamental to social adaptation, and a warm and emotionally secure atmosphere seem to be intrinsic elements in successful care of the mentally ill. Small collectives where a limited number of persons can live in close contact could be the most appropriate link for the mentally ill in their return to life in society after a period of illness.

The patients and relatives claim their rights to an active role in the planning of future mental health services and programs. For long periods of their lives, many patients live in various types of institutions and, therefore, their experience makes them well-fitted for involvement in the planning of institutions. Many professionals, however, do not consider this and instead, view patients as persons who are expected to be grateful to society for having provided their basic needs.

What is the role of the consumer in planning mental health services and institutions? Can the mentally ill seriously be expected to contribute to the planning of expensive institutions? The critical attitude of patients, ex-patients and relatives towards established psychiatry must not provoke the opposition of professionals but rather be accepted as a challenge to initiate fruitful co-operation for a more humane treatment and care of those who require help. For professionals and politicians, this point of view has been difficult to accept and to understand but the demand from patients and relatives is growing stronger and must be accepted.

Presentations to this workshop were given by three delegates from Denmark, two patients and a psychiatrist. The patients had from 7 and 14 years respectively been under treatment in Danish psychiatric departments, and one is still in treatment as an outpatient. Speaking from experiences as consumers of mental health systems, they stressed the value of both the psychopharmaceological and the psychotherapeutic approach to the treatment of mental diseases. They accept the occasional need of forced treatment of psychotic patients who lack

Richard C. Nann, Dorcas Susan, Butt, and Lourdes Ladrido-Ignacio (eds.), Mental Health, Cultural Values and Social Development, 236–237.

insight into their illness, but also emphasized that it is a must for successful treatment that a sincere mutual sympathy and respect is present between patient and therapist. There is a need that psychiatry changes from being only disease-oriented to being more problem-oriented. The risk for relapse of disease when discharged directly from hospital to unchanged social conditions was discussed, and the importance of intermediate institutions (half-way institutions) was stressed.

Patients in stable psychotic phases often are able to take responsibilities in official duties both in organizational work, in committees for patients rights, etc. One of the workshop participants, for example, had for three years been a representative in the Danish Social Supreme Court, and also on the managing board of a condominium, in addition to filling leadership positions in a local division of the Danish National Society for the Welfare of the Mentally Ill. In stable psychotic phases, patients also are able to cope with common working situations in earning their own income. Thus, patients are capable of taking responsibilities not only for themselves but also for mutual interests in society.

Mr. P. Okura drew attention to plans for a citizen board in the U.S.A. from which manuals are now available. In conclusion, it was emphasized that our attitude towards patients' ability to cope with responsibilities has to be changed radically.

Faculty: Dr. Knud Jensen (Denmark)
Chairperson: Mr. Patrick Okura (U.S.A.)
Facilitator: Mrs. Consolacion Cazenas (Philippines)

Dr. ALAN STOLLER (Australia)

MENTAL HEALTH RESEARCH AND THE DELIVERY OF SERVICES

INTRODUCTION

This workshop is concerned with the development of psychiatric services and their delivery in terms of the milieu in which they arise – as expressed through the biological, socio-economic and cultural factors. It will address itself to the overall principles involved in planning, organizational development and evaluation. It will aim to deal with the epidemiology of psychiatric disorders in both developed and developing countries. Regular monitoring of services with regard to intake and outcome and the changing patterns surrounding these phenomena will need to be considered, as well as changing patterns of psychiatric practice and the levels of expectation of patients, relatives and the community in general. Psychosocial factors such as are inherent in family structure, social networks, supportive community institutional practices, diagnostic process, care-seeking, social discrimination, patterns of utilization of existing service, and the realization of unmet and future needs, will need to be brought into the picture. The interaction between physical and mental ill-health will vary from one community to another and requires elucidation. The general principles of legislation for the mentally ill will need to be determined and applied to countries at different stages of development. Various research methods are being used to bring out the picture of mental health services and, in this regard, emphasis will be laid especially in the burgeoning skills of social psychiatry.

I propose initially to indicate the principles which are being followed in developed countries with regard to the production of mental health services for preventing and ameliorating mental ill-health and relate these to ongoing activities in developing countries, so that clues may be obtained as to how best to deal with mental health problems. The basic tenets which have emerged are that services should –

(i) be appropriate to the cultural and socio-economic circumstances of the community involved;
(ii) be readily accessible and hence locally and regionally planned;
(iii) operate through a wide range of resources, primarily community-based and extending from early treatment facilities through to long-term care;
(iv) be extended to those mentally ill persons who are being treated in Forensic Services, in Social Welfare facilities and, indeed, living free in the community; and
(v) be subject to legislation which essentially protects the rights of the individual but does not neglect the necessary reciprocal rights of the community.

Richard C. Nann, Dorcas Susan Butt, and Lourdes Ladrido-Ignacio (eds.), Mental Health, Cultural Values and Social Development, 238–245.

It is recognized that, historically, developed countries have passed through a phase of rapid urbanization, accompanied by the extrusion of severely mentally ill patients from the community into large institutions where they tended to become desocialized, and are now in the process of reversing this trend and encouraging greater degrees of self-help and community participation. In the latter process, a number of professions have become involved in the management of mental illness and the promotion of mental health and an inter-disciplinary and multi-professional approach is currently in operation.

Research has moved extensively away from a pure biochemical model, incorporating sociology and other disciplines such as economics and even political science, whilst additionally examining the individuals within a biopsychosocial framework.

The task to which we are addressing ourselves concerns research methods and practices which need to be fostered to illuminate the social issues which are intimately bound up with our search for those basic principles which will enable us to foster the best possible service for a community irrespective of its socio-economic development.

EPIDEMIOLOGY

A fundamental discipline in the examination of service delivery is epidemiology but, within a particular community, for this to be effective, consideration needs to be given to its definition of mental illness and mental health, diagnostic categories (which vary with philosophical and cultural differences as well as with historical change), legislative and organizational patterns and treatment procedures. Patient and community attitudes are highly significant in determining the kind of services provided.

As already stated, there are problems of diagnostic consistency in the face of the effect of social and ethnic differences on patient-doctor communication. Besides equivalent population sampling, sociodemographic and mental health data need to be comparable. Data from public records alone is insufficient, especially as developed countries are moving towards the greater usage of general hospital and community programs with public services handling the more severe and more easily recognizable cases. There is additionally considerable morbidity in the community which needs to be monitored.

The uses of epidemiology are considered to be sevenfold:

(1) Study of historical trends.
(2) Community diagnosis of mental health problems.
(3) Completion of the clinical picture of mental illnesses.
(4) Psychosocial influences.
(5) Factors influencing outcome.
(6) Discrimination aspects.
(7) Cultural differences.

I have been concerned with a number of community health surveys and the issues which emerge are:

(i) how far discomfort can be labelled as mental illness?

(ii) how short-lived are many mental health symptoms?

(iii) how far are such symptoms temporary defences which lead to personality growth?

Our surveys, covering both rural and urban areas, have shown an overall rate of around 18% of the total population exhibiting symptoms which could warrant psychiatric attention. There is, however, an obvious difference between "count surveys" and "service surveys"; thus, although 3% of children are said to be born mentally retarded, administrative prevalence is 1%.

It has been shown that social disabilities are more important than symptom severity in determining community functioning. In one community survey, it was shown that 11% were impaired but this group declined to 6% after one month, indicating a normal defense to adversity in 5%. It was shown further that spontaneous remission was less likely after three months duration. A minimal estimate of 3% persistently severe impaired, both symptomatically and socially, was found, predominantly neuroses and minor depressions, with a sizeable number of schizophrenics and a lesser number of manic-depressives. A further 1% showed disability habits (such as tics and stuttering) and another 5% with personality disorders, drug addictions, mental retardation and chronic brain disorder. The latter were extensively involved with general health, social and forensic services. It is necessary to determine how far these contribute to long-term health and social services, as well as accidents, homicides and suicides. Bound up with all community surveys is the question of cost and the cost-effectiveness of the various services involved.

MEASUREMENT OF MENTAL ILL-HEALTH

Rating scales and questionnaires are used in the various surveys and in psychosocial investigations in general. One of the problems with these methods is how to incorporate a severity factor, eliminate individual biases and make them value-free? Besides those published, numerous *ad hoc* scales are used by individual researchers for their studies. The choice of a scale is often arbitrary and must account for many of the conflicting results.

The three main uses of questionnaires and rating scales are:

(i) screening devices for determining incidence and prevalence;

(ii) method for determining patterns of symptoms in individuals or in a group of patients;

(iii) measure of severity of disorder.

These measuring methods may be administered through a trained observer or be self-administered by the patient. In the latter case, adequate comprehension and literacy is required and this is not good at the beginning of a trial, anyway; whilst, in the former, inter-rates correlations are necessary.

Depressive scales show differences in terms of emphasis on somatic symptoms, reflecting the clinical orientation of the originator. There are also variations in the sensitivity of scales; how far information access is determined and how patients can utilize them accordingly. Specificity is affected by the fact that psychiatric symptoms tend to overlap in various psychiatric disorders and this, of course, casts doubts on the degree to which mathematical treatment of symptoms can be regarded as satisfactory as, for instance, in global severity scales and visual analogue scales. Careful use of words in describing aspects of the illness are necessary.

One development, the Personal Questionnaire Rapid Scaling Technique (PQRST), requires the therapist and patient together to work out what areas are to be monitored to determine progress, and these are evaluated separately. The problem, of course, resides in the difficulty of replication by other investigators.

It is felt that the time has come to carefully look at existing scales, how they compare, and how they may be amalgamated and improved. As things are at present, the assessment of the severity of a disorder should be based on two or more different types of measure; e.g. nurse, researcher, self-assessment. Socio-demographic factors as well as symptom complexes need to be evaluated.

PSYCHIATRIC TREATMENT

Clinical reorientation leads to changes in organizational systems, but these will not come about unless the socio-politico-economic climate is favourable. Short-term treatment is more indicated in depressive states and acute onset neuroses but many chronic neuroses are more resistant to treatment than psychoses. Personality disorders and schizophrenics with poor pre-hospital history will also require long-term therapy. Long-term residential care is having to cope with larger numbers of brain-disabled persons through aging of the population, increased accidents with advancing affluence and industrialization, and mentally retarded persons who are surviving longer. This needs to be continuously monitored within a particular community where services are being organized.

Short-term cases require continuity of care from hospital to out-patient and day-patient facilities and much work still needs to be done as to how far chronicity can be prevented or ameliorated by particular professional pharmaco-therapeutic or social interventions.

Resources are being fed into early treatment facilities and community after-care and, accordingly, patients in chronic wards tend to be relatively neglected. There is still much to be known as to how far chronic patients can be motivated.

The term "Social Breakdown Syndrome" was coined in 1972 to indicate that patients in the community can be just as decompensated and dependent as those patients in institutes whose passive dependency has been fostered by drugs and poor, unstimulating milieu. The concept implies sociogenic factors affecting the illness to produce disability (impaired function) and, finally, impairment (disability interacting with adverse social environment). The longer decompensation is allowed to develop (over a year), the poorer is the prognosis and the more social life is damaged. There is a high rate of spontaneous recovery from the acute social breakdown syndrome but not for the chronic "Social Breakdown Syndrome". If improvement is to occur in the latter, early rehabilitation programs are necessary; but, even here, it is not known how some cases respond. It would appear that continuity of the therapeutic team's influence outside of hospital is necessary, as is a wide range of resources.

One cogent opinion expressed is that the young adult chronic in the community is to be the major mental health challenge of the 80s. There is a need to identify more precisely the individual and group characteristics of those 18–30 year olds of whom, currently in one U.S. area, 60% were estimated to be schizophrenics, 10% affectives, 20% personality disorders, 5% drug abusers and 5% organic brain syndromes. How these are to be handled, what supports will be required, what facilities will be needed has to be worked out for each geographical area.

Research into the psychosocial treatment of schizophrenic may be taken as a paradigm for psychiatric disorders of some degree of severity.

In general, rapid dramatic results cannot be expected; therapy needs to be individualized for the patient and outcome measures defined. Rehospitalization is not a good indicator of relapse as this may be due to administrative measures, the non-hospital resources available, the type of living arrangements and the family climate. Such variables as ability to work and social and interpersonal skills are significant with regard to adjustment. Individual psychotherapy cannot be seen as separate from the environmental milieu of the schizophrenic, but the situation has to be set up by which it may be compared meaningfully with group therapy and family therapy. If comparisons of treatment programs are to be made, patients should be relatively acute, therapists experienced, treatment and follow-up should be for a prolonged period, outcome measures should be appropriate, and drugs should be controlled. Samples of patients for this type of evaluation should be sufficiently large to allow for analysis and comparison of sub-groups. Family therapy effects are by no means clear-cut; whilst there is value in preventing hospitalization and readmissions and allowing more rapid discharge from hospital, prolonged studies with well-defined methodology are needed to examine not only positive, but also negative, effects of family involvement.

There is much in the way of research into the contention that psychosocial factors cause mental disorders, and do not just influence course and outcome for which there is no firm foundation in fact. Life events research still needs systematic analysis into stable and interactional preceding events; vulnerability research needs to be analyzed in biological, psychological and social terms and the specific factors teased out that produce vulnerability; pathogenesis needs to demonstrate how psychosocial systems upset cerebral systems and, additionally, how this produces abnormal behaviour; and finally, how individually, or in conjunction, pharmacotherapeutic and psychosocial therapeutic methods influence the latter. Taking a simple matter such as depression, multivariate statistics has as yet been unable to define the types of syndrome which would best be treated by particular antidepressant drugs.

SERVICE ORGANIZATION

As indicated already, there has been a movement away from long-term incarceration of severe forms of mental disorders to shorter stay, with improved pharmacological and social therapy, enhanced physical environment, increased staffing, greater freedom and more individualized treatment regimes. Coincidentally, there has been growing psychiatric involvement in a wider range of human problems through a spread of community facilities. The contention that these innovations have reduced the cost of patient management overall has not yet been validated. More refined definitions of the specific and non-specific ingredients of each program, and their relationship to optimal functioning, need to be produced and evaluated. Comparative studies are needed on patients with relatively acute disorders, utilizing particular facilities and subjected to different therapy regimes.

There is little doubt that pharmacological and psychosocial improvements in the treatment of psychiatric patients has produced great benefits but there are still negatives in the current scene which require attention. The question still needs to be asked: "have we reduced chronicity?"

Patterns of utilization of particular facilities need to be evaluated on a regular basis, in terms of such factors as community and patient attitudes and legislative provisions. Different social and cultural groups have been shown to vary in the way they use different types of facility, and, in many cases, ignore medical practitioners in favour of non-medical healers. It is necessary to research more definitely into the current extrusion of chronic patients into the community, with a not inconsiderable dumping of such patients in prisons, vagrant hostels, sleazy hotels, or compelling them to "live free".

The trend towards short-term residential care has been based on prevention of chronicity. The establishment of patterns of triage (3–21 days), short-term care and long-term stay (up to six months) in acute psychiatric hospital units, with active patterns of milieu and individual treatment, and continuity of the multidisciplinary professional team in follow-up is seen as desirable. The encouragement of family support and work experience are also seen as necessary accompaniments. Yet, withal, are we preventing chronicity in a condition such as schizophrenia? Are we over-capitalizing on resources which are of unproven value? We still have to find the answers to these questions, if at all possible. But the process must be an arduous one in view of the large number of variables involved and the difficulty of making individually meaningful what are biopsychosocial complexes. We have yet to determine how far hospital care can be eliminated and patients maintained through a supportive social network in the community, with special professional consultation for crisis situations. One still has to research into how one can adequately define dangerousness (harm to self or to others) and prognosticate on this basis in terms of placement in the home, in open ward, or in closed facility.

The process of evaluation of a particular therapeutic centre requires firstly that data collection take place so that hypotheses be constructed from analysis of the data: e.g., type of persons involved, sociodemographic groupings, value systems, neighbourhood supports, and patterns of illness in particular groups. On such a basis, programs can be planned, meaningful questions can be asked, and applied research programs can be directed to management and outcome. This process can take up to three years, after which, more theoretical inputs for research might be meaningfully formulated. The data collection is useful in providing a sampling frame for random sampling of sub-groups and, if definable in terms of statistical census areas, can be more widely generalized. Such a program has been in operation for the entire State of Victoria, Australia, since 1961 (Pop: 3,600,00 currently) and its case register and regular annual analysis of data is still ongoing.

DEVELOPING AREAS

The majority of persons in developing areas will tend to seek out the aid of a traditional healer before considering western psychiatry and this applies to literate as well as illiterate citizens. With increasing urbanization, education, and upward socio-economic mobility, the practice is diminishing in the latter. Access to traditional healers is also a factor since medical practitioners are in short supply. In a few areas, western practices are juxtaposed on traditional treatment, and the two work in conjunction. Research needs to be undertaken in each area to see how the best elements of both can be incorporated within a range of psychiatric services, developing an ideological orientation which will be relevant to the sociocultural context of the population and provide for effective rehabilitation. It has already been postulated that schizophrenics in developing areas are less likely than their counterparts in western countries to suffer long-term impoverishment of personality. Social factors would necessarily be important and should be thoroughly teased out to the advantage of Western psychiatry.

Full support needs to be given to the training of native-born psychiatrists operating within their own sociocultural system and developing theoretical structures appropriate to the life views inherent in the community within which they reside. The establishment of services, involving local communities and relatives, such as the Aro Mental Hospital community villages project in Nigeria, indicates how, at certain stages of community development, certain patterns of organization are viable. Comparative studies of such projects need to be compared and adequate criteria determined for evaluating them as a preliminary to such comparison. In actual fact, developing countries have a wide range of healing services. With progressive urbanization and sophistication, western-type practices are utilized to greater degree, but there is a vast migratory population from rural into urban areas which invites research as to the effect of social influences on the production of mental disorder. It is essential, in such studies, not to operate through a negative bias but objectively estimate positive growth as well as the development of pathology.

CONCLUSION

The author has been privileged to found and be associated with the Victorian Mental Health Research Institute in Australia covering a State population of 3,500,000. The results of 25 years of research indicate a primary focus as the analysis of data concerning the intake of a wide range of psychiatric disorders of varying severity, from community treatment to long-term mental hospitalization. This data has been supplemented by community surveys which have related this data to the existence of psychiatric problems in the community-at-large and facilitated the delineation of groups-at-risk. The next phase was the study of social and familial factors relating to mental illnesses and specific studies of psychosocial disorders. Associated research has been concerned with assessing the perceptions of patients and the attitudes of the community in determining their influence on behavioural aspects of such illnesses. The latest stage has been the development of methodology for the evaluation of psychiatric facilities and their programs.

It is essential, in my view, to avoid institutionalization of mental health institutions and practices and, above all, to avoid over-professionalization. In this latter regard, the developing areas may be of significant value to what may prove to be "over-developed", or skewed organization of psychiatric services in developed areas.

Faculty: Dr. Alan Stoller (Australia)
Chairperson: Dr. Kusumanto Setyonegoro (Indonesia)

CORAZON JULIANO-AGRAVA and LOREN AMOR

YOUTH WORKSHOP: FOR THE YOUTH BY THE YOUTH

The youth of today, possess vision and ideals for the future. They also possess the character and mental health to enable them to meet the problems that beset their environment. They have a commitment to make the future brighter.

However, in consideration of the problems that affect some sectors of the youth, the following recommendations are presented:

(1) Creation of youth development centres at the community level to extend services for the enrichment of youth in the search for identity. Among the activities and services which such centres should provide are the following: a forum for parent-child encounters; a centre for information dissemination on available services to understand and to help the adolescent who encounters a crisis; a base for crisis-intervention such as the provision of telephone or personalized counselling; and a network to follow up on such encounters, and to conduct further activities in meeting problems of youth and disseminating relevant information to the community.

(2) Encouragement of a love of work to instill a sense of responsibility among the youth by: providing work-related activities in early childhood; promoting apprenticeship programs for youth; and conducting more career-development programs for youth, especially for those in high school and for the out-of-school.

(3) Provision of more scholarships from both private and public sectors for needy and other deserving students.

(4) Provision of more rehabilitation programs for youths in trouble with the law, with a more person-centred approach that emphasizes respect for human dignity.

(5) Provision of services to the youth who go to the cities to study or work. These should include housing facilities and transportation.

(6) Creation of a civic-action body that will help monitor television programs and advertisements, and enable parents to exercise more supervision of T.V. programs available to the youth.

(7) Encouragement of more spiritual retreats and related activities.

(8) Development of a plan of action for participation of youth in government programs that directly or indirectly affect the youth.

(9) Urging of governments to promote family programs with emphasis on moral values.

(10) Urging of governments to consider the above recommendations from the youth participants to the World Congress on Mental Health.

Richard C. Nann, Dorcas Susan Butt, and Lourdes Ladrido-Ignacio (eds.), Mental Health, Cultural Values and Social Development, 246–247.

Chairman: Justice Corazon Juliano Agrava (Philippines)
Co-Chairman: Dr. Cornelio Banaag (Philippines)
Co-ordinator: Dr. Odita D. Yatco (Philippines)
Facilitator: Ms. Loren Amor (Philippines)
Participants: Marcy Rohn (Canada); Alexandra Guest (Canada); Marissa E. Estuaria (Philippines); Liza E. Lagdameo (Philippines); Josephine M. Cristobal (Philippines); Faith Lilyvic R. Canoy (Philippines); B. Dave Feliciano (Philippines); Blesilda D. Tan (Philippines); Ferbian T. Penaflor (Philippines); Mary Jocelyn F. Somera (Philippines); Erlinda R. Nale (Philippines); Victoria M. Aspiras (Philippines); Raquel Fausta O. Cordero (Philippines); Nanette Vina Amor A. Melosantos (Philippines); Virma D. Gutierrez (Philippines); Shirley L. Panganiban (Philippines); Ignacio C. O. Sison (Philippines); Shelah Hozel I. Navarro (Philippines); Aurora P. Bersamira (Philippines); Laurel Johnston (Canada); Flora May Pinto (Philippines); Joyalita Tajonema (Philippines); Lorelie B. Sanchez (Philippines); Deanna Angeli B. Jison (Philippines); Danny G. Yap (Philippines); Miriam B. Villarmenta (Philippines); Romualdo Mescua (Philippines); Gemma Panganiban (Philippines); Cecilia I. Robang (Philippines); Estrellita A. Nillo (Philippines); Armina Amatong (Philippines); Zinia G. Cruz (Philippines); Maichie B. Acantilio (Philippines); Cecile R. Borja (Philippines); Christine Mary Dingcong (Philippines); Esther Anor (Philippines); Carmen Aramburo (Philippines); Brendan/Vincent/David Beiser (Canada); Rosita Diago (Philippines); Minerva Felipe (Philippines); Ruby Reyna Chan (Philippines); Noli Laforteza (Philippines); Jules Estacion (Philippines); Noe Esguerra (Philippines); Margarito Hernandez (Philippines); Imelda Lim (Philippines); Cristia Manangsang (Philippines); Amanda Ricks (Canada); Leo Ciriaco B. Viajar (Philippines); Rolando San Miguel (Philippines)

THE AGE OF TRANQUILIZERS

This workshop took the form of a panel discussion on the medical, sociological and legal issues relevant to psychoactive drugs; their effects on society; and the current controversies on their use and misuse. The panel comprised the following speakers: M. Klingler, M.D. (Switzerland), John Marks, M.D. (United Kingdom) and Manuel Flores Bonifacio, Ph.D. (Philippines). This summary presents a synopsis of their comments.

PROF. KLINGLER

The development of three main classes of psychotropic drugs, the neuroleptics, the antidepressants and the tranquilizers, will be described. It happens that decisive progress for all three classes took place between 1950 and 1960.

Neuroleptics

Histamine had been synthesized as a chemical curiosity in 1907. The attempt to use it as a therapeutic tool proved to be unsuccessful. However, around 1940, antihistaminics were discovered and used progressively. One of their side-effects was sedation. Following up this side-effect, Chlorpromazine, the first neuroleptic, was discovered and introduced in the fifties. It revolutionized the therapy of many psychotic patients and made it possible to release them from institutionalized therapy.

Antidepressants

Isoniazid and Iproniazid were introduced antituberculous agents at the beginning of the 1950s. A mood elevating property was soon observed in tuberculous patients. Thus was discovered the antidepressant action of monoaminooxydase inhibitors.

Nowadays, the most important antidepressive medicaments are tricyclic substances.

Tranquilizers

In the screening of an entirely new class of chemical compounds, the Benzodiazepines, their taming action in fighting animals, their anxiolytic, anticonvulsant, muscle-relaxant and sedative properties were found. Chlordiazepoxide (Librium), the first minor tranquilizer of the Benzodiazepine series, was introduced 1960.

Richard C. Nann, Dorcas Susan Butt, and Lourdes Ladrido-Ignacio (eds.), Mental Health, Cultural Values and Social Development, 248–252.

Sources for New Drugs

New drugs can be developed along four main lines:

(1) *Rational*: We know a precise physiological mechanism that goes wrong in illness and can be corrected. Examples are Insulin in Diabetes and 1-Dopa in Parkinsonism.

(2) *Tradition*: The 19th century saw the development of many alcaloids from traditional sources, for instance morphine and atropine.

(3) *Screening of New Chemical Entities*: This has given rise to the majority of the modern drug classes. Benzodiazepines are one example.

(4) *Molecular Variation of Known Drugs*: This can give rise to better prolifera-tion of individual effects of a substance. But molecular variation can also lead to entirely new fields of activity. Starting from the sedative side-effects of antihistamines the neuroleptics were developed by molecular variation, the first being Chlorpromazine. The mood elevating side-effect of antituberculous treatment gave rise to the first antidepressants. The tricyclic antidepressants have been discovered when other therapeutic objectives were pursued.

Guidance of Research

History teaches that the main roads of new drug development, synthesis and screening of new chemical classes, and molecular variation of known drugs, can rarely be guided by nosological or social objectives. Often there is a strong element of serendipity involved in these discoveries. The first step is usually an unexpected empirical finding like the mood elevation of tuberculous patients in certain treatments. This can then form a lead for systematic investigation in new fields of therapy.

DR. MARKS

The term "misuse" of drugs implies their use and inappropriate use in therapy rather than abuse within the drug 'street scene'. We are really broadly concerned with the neuroleptics, the antidepressants and the tranquilizers.

Neuroleptic drugs are now primarily used for the severely psychotic. Although there are problems with side effects, the merits of this group of drugs in therapy is not in serious dispute.

Although medical misuse of antidepressants can occur with a wrong diagnosis, it is much more common for a misdiagnosis of anxiety to be made in a case of depression. In consequence, it is clear that there is much more likely to be under-use of antidepressant drugs than overuse. Abuse of antidepressants is virtually unknown, though withdrawal reactions can occur on abrupt withdrawal.

The remaining group is that of the tranquilizers and in the light of medical and lay press comment it is important to examine these carefully. Firstly, what is their level of use, and is this level justified?

Studies reported in the earlier part of the last decade found that tranquilosedatives were used by approximately 15% of the population in any year, with benzodiaepines used by about 9%. The total use was increasing at that time, but evidence from many countries, including for example the United States, United Kingdom, Scandinavia and Czechoslovakia suggests that a peak was reached about 1975 and, since this time, the total use of the tranquilosedatives has remained level or usually fallen. Taken overall, it appears that perhaps a maximum of one in ten of the population now receives a new prescription for a tranquilosedative in any year.

Various recent studies have shown a level of significant psychiatric morbidity in the population of industrially developed countries of some 20 to 30%, of which anxiety accounts for the major share. Nor is this situation restricted to the industrially developed countries, for in a recent study in four developing countries, one of which was the Philippines, the estimated overall frequency of psychiatric morbidity was 13.9%, with the majority suffering from neurotic illness. Thus, the level of psychiatric morbidity is higher than the level of use of the tranquilosedatives, and these figures suggest under rather than over prescription. It is important, however, to determine whether the right patients are receiving treatment.

With this level of justified use, is there any misuse? The answer is undoubtedly yes. Firstly, the drugs may not be used for appropriate cases. While tranquilosedatives can reduce the anxiety component in patients with anxiety and depression, they have no effect on the depression. Indeed, with the relief of the anxiety, the depression may appear to get worse.

Moreover, there may be inappropriate use of the tranquilizers. These drugs, indeed any psychoactive drug, should not be regarded as the only form of treatment. They form one component of total therapy, and psychotherapy, help with environmental causes by psychiatric and social workers, etc., must all be regarded as vital components of the overall treatment. The best results are achieved with the appropriate use of all forms of therapy.

Thirdly, there is evidence that the drugs can be used for too long a period. Drugs should be withdrawn as soon as they are no longer required for therapeutic purposes and the current evidence suggests that at least a proportion of patients continue with their psychoactive drugs for a longer period than is necessary.

Fourthly, is there misuse of these drugs as a result of dependence? The answer to this is also yes. Dependence can occur when the drug is taken for a long period at therapeutic dose levels. Some members of the tranquilosedative group, for example barbiturates, methaqualone and perhaps some of the short-acting benzodiazepines, appear to have a higher dependence risk than do the longer acting benzodiazepines.

DR. BONIFACIO

The following comments stem from the point of view of a social scientist from a developing country, the Philippines. From this perspective, it appears difficult to respond directly to the issue of psychoactive drugs in terms of social crisis. Treating psychoactive drugs in terms of a social problem appears to be the more appropriate in a developing country.

There is no denying that psychoactive drugs have important therapeutic value in solving the various emotional problems that affect some members of a given population. With the rise of mental illness in the Philippines, the use of psychoactive drugs will be indispensable. It is because of this that we want to voice a plea for the use of judgment and caution in the administration of psychoactive drugs. Such a plea is made because the use of such drugs will not always lead to a total rehabilitation of the patient. Studies have shown that patterns of rehabilitation are generally affected by a number of non-specific factors which must be accounted for in any attempt to demonstrate the full value of psychoactive drugs. Thus, the role of non-specific factors in the administration of psychoactive drugs cannot be avoided but must be confronted directly.

It is because of the complex nature of mental illness that a thorough understanding of the various sociopsychological factors contributing to the generation of such a disease must be carefully documented. A search for the solutions to these problems is more important than the simple and direct administration of psychoactive drugs. The administration of the drug must be supplemented by a carefully designed program of social psychological therapy. In other words, the management of the patient and his social environment is totally indispensible in the treatment of mental illness.

It is in this connection that psychoactive drugs can be a social problem for the simple reason that drug administration is more convenient than overcoming the complex social psychological basis of mental illness. Unwittingly, the patient in turn may resort to continuous drug use since it generally relieves him of his problems. This is perhaps the genesis of drug dependence. Another implication of drug use is the potential depersonalization of the relationship between doctor and patient. In view of the convenience of administering drugs, the doctor may unwittingly ignore the sociopsychological sources of the problem. There is also the danger that the family of the mentally ill patient may avoid participating in the therapeutic process by encouraging the patient to take his regular dose of medicine. In other words, we must recognize that the use of psychoactive drugs can never replace the need to unravel the sociopsychological components of mental illness.

Regardless of the structural set-up of the community health program, what must be recognized and emphasized is the fact that mental illness is influenced by physical, social and psychological factors. Consequently, a more careful delineation of how these factors contribute to the generation of mental illness is in order. Such a consideration is crucial in developing countries where widespread poverty and the lack of access of many people to opportunities greatly enlarge the source of stress. The physician situated in the local communities must be fully oriented to the sources of mental illness and what drugs he or she can administer to the patient. However, we wish to reiterate that teaching the physician to administer psychoactive drugs does not remove the main responsibility of understanding the sources of the illness.

Considering the lack of adequate mental health services in many developing countries, the use of psychoactive drugs is in order. However, such drugs are not the panacea for these human problems. The active interplay of physical, social and psychological factors must always be taken into serious consideration in any form of therapeutic encounters.

SECTION THREE

THE PRE-CONGRESS INTERNATIONAL SEMINAR
ON
THE DISABLED AND MENTAL HEALTH

INTRODUCTION

In observance of The International Year of Disabled Persons, the 1981 World Congress on Mental Health included a special Pre-Congress International Seminar on "The Disabled and Mental Health". This seminar was sponsored by the following four organizations: The Philippine Foundation of Disabled, Inc., Rehabilitation International, The Philippine Mental Health Association, and The World Federation for Mental Health.

The seminar met on July 24–26 at The Development Academy of the Philippines in Tagaytay City, Cavite, Philippines. In addition to presentations from key-note speakers, two panel discussions highlighted this seminar. The first focussed on the theme, "Coping With My Disability", with presentations from four speakers. The second concerned the theme, "Attitudes Towards Disabled Persons", with presentations from an expert in the field of Special Recreation, a service provider, an architect consultant, and the mother of a disabled child.

Richard C. Nann, Dorcas Susan Butt, and Lourdes Ladrido-Ignacio (eds.), Mental Health, Cultural Values and Social Development, 255.

LIST OF PARTICIPANTS

CANADA
Gowan Guest

FRANCE
Dr. and Mrs. Roger Amiel

GUAM
Del Basa
Adelaida P. Bellin
Lourdes Bitanga
Kim Bottcher
Michael F. Caldwell, Ph.D.
Lourdes Camacho
Rosalia T. Castillo
Marilyn Chargualat
Tom Guest
Lrrain Horton
George Kallingal, Ph.D.
Maria D. Leon-Guerrero
Fidela F. Limtiaco
Pacita Mangulabnan
Pete M. Marcial, Rev.
Irene Moody
Louis Reyes
Albert San Agustin
Claire Virata
Leonisa Untalan

HONG KONG
Lina Yuk-Shui Wong
Tse Tsun-Him

INDIA
Anil Bhuson Dutt, Dr.

JAPAN
Kunihiko Asai, M.D.
Yoshiro Asai
Sanjo Bunai
Mine Ito
Midori Kawazu
Setsuko Matayoshi
Tomohiko Matsushima, M.D.
Masao Matsushita, M.D.
Eiko Miyata, M.D.
Koichei Naka
Nobuo Namikoshi
Tadao Ryuchi
Shozo Shimada
Yoshitomo Takahashi, M.D.
Mariko Uehara

MALAYSIA
Edward Durin
Catherine McDonald
Kumaresa Al Orme
Dipu Sarbadhikary

NEW ZEALAND
Gay Alexander
Nick Higginbotham, Ph.D.

NORTH MARIANAS
Manuel Villagomez

PAKISTAN
Mohammed R. Chaudhry, M.D.

PHILIPPINES
Mercedes Adorio
Belen Almonte
Miguel Balbin, Sr.
Trinidad Baldo
Diwata A. Baluyut
Julita C. Benedicto
Purita Cajuiat

Richard C. Nann, Dorcas Susan Butt, and Lourdes Ladrido-Ignacio (eds.), Mental Health, Cultural Values and Social Development, 257–258.

Felicula Castaneda
Aurora G. Corpuz
Orisonia Datuin, M.D.
Nenita Davadilla
Danilo Delfin
Rodrigo Esguerra
Elmer Estrella
Rachel E. Fidelino, Atty.
Abner Fronteras
Ligaya Gamez
Aida Gonzales
Rebecca Jacinto, M.D.
Erlinda Lolarga, Ph.D.
Arcadio Lozada, Gen.
Leonida Mariano, M.D.
Azelvita Navarro
Joselina Noda
Marcelo Ordoñez
Dolores Ramos
Sylvia Reyes
Carmen B. Seña, M.D.
Aurora T. Tiu, M.D.
Carina A. Valle
Narcisco Varona
Natividad Yasay

STATES OF MICRONESIA
Godaro Lorrin
Nory Onietam

TAIWAN
Robert Ronald, Rev. Fr.

UNITED KINGDOM
Kenneth Bayes, Arch.

U.S.A.
Richard Hunter
John A. Nesbitt, Ed.D.
Chester M. Pierce, M.D.

ORGANIZING COMMITTEE
Charlotte A. Floro, Prof.: President, Philippine Foundation for the Rehabilitation of the Disabled, Inc.; Rehabilitation International Vice President for Asia and the Pacific.
Eleanor T. Elequin, Ph.D.
Olga Ruiz de Arana, Dr.: Psychologist Consultant, Philippine Mental Health Association.
Curie C. Rubio, Community Development Co-ordinator.
Grace Cabanos: Chief Psychologist, National Mental Hospital.

Mr. S. D. GOKHALE

THE DISABLED AND THE THIRD WORLD

BACKGROUND

Handicaps, whether of body or mind, sometimes result from accidents, but they are often the consequence of failings – war, hunger, disease – of the societies in which we live. The victims emerge bearing the stamp of a profound difference from their fellow, a difference which too many people believe to be irremediable. Thus, in both the industrialized and the developing countries, the handicapped find themselves under sentence of exclusion from society. Our laws and, more generally, our everyday life, even in its simplest acts, seem to overlook the very existence of the handicapped. The fact that they are in many cases shut up in special institutions, kept dependent on assistance and cut off from the rest of the community perpetuates society's ignorance of their real needs and aspirations. Yet they ask for nothing more than the means of joining in the various aspects of social life and, as a corollary, for society to fully accept their participation.

The satisfaction of this legitimate demand requires, however, a two-fold line of approach. It is necessary to mobilize all the material, scientific and human resources needed not only to prevent peri-natal accidents and to cure the disabilities of the handicapped, but also to enable them to take their share of responsibilities and enjoy their rights on an equal footing with all members of society. Such is the objective of rehabilitation, whose primary aim it must be to ensure their social integration.

THE PROBLEM

Disability is among the major causes of dependency and deprivations in most nations. The resulting losses are expressed in increasing measures and all this adversely affects the labour market. With prolonged disability, families often are broken up; welfare costs are increased; essential skills are lost to agriculture and industry; and, in this vicious circle, purchasing power and tax revenues are reduced. In human terms, the cost is even greater in the loss of pride and self-respect. Millions of disabled people in the world are not living normal productive lives because of neglected disability.

WHAT IS A HANDICAP?

Impairments: Concerned with abnormalities of body structure and appearance and with organ or system function, resulting from any cause; in principle, impairments represent disturbances at the organ level.

Richard C. Nann, Dorcas Susan Butt, and Lourdes Ladrido-Ignacio (eds.), Mental Health, Cultural Values and Social Development, 259–271.

Disabilities: Reflecting the consequences of impairments in terms of functional performance and activity by the individual; disabilities thus represent disturbances at the level of the person.

Handicaps: Concerned with the disadvantage experienced by the individual as a result of impairments and disabilities; handicaps thus reflect interaction with the adaptation to the individual's surroundings.

MAGNITUDE

It is estimated that about 450 million people – roughly 10% of the world's population – suffer from some form of physical, sensory or mental handicap. The figure may be even higher – around 13% – according to recent estimates by the World Health Organization (WHO). Still more serious is the fact that the problem, seen in both quantitative and qualitative terms, shows no signs of diminishing.

A survey conducted in 1968 by Rehabilitation International, an international agency with 105 member organizations, which serves disabled persons in 65 countries, produced the now familiar estimates that there were some 450 million people in the world with significant disabilities, and that the number was increasing by approximately three million per year. Subsequent calculations substantiate that the total is probably in the range of the original estimate. If the increase has been at the rate estimated, then the total today is nearly 500 million.

This is also true of the blind, orthopaedically disabled, leprosy affected and disadvantaged.

RIGHTS OF THE DISABLED

At the XIXth session of the UN General Assembly in 1975, the Declaration on the Rights of Disabled Persons was adopted, which proclaimed that the "disabled persons have the inherent right to respect for their human dignity", they "have the same civil and political rights as other human beings", they "have the rights to economic and social security and to a decent level of living . . . , to secure and retain employment or to engage in a useful, productive and remunerative occupation and to join all trade unions". It adds that "disabled persons shall be protected against all exploitation, all regulations, and all treatment of a discriminatory, abusive or degrading nature".

The movement towards Rehabilitation of the Disabled arises out of the understanding that the handicapped person is an individual with full human rights, entitled to receive from his country every possible measure of protection, assistance and opportunity for rehabilitation. With opportunities for development, the disabled person can become an economic asset to the country instead of being a burden on the State. It is an important consideration that the handicapped person can best be rehabilitated by achieving economic and social independence within the community, and not by being segregated in an institution, spending his life in a sheltered environment as an economic burden and a social parasite.

GOALS OF REHABILITATION

Rehabilitation has two goals:

(1) To provide every person with services aimed at preventing the appearance of possible disabling conditions and to give all necessary treatment to lighten any disability, to develop the patient's remaining abilities to the highest possible level.

(2) To provide society with a means of regaining the disabled person's economic contribution and/or reducing the cost of institutional care, sickness benefits, disability pensions, etc.

It is important to realize that rehabilitation does not only arise out of mere humanitarian goals, but also has significant economic benefits, arising out of efforts to enable the disabled to maximize his potentials for leading an independent life.

WHAT CAN BE DONE

A great deal can be done in terms of legislation, assistance, education, employment and prevention. There is much to learn from the experience of other countries through exchange of information and findings. If we are to be aware of the problem, we must be informed about it, and if we are to become involved, we must be aware.

The year 1981 must usher in an era in which increased concern is shown for all disabled persons and in which national and international endeavours are co-ordinated. How can this be done? At the national level: (1) through the work of various associations in the creation of mobilization of effectively run scientific and public information systems; (2) through the introduction of preventive measures (such as genetic counselling, vaccination, early diagnosis, the laying down of standards in order to prevent or reduce accidents on the roads and in industry, etc.); (3) through the development of social education characterized by integration and individual approach consistent with the nature and severity of the disability; (4) through full rehabilitation and incorporation into the workforce; (5) through full participation in cultural, political, social and economic life; and lastly, (6) through the dismantling of architectural or social barriers.

As the United Nations representative of IYDP has said,

> A handicap is not simply the corollary of a disability, it is also in part imposed by society. Furthermore, the definition of a handicap varies according to a country's culture, traditions and level of development. In a rich country a blind person can, for example, obtain a

complete education giving access to a profession, whereas in most developing countries he or she may not have access to education, such a person would be handicapped not only by a disability, but by an additional handicap imposed by the social and economic conditions. One of the major objectives of the IYDP is to encourage governments to eliminate progressively all such forms of handicap, of which disabled persons are the victims.

CATEGORIES AND PROBLEMS

No amount of straining the imagination can adequately convey to persons of normal hearing what it feels like to be deaf from birth or in early childhood. Deafness deprives an individual of the ability to enjoy, not only music, but even more important, environmental sounds such as those made by singing birds, rustling wind, croaking frogs and running streams. Great as these deprivations are, they are nothing compared to language retardation, which early profound deafness imposes upon its victim. Edna Lavine, a notable psychologist who had studied extensively the problems of deafness, once lamented: "Not to hear the voice is not to hear spoken language. Not to hear spoken language means that the child remains in complete ignorance of this basic verbal tool for human communication."

Social factors are related to the occurrence of mental illness in a number of ways. It often happens that social events or conditions are largely responsible for precipitating a mental illness, while social conditions may combine with psychological or biological factors to predispose an individual to illness. Social factors can also influence the course and outcome of a mental illness, since the effectiveness of treatment will depend largely on the social context in which it is provided. Moreover, cultural attitudes and beliefs also play a part in defining who in a society is to be labelled mentally ill, in the process by which a person is recognized as needing treatment.

THE DEVELOPING COUNTRIES

It is a sad fact that in the developing countries, a majority of the disabilities are preventable, and are generally related to poverty, disease, malnutrition and ignorance. Most of the population in these countries is rural, agrarian-based. Poor sanitary standards, crowding and insufficient resources for medical prevention and care result in a high prevalence of infections and diseases, leading to physical or mental impairment and disability. Particularly, in the remote areas, even basic services such as clean drinking water facilities are unavailable.

In the developing countries, less than 20% of the population constitutes the work force that actively contributes to the economy by production of goods and services. The majority of people live on subsistence economics, agriculture being the chief occupation. It is alarming to know that a very large number of people, even up to 50 percent of the population in some countries, live below the poverty line, where even their basic needs in terms of sheer calorie requirements remain unmet.

A major portion of the work force is unorganized, including farmers with small land holdings, landless labourers, village artisans and craftsmen, and in the cities, the large shifting population of migrant labourers, construction workers, domestic servants, and so on. These workers are not covered by any legislation, social security, or statutory protection, and consequently, along with their families, are very vulnerable. Usually in such cases, diseases and disabilities directly result in rehabilitation.

In developing countries, rehabilitation services should be closely related or attuned to the total environment of the disabled person. An appliance is only a tool to restore a lost function, it is not the function itself. For the appliance to serve truly as a function, much depends on the social values and social relationships surrounding the disabled person. It must be assessed to what extent this physical redress will prejudice or hamper the assimilation process of the disabled individual. Hence, there is a need for application of appropriate technology to rehabilitation in the rural setting. Rehabilitation efforts in the rural sector are grossly prejudiced, not only by a simple arithmetical lack of adequate detection prevention and treatment services, but also by insufficient appreciation of the need to treat functionality and its restoration in a societal rather than a purely physical context.

Another essential perspective when considering rehabilitation in the rural sector is that the core disability problem manifested in rural areas is vastly different from that prevailing in urban areas. Road and industrial accidents, environmental hazards, etc. may create a different disability syndrome than domestic fires, farming accidents, ill-informed use of agro-chemicals, etc. The virtual absence of timely medical aid at the time of birth, during the early years, at the time of unforeseen accidents during old age, etc. creates another set of disability-leading variables that are peculiar to the rural situation.

Since the causative syndrome of rural disability is different, it naturally calls for specialized approaches in rehabilitation covering all its basic component areas with regard to prevention, detection, diagnosis correction, restoration, and socio-economic rehabilitation.

CAUSATION

In the world's industrially developed countries, the scale of the disability situation is just the same as in the developing world, but the nature of the problem is different. There is no trachome, no anchocerciasis, no severe quantitative malnutrition, but alcoholism and drug addiction are on the increase, and road accidents and accidents at work – those characteristic features of industrial society – are claiming a rising toll of victims.

It is estimated that some 40 million persons are handicapped as a result of alcohol or drug abuse. In 14 of the 16 countries where WHO has carried out surveys, over two percent of the population are alcoholics. It should be noted that alcoholism is a cause of many psychiatric disorders, as well as accidents on the roads and at work.

Cardiovascular and cerebrovascular illnesses, which have major disabling effects, are particularly widespread among those who live the hectic pace of the industrially developed world.

The various afflictions resulting from peri-natal accidents (some 110 million births take place each year) are found in all countries, but they are most prevalent in the developing world. This is not only because of insufficient medical attention during pregnancy and confinement but because some 75% of all births take place in the developing countries where peri-natal risk is higher.

Nutrition during pregnancy and the first months of life is vitally important, yet some 800 million persons today go hungry and 800 more suffer from dietary deficiencies. In 1978, at least 20 million children under five perished because they were deprived of the minimum conditions necessary for survival.

COMPONENTS OF PLANNING

It is evident that in rehabilitation planning for the rural sector, this evolutionary process transforming rehabilitation from an individual 'aid' to a community 'service' must be hastened since that is the principal way in which to overcome the gap created by absence of even minimal conventional service.

A sequel component to the above would be to ensure adequate intersectoral (both cross sectoral and intra-sectoral) linkages. The useful linkages, for instance as have been drawn between paediatric and public health, between health and nutrition, between all these and education are not yet reflected in rehabilitation. Nor are preventive and public education elements given appropriate attention as complementaries to rehabilitation.

Only the broadest possible approach that meaningfully reflects such reinforcing links would be helpful in putting the limited service resources available to a developing country to optimum use. It would also enable disability to be treated in its totality rather than in isolation.

A third component would be to redress the present imbalance between rural-dominated need and urban-dominated service. This means reversal of priorities not only in planning and budgeting, but also in the evolution of the service itself. At present, the phenomenon common to all social sectors is that there is a wide gap between the two ends of the service spectrum. In the cities and metropolitan areas, the very best and costliest facilities exist for rendering care. At the other end are remote rural and tribal areas, or other backward regions where the service is either non-existent or terribly sparse. In the middle somewhere are the rural and peri-urban areas, as well as the urban slum-dwelling population for whom a skeleton service operates, which is generally free of heavy subsidies but, on account mainly of over crowding and insufficient resources, is highly unsatisfactory.

While such service imbalances can be contended with by the normal population, for the disabled who have difficulties in commuting, gaining access to distant services, it is virtually impossible. In their case, the adage of 'reaching the service to the people' becomes much more than a slogan. It becomes an unavoidable need. This is also a component that distinguishes rural rehabilitation planning from planning in any other sector. In further amplification of this distinction, I would like to recall a quote from Karl Marx, which he made while comparing two revolutions:

There, the phrase went beyond the content;
Here, the content goes beyond the phrase.[1]

HOW TO REACH THE LOWEST OF THE LOW

Even when rehabilitation programs are in operation, as they are in many cities in the developing countries, their services rarely reach the residents of the rural areas and the urban slums.

The implications of this combination of disability and poverty are dreadful and tragic. We have not come to grips with the interactions between these two forces – the frequency with which untreated impairment starts or accelerates the collapse of a family's already fragile economic base, the degree to which social and economic deprivation are fundamental causes of impairment, and of the isolation of impairment into permanent disability.

We are finding that, when programs to assist the development of the community are planned, the benefits go lastly and least to those families that are burdened with both poverty and disability. Many a time it is observed that governments are happy to establish a service, but are not always careful to see that the service reaches the doorsteps of the poor disabled.

ATTITUDES AND STIGMA

Within the family, it is too often the child with the impairment who is denied the chance for education and intellectual stimulation. Attitudes and patterns of individual and social behaviour that are themselves important causes of disability and of handicapped lives in the developing countries. These social forces are not unique to developing areas; they are well-known in every part of the world. When, because of the functional limitation associated with an impairment or because of the stigmatization of the disabled person, he or she is not permitted to grow and fulfill the traditional role, the individual is very likely to become a non-person, an outcast without value to self, to the family or to the community.

THE ASIAN SCENE

In the last 20 years there has been, all over Asia, a fresh and dynamic awareness of the rights of handicapped people. New laws have been passed and new institutions created to make it possible to restore to handicapped people their inherent right to a self-respecting, independent life. Some of the countries, like Malaysia, have had traditions in social welfare which had either to be modernized or supplemented by scientific-modern methods. The catalytic agent in many of the countries of this region has been either war (Korea, India, Bangladesh, Japan) or a ravaging epidemic (Indonesia, Micronesia). But, from that point on, the countries concerned have moved ahead, expanding services so as to offer the facility of rehabilitation to many types of disabilities.

Almost in every country in the Asian region – and this is true of western countries also – it is the volunteer, social welfare workers who have been the first to become aware of the needs of deprived people in society. Later, slowly, the official agencies and government departments have entered the picture to give financial, legislative and structural support to the work begun by the volunteers and to promote new ways and means of improving and extending services. Perhaps, because of the political and economic conditions in the whole region, many of the countries of Asia have relegated to second place handicaps such as mental retardation, deafness or dumbness and concentrated on the orthopaedically handicapped or the blind, which are more visible.

REHABILITATION MODEL

The rehabilitation model that has dominated the scene, both in the industrialized West and in our international assistance activity, has three working parts: fancy buildings, elaborate equipment and highly specialized professional personnel. We have evolved standards for each of these components in the most sophisticated setting with unlimited research and development funds, and have cloaked these standards in an aura so sacred that we in the developing world are led to believe that anything different is unacceptable.

Our emphasis has been on services that the professional will give to the disabled person and, to a lesser extent, to the family. Initially, because the fashions of our epoch have led us to believe that we can solve anything by an operation, a pill, a pad, an exercise, or a diet, we have projected rehabilitation as an essentially medical exercise. Educational and vocational rehabilitation have been close behind and, in the cities of developing countries, the numbers of centres specializing in the medical rehabilitation of a few people are followed closely by other centres dealing in what is called special education, vocational training and sheltered employment, but which too often carry out primarily custodial functions.

In developing countries, virtually all the techniques used for rehabilitation are either copies of, or derived from, techniques in use in developed countries. While they deal in the main with essentially similar problems, in a village setting some of them may be unsuitable unless they are altered to fit rural needs. Limited work has been done along these lines in some countries.

While it is possible to design simple aids and appliances for the disabled, there is always a need for repairs or replacement, facilities which exist in mainly urban centres. The use of specialized equipment is an even more difficult proposition.

Beyond this basic and possibly most important motivation for action is the fact that no society, developed or developing, can carry forever the burden of an unproductive, impoverished section of its population – or, to put it differently – society as a whole stands to benefit economically and socially if the disabled are educated and trained and fully integrated into the social and economic life of the community.

The different aspects of the rehabilitation of the disabled leads me to a particular concern I should like to share with you. In rehabilitation efforts that have been made so far, the tendency has been to isolate the disabled: special institutions, special classes for children and special places of work – the techniques and rehabilitation methods used have taken them away from the community and its activities. Added to this is the expression of attitudes in our day-to-day living which are based on the assumption that the disabled do not exist: public transport, public facilities, shopping centres, roads, pedestrian crossings and so on have been so designed that they succeed in preventing the disabled from using them or at least in making them difficult for the disabled to use. This kind of prejudice cannot be eradicated in a day, or by government decree alone. It has to be worn away from within, and this change can be effected only if the community is exposed to well-planned publicity and information campaigns using all the media as well as person-to-person contacts.

Particularly in developing countries, prevention programs are a crucial part of any general health program and, again, this is an area where intervention programs have not succeeded in covering the population fully. A good deal of excellent work has been done with the help of United Nations specialized agencies and non-governmental organizations, but the aim surely must be to make prevention programs reach out to the inaccessible areas of each country and to population groups who have not yet been covered. Funds represents a major constraint; personnel another. Yet inadequate action here has its own cost, which society will have to bear, in some form or other.

International co-operation and assistance has produced some islands of excellence – centres, schools and programs that are functioning as well as the models from which they have been derived. But the totality of existing services reach at best a few thousand people in these areas. We may therefore question whether the concepts of rehabilitation services which have evolved in the industrialized West are necessarily appropriate for areas with quite different economic and social situations. What we need is to evolve rehabilitation services to suit local conditions.

It has been the western model and practice, to lift both the problem and the person with the problem out of the social context in which they exist and to attempt to find a solution in a new context. We have only slowly learned that a person with a disability is also a person with a lot of other things: with a family, with tradition, with tastes and appetites, with fears and apprehensions, with pride and ambition, and with a culture through which these elements are integrated. Therefore, to uproot a disabled person from his family context, to live in an institution, is likely to endanger his future.

WHAT CAN WE DO?

What can the community really do for the disabled? The two basic issues are to understand the disabled and to accept them as equal partners in society. The disabled persons do not want pity and charity. They want equal opportunity.

Whenever services are organized by the service club or by government, these services very often reek of patronage and charity. I think the community could do well to see that, at no stage, are disabled persons humiliated by this kind of patronage. As an action plan, the community could really concentrate on the following services:

(1) To overcome the physical *barriers* for the disabled in public utilities such as theatres, banks, temples. The service clubs could undertake to provide a private ramp in addition to steps so that a person in a wheelchair could have access to the building.

(2) Every disabled child has a right to education. The community should develop a movement of integrated education so that the blind, deaf and orthopaedically handicapped could join the mainstream of education. To do this, we may have to persuade the schools and, if necessary, provide for a special remedial teacher. We may also have to provide for the cost of education of some of these disabled children.

These children need support in terms of health, education and welfare and one of the best programs is to sponsor a child. Sponsorship does not mean doling out of money. It means creating a bond of affection between sponsor and child. The Community Aid and Sponsorship Program has so far sponsored over 7,500 children and the community could provide generous and massive support to the campaign. The Prime Minister of India has supported this program along with the Government of India and Government of Mahsrashtra. Private institutions, industries, banks and service clubs could surely participate in this project.

(3) To assist orthopaedically handicapped children, rural camps should be organized for the disabled, where the nature and extent of disability could be identified and appropriate *referral services* for treatment offered. These camps are not very costly. If service clubs could sponsor one camp at the cost of Rs. 5000/ – every once in a quarter, it would make a major contribution.

(4) Service clubs could also undertake to develop a bank of *artificial aids and appliances*, as well as aids to daily living. It is a fact that, in many cases, artificial limbs have to be tailor-made, but some of the appliances could be standardized. The bank of this kind is not a very costly project but,

with the help of industries, it may be possible for service clubs to organize such a bank.

(5) *Recreation* and leisure is one of the basic needs of a healthy life. To organize Sunday recreation for the disabled, such as taking them on a picnic or to a beach, taking them for a film show, providing them with toys, libraries or libraries of talking books for the blind, even a simple story-telling session could be organized. There are professional story-tellers and their services could be utilized.

(6) The disabled are not only the young. *Senior citizens* or people above 60 years also become disabled for one reason or the other. Because of adjustment problems; some of them become kind of a parasite in family structure. To provide daycare centres for the elderly disabled could be one of the activities of a futuristic nature. The Indian family is still strong as an institution. However, this problem is appearing in urban areas and, therefore, it is necessary that such projects for the disabled elderly are undertaken by service clubs, especially in view of the International Convention on Aging in 1982.

THE AREA OF ACTION

The population of countries within the ESCAP region was estimated to be more than 2,289 million in 1978, of whom over 70% lived in rural areas.[2] While accurate data on the disabled among them are not available, a report, "Childhood Disability: Its prevention and rehabilitation" prepared by Rehabilitation International for UNICEF (E/ICEF/L.1410) indicates that one child out of every ten is born with or acquires a physical, mental or sensory impairment. The information collected during the field surveys made for the report indicated that the percentage in developing countries was, if anything, higher. Most studies have shown that, in general, a tenth of the world's population is disabled in one form or another and in varying degrees.

The study made by Rehabilitation International noted some facts relevant to our purposes, among them the fact that while it is in the developing countries that most of the disabled live, little or nothing is being done to prevent either the occurrence of impairment or its damaging consequences. The need for action in this field is, admittedly, recognized by all countries; in keeping with the Declaration on the Rights of Disabled Persons (General Assembly Resolution 3447 XXX), the Declaration of the Rights of Mentally Retarded Persons (General Assembly Resolution 2856 XXVI) and Resolution 1921 (LVII) of the Economic and Social Council on the prevention of disability and rehabilitation of disabled persons, most countries have taken some steps to provide preventive and rehabilitative measures in varying degrees. Personnel are trained in some countries for specific areas of work in this field and research is also being undertaken in a number of countries in the field of prevention of disability, education, vocational training and social rehabilitation.

The main reasons for the inadequacy of services in developing countries are two: one is the general ignorance at all levels of the conditions of the disabled and the other, which stems from the first, is the very modest amount of money allocated for such services. To some extent, this is understandable. In some countries where living standards are very low and where there are a host of problems to be faced, such as scarcity of food and essential commodities, lack of irrigation and power, high prices, unemployment, etc., the allocation of resources for disability prevention and rehabilitation tends to be modest. The argument usually given by planners and administrators is that nothing more can be done – a view which is conditioned by their having to make difficult choices between competing areas of the developing spectrum.

The minute amounts earmarked in most developing countries for disability prevention and rehabilitation are unfortunately based on a lack of a true understanding of the reasons why programs for disability prevention and rehabilitation are essential in a development program. Ignorance and an almost total absence of information were found during the study made by Rehabilitation International to be not only true of illiterate villages, but also of community leaders, professional people, government officials, and international planners and administration.[3] Perhaps the greatest handicap that a disabled person has to face is the complete lack of knowledge and information among the able-bodied concerning the disabled, of their ability to learn and train and to engage in economically useful occupations. Indeed, this ignorance very often develops into prejudices and fear, and in a number of countries into superstitions, which highlight the disability and even rob the person affected by it of the attributes of a human being. In the words of Norman Action, the Secretary-General of Rehabilitation International, at a symposium on "Disability and the Developing World" held in Washington DC in September 1979 (E/ICEF/Misc.318):

" . . . there is an abysmal lack of accurate information about disability; its causes and consquences, and about what we can do about these things; and an equally appalling wealth of misinformation, prejudice, superstitution and fear. This is a major factor in the family's inadequate reaction to the problem when it arises; it is a fundamental reason for the community's ostracizing individuals and families that are affected with disability; it exists in the institutions that might be helping, but aren't – the health centre, the school, the religious groupings; it permeates all echelons of government from the village chief to the ministers of health, education, welfare, labour, and it is endemic in the representatives of international and other organizations who are advising on the procedures and priorities of development, and administering international assistance. This absence of information and understanding, and the manner in which it reinforces the traditional distorted concepts of disability which flourish throughout the world, does much to conceal the real magnitude of the problem and to confuse everyone's thinking about the solutions."

The enormity of this ignorance is so pervasive and has been so ingrained in society that it includes the disabled themselves. Born into or living within societies permeated by ignorance, prejudice, fear and superstition, a disabled person comes to look on himself as an outcast, as someone incapable of useful work, a person who must depend on charity and remain cut off from a normal social life to the end of his days. This is particularly true of those who are disabled owing to a "stigmatized" disease such as leprosy, epilepsy, etc.

NEED FOR NEW PERSPECTIVE AND STRATEGY

It was assumed in the western model that, by stimulation and assisting the establishment of showplace institutions in capital cities, we would start a percolating process that would eventually diffuse appropriate levels of services to the smaller communities. It has not happened, and we should now know that it will not happen unless there is a very hard-headed plan. The whole process is a continuum of prevention, rehabilitation and social action. These are not separate crusades, they are inter-acting components of a system whose only purpose is to support the optimum development of each individual's capacity and personality. A high priority must be given to convincing everyone who deals in policy that *disability is an important cause and consequence of under-development*, and that dealing with it must be a priority item in any intelligent development plan.

The most important asset for any program for disability prevention and rehabilitation is the family, and in most developing areas the ties and functions of the family are strong components of the social context of the individuals. Successful work at this level, by remaining within the family and the existing social framework of the individual's life, can do much to maintain normal human development, whether or not the impairment can be eliminated or reduced.

Asst. Secretary-General,
International Council on Social Welfare,
A-2, Rasadhara Co-op. Housing Society Ltd.,
385, S. V. P. Road,
Bombay-400 004, India

NOTES

1 Karl Marx, from the Eighteenth Brumaire of Lois Bonaparte, 1869.
2 "1978 demographic estimates for Asian and Pacific Countries", Population Division, ESCAP.
3 See WHO Program and Policy.

NICK HIGGINBOTHAM, Ph.D. (New Zealand)

CULTURAL SENSITIVITY OF HELPING SERVICES FOR PSYCHOLOGICALLY DISABLED IN DEVELOPING NATIONS

Human service planners are becoming sensitized to the manifold inadequacies of transporting Western biomedical systems of health care to the developing world (Benyoussef, 1977; Kleinman, 1980; WHO, 1975); Modern psychiatry's promulgation as a preferred model, with its attendant technological trappings and highly structured organizational characteristics, has particularly drawn sharp questioning in recent years (Carstairs, 1973; Higginbotham, 1976; Marsella and Higginbotham, 1979). Two issues are salient: First, is it feasible (politically, socioeconomically) for developing regions to embrace the standards of modern psychiatry in the design of mental health systems? Second, does an essentially Western model of service delivery manifest cultural sensitivity to these societies as measured by community acceptability and agency accommodation to "fit" unique cultural patterns? The author has addressed these important questions through a review of the international psychiatry literature and field research involving 200 interviews of mental workers in 45 facilities in Japan, Taiwan, and the ASEAN countries (Higginbotham 1979a, b, c).

FEASIBILITY OF DESIGNING MENTAL HEALTH CARE ACCORDING TO CRITERIA OF MODERN PSYCHIATRY

Operational criteria of modern psychiatry are achieved when a nation allocates sufficient resources to secure a system of comprehensive services, preventive programs, continuity of care within and between institutions and into the community, and accessible care. From the case analyses for Taiwan, the Philippines and Thailand (Higginbotham 1979c, pp. 111–511), it is evident that powerful forces are extant which severely limit the development of viable programs. These forces operate at the national level, involving government priorities and economics, and at the level of agency functioning. National level barriers are reported first.

BARRIERS AT THE NATIONAL LEVEL

(1) Government attention in developing nations is on agricultural growth and industrial capabilities, and the elaboration of infrastructure supporting them. Social welfare and public health matters are assigned priorities well below these main concerns. Mental health services are given lowest priority within public health administrations preoccupied with establishing health infrastructure (building hospitals, training physicians) and targeting

Richard C. Nann, Dorcas Susan Butt, and Lourdes Ladrido-Ignacio (eds.), Mental Health, Cultural Values and Social Development, 273–286.

programs for nutrition, environmental sanitation, maternal and child care, infectious disease control, etc.

(2) The absence of active national executive bodies for planning, policy making, co-ordinating, and evaluating mental health programs hinders crucial processes: (a) creation of legislation strengthening and regulating psychiatric services; (b) co-ordinating of University training with community and institutional needs; (c) recruitment and deployment of manpower; (d) planning for nation-wide coverage and integration of local with regional service units; and (e) inclusion of psychiatric intervention in government health insurance, to ease client entry and attract more qualified staff.

(3) Independent University psychiatry departments are quite rare as are parallel courses for allied professionals. Present departments educate students according to disease patterns and medical specialties appropriate to affluent societies. Graduates move in disturbing numbers to Western industrialized nations where they can take advantage of attractive economic opportunities.

(4) Overall, there remains an inadequate mapping of the incidence and prevalence of psychological impairment. Empirical documentation of community needs, characteristics of potential service users, treatment effectiveness, and the sociocultural origins of dysfunction is required to focus government attention to these concerns and guide new program creation.

(5) Of singular significance is the extreme maldistribution of resources following the dichotomy between urban and rural living conditions. Hospitals, after-care units, training and specialty programs of all descriptions, and manpower are concentrated almost exclusively in one or two urban centres approachable by city-dwelling Westernized elite. Rural people are cut off from psychiatry by barriers of geography, transportation, communication and social distance.

BARRIERS AT THE AGENCY LEVEL

(1) Individual agencies do not provide a comprehensive array of functions and treatments beyond core elements – inpatient, outpatient, diagnostics, neurological assessment. Services for special groups and alternatives to inpatient care are rare (e.g. suicide crises, substance abuse, transitional living, autism and childhood disorders). Only one or two community-level centres are available. Most agencies over-rely on drug and ECT management excluding alternative therapeutics.

(2) Preventive and indirect mental health services are given low priority because they demand additional manpower in a system overloaded with existing cases. Prevention through ecological change – redirecting harmful sociopolitical institutional practices and stress amelioration – was not deemed within the purview of any agency visited.

(3) The large residential programs could not maintain sufficient multidisciplinary staffing to allow either meaningful professional/patient contact or fluid transfer from one psychiatric team member to another based on diagnosis or changing needs. Non-medical personnel are gravely absent throughout these systems dominated by nursing and physician personnel. At provincial institutions, treatment is custodial at best. The sheer weight of outpatient contacts – sometimes numbering several thousand per month – dictates that professional contact be restricted to prescribing and monitoring drug interventions.

(4) Continuity of care between institutions, has two weak points: (a) the inadequate linkage between the mental health and public health systems; and (b) the proliferation of "dumping ground" institutions: those with multiple referral sources into them but few, if any, referral pathways leading back out into the community.

(5) Institutional action aimed at permitting smooth patient transition back into the social environment is another low priority. Manpower is deemed too precious for delivering after-care services at the home or village level nor are staff deployed to liaison with relatives in co-operative case management. Insufficient alternatives to inpatient care hinders the flow of patients from highly restrictive environments to those with minimal supervision forcing an over-reliance on institutionalization.

(6) Lastly, access is impeded because those without financial resources can neither afford to travel to these few metropolitan clinics nor pay for private care and the minimal fees for public-funded institutions. Furthermore, waiting lists and chronic overcrowding of the few respected inpatient units frustrate potential users and are nightmares to outpatients waiting long hours for brief physician consultations. Rural and low-income citizens are thus shut out from public mental health care.

Despite these overpowering restrictions, a critical mass of service units and professionals has emerged in the capital cities. Psychiatry is accessible to select urban dwellers and achieves a measure of comprehensiveness when diverse agencies function in a co-operative manner. Furthermore, historical interchange with foreign training centres and expertise from international consultants have undergirded the creation and expansion of national mental health programs. Despite the continual infusion and updating of mental health technology by international sources, the overall impact is imperceptible. These nations simply cannot allocate sufficient political, economic, educational, and manpower resources to generate a fully functioning delivery system beyond one or two metropolitan enclaves. In brief, the Western model of psychiatry cannot be lauded as even remotely feasible as a standard for nationwide mental health service delivery.

CULTURAL SENSITIVITY OF EXISTING PSYCHIATRIC SYSTEMS

The second issue addressed by the case studies concerns the interface between sociocultural context and agency operations. Succinctly stated, to what extent do programs reflect prevailing community ethos?

This next section summarizes the case study findings regarding agency acceptability and accommodation – two indices of cultural sensitivity.

EVIDENCE OF NON-ACCEPTANCE

(1) The community/agency gap is bridged through active institutional liaison with responsible persons from the patient's natural environment. Yet, there are few formal ways in which community members close to the patient are brought into the procedures for goal setting and therapy administration. Treatment planning and case management are the purview of the medical staff, especially the physician, who remains the final authority.

(2) Acceptability is also strengthened by formal avenues of agency accountability to the opinions of social leaders and service recipients. However, the concept of a community advisory board was alien to nearly all agencies. Needs assessment surveys, establishing accountability by identifying under-served users, were also absent from program priorities.

(3) In the eyes of service providers, mental institutions are disturbingly alienated and isolated from the ongoing stream of community life. They see their clinics as unknown or mostly misunderstood and stigmatizing. Psychiatry is thus reserved as a last resort when all other methods of help have failed. In short, programs are rejected by traditional-minded citizens whose beliefs and health customs are incongruent with what is offered.

INSTANCES OF COMMUNITY ACCEPTANCE

(1) Agency penetration by the community was noted at a few key points of contact involving family members. Examples were recorded of family therapy, family education seminars, and spouse counselling. Relatives were sometimes assigned the responsibility of watching for new symptoms, giving medicine, and making sure the patient returned for follow-up visits. The most significant correspondence between clinic and patient's social group occurred in Taiwanese and Philippine institutions which allowed relatives to "live in" and take part in the day-to-day management routine.

(2) Agency acceptance was not considered a problem, after the family made the commitment to bring their impaired member for help. Once surpassing this threshold, rejection of treatment approaches and disbelief in therapeutic efficacy are no longer thought to be the issues. It may be that agency contact mobilizes hope in a positive outcome, especially in light

of the trials and tribulations endured by the family prior to their seeking clinical asistance.

However, these admirable gestures at community integration cannot begin to offset the profound stigma and alienation experienced by agencies, especially with regard to provincial client populations not exposed to modern education. Stated tersely, psychiatric institutions are unacceptable to most except when all other avenues have failed and desperation reaches its climax.

CULTURAL ACCOMMODATION IN AGENCY OPERATIONS

The second index of culture sensitivity is measurable through efforts to incorporate key customs of community health behaviour into institutional environments. Staff reported five critical dimensions for culture accommodation: family role, popular conceptions of disorder, expected therapist manner, expected therapeutics, and ward activities.

KINSHIP ROLE

The pre-emininent position of Asian kinship groups in controlling the lives of individual family members is generally recognized among mental health workers. The initial point of clinic contact with the family is crucial for engendering their co-operation and respect, and halting the widening patient/family chasm which may result in abandonment to institutional care. Preliminary accommodation to gain kinship confidence was undertaken in a variety of ways: entire families were invited in for the intake interview; physicians sought to relieve unspoken fears by fully explaining treatment approaches and asking permission prior to shock therapy; quick demonstrable improvements via drugs were sought before asking family participation in rehabilitation efforts; and family attendants are allowed to live in on certain wards and offered formal staff contact in some cases.

FOLK THEORIES

Sensitivity to popular and folk theories of psychological impairment is another requirement of a culturally responsive organization. The most dominant form of accommodation to traditional concepts is non-judgmental acceptance of them. When confronted with such beliefs, it was recognized that attacking them directly would only serve to alienate the patient. One strategy was to simply ignore folk notions or gently point out the difference between traditional and "scientific" concepts. Seasoned therapists recognized that knowledge of folk nosologies and culture-bound syndromes was useful in working effectively with traditional clients. Most workers manifest a permissive attitude toward aherence to folk healing customs as long as it does not interfere with their approach to therapy. A few even permit visitation to priests or herbalists during hospitalization. At minimum, there is a general awareness that patients take a circuitous route to the hospital, arriving only after a variety of local healers and self-cures are exhausted.

WARD ACTIVITIES

Ward-level activities provide a rich arena for accommodation to the patient's social background. Linguistic matching – the assignment of patients to staff who speak the same dialect – was prevalent. Often, relatives of ill, elderly, suicidal, or unmanageable inpatients were asked to reside on the ward as "watchers" or "amahs". Bangkok's Buddhist Priest's Hospital was set up in harmony with the culture of its residents: all attendants there are male and physicians are careful to accord full respect to the holy men they treat. Recreational, occupational and vocational therapies were aimed at familiar pastimes. Occasionally practical skills are taught enabling the person to return to his family capable of making an economic contribution. Ethnic and religious minorities such as Thai Hill Tribe groups were sometimes permitted to stay together in the hospital and observe their own customs of worship and diet. Practitioners deemed it urgent to stabilize minority patients with drugs and return them quickly to their families, because hospitals were more alien to them than to other groups.

THERAPIST'S MANNER

Persons seeking clinic aid appear to hold well-defined expectations of what the therapist's manner should be in order to make them feel confident and secure. The most commonly described attribute was that of an authority figure – "fatherly", in command of the situation, and almost godlike. Yet, equally important, the authoritarian stance should be tempered with a warm, human side. He/she should allow emotional dependency, be cheerful, friendly and helpful. It was also best for the therapist to give direct, concrete advice and exude confidence that the intervention will assuredly work. In all cases, one should avoid shaming the patient and mentioning embarrassing topics until the relationship is well-established.

EXPECTED THERAPEUTICS

To an overwhelming extent, patients admitted to psychiatric clinics construe their presenting problems to doctors in somatic terms. They expect curing measures to be physical rather than psychological. The medically-oriented institutions are well-suited to accommodate to these expectations. The uniform components of hospital care are psychotropic medication, electro-convulsive shock, bed rest, and vitamin supplements. Very few receive talk therapy apart from explicit advice from the physician on how to handle specific problems. Non-medically oriented centres must sometimes provide orientation sessions to teach clients what to expect. Therapists interested in applying psychological interventions first meet their patient's medical expectations in order to build rapport and compliance before shifting to alternative strategies.

INSTANCES OF NON-ACCOMMODATION

Over 80% of those completing an attitude questionnaire positively endorsed 12 of the 16 accommodation items. Such statements as: "Staff should adjust their personal manner to fit the expectations of patients from different social backgrounds", and "staff should know the traditional names for mental disorder", were nearly unanimously agreed by the respondents. Yet, there are clear discrepancies between these apparent positive attitudes toward culture accommodation and actual practices found in or missing from clinic procedures. Below are listed five examples of non-accommodation to community customs detracting from agency cultural validity.

PATIENT RE-EDUCATION

Many staff consider it proper, even mandatory, to re-educate those patients maintaining traditional conceptions of psychopathology. Personnel strive to teach traditional-minded individuals to view their problems in psychiatric terms. Even those ethno-psychiatrists who have documented the influence of indigenous theories on symptom expression maintain that the effective psychotherapist, while accepting the patient's scheme, must reinterpret it for himself in modern concepts.

NATIVE HEALER REJECTION

Although there was solid agreement that staff should know the folk healing practices, in no instance was native healer participation sought in case management. They view native healing as a waste of finances, a delay from proper care, or even harmful: Staff ask that families stop taking their ailing member to indigenous practitioners while under psychiatric care.

SOCIAL STATUS DIFFERENCES

Even though it was clearly recognized that social differences between staff and clients was a moderate problem, there was seldom any policy that personnel be hired whose backgrounds closely matched those of service users. This problem was most acute in Thailand. Rural Thai are extremely reluctant to approach persons of the physician's status. Communication barriers arise from differences in social status and differences in education, thinking styles, and basic values between the two groups. Patients are put off by the business-like, arrogant, scolding and inattentive manner of clinic doctors. They much prefer local healers who spend a lot of time with them, explaining what has caused their illness and expressing genuine concern.

LIMITED FAMILY PARTICIPATION

As a rule, institutions prefer minimal "interference" by family members in the treatment regimen. With pressing shortages of personnel, it is simply too great a luxury in most cases to take the time to permit community members meaningful involvement. Families are invited to visit and staff do encourage their continued contact with the patient to avoid abandonment, but any treatment role relatives do play is generally circumscribed.

NEGATIVE STEREOTYPES

Lastly, mental institutions not only carry the negative connotations of custodial care – confinement places for the "mad" and hospitals from which no one returns – but are also associated with poor souls dying away from home. In Thailand, such places are filled with the wandering spirits of persons who did not have a peaceful death in their homes. These spirits themselves are looking to possess the living and cause illness.

SUMMARY

The survey of mental health resources in Taiwan, the Philippines and Thailand was intended to learn whether or not the standard of Western psychiatry is feasible as a model for service delivery among developing Asian nations. A second phase of the survey assessed the degree to which Western-derived institutions are integrated into the sociocultural milieu of their intended recipients. A guiding premise is that continuity with client culture builds agency acceptability and establishes the cultural validity of mental health programs.

On the issue of feasibility, the case study findings are unequivocal. At national or even regional levels, these countries are unable (unwilling) to allocate economic, education, administrative, research and manpower resources to secure the standards of care prescribed by contemporary criteria of psychiatry. Extant psychiatric systems, functioning in an integrated fashion, are capable of providing sufficient intervention resources to meet the needs of a circumscribed number of middle and upper class residents of these nations' capital cities.

The question of cultural sensitivity of mental hospitals and clinics is less straightforward because community attitudes were not directly assessed. Nevertheless, staff perceive their clinics as alien entities in the ongoing stream of community life. Psychiatric treatment is stigmatizing; it is unacceptable except at the last possible moment as a desperate gesture to relieve suffering. A full range of accommodation tactics were noted, but most tended to be informal and makeshift. Accommodation *per se* was not elevated to the level of policy or program objective. For example, accommodation undertaken at the initial point of agency contact was intended to win over family confidence and co-operation. Once staff secured the family's commitment to treatment, then clinic-preferred therapy modes were introduced. Traditional-minded patients were re-educated to acquire a more psychological view of their problems and appreciate the advantage of psychiatric methods.

In brief, the sites visited were culturally insensitive and isolated in relation to the healing customs and beliefs of the general population. Their range of appropriateness and accessibility was narrowly restricted to the urban elite. The following section considers in detail the implications of culturally unresponsive services and describes an approach for designing new services contiguous with cultural values and behaviour.

TOWARD AN INTEGRATION OF CULTURAL CONTEXT WITH THE DESIGN OF MENTAL HEALTH SERVICES: THE CULTURE ASSESSMENT AND ACCOMMODATION MODEL

INTRODUCTION

The implications of cultural insensitivity or discontinuity between formal helping services and sociocultural context are profound. Host culture incongruity with Western mental health technology brings impetus for sociocultural adaptation or even disintegration. Yet, the case studies found no community-level review of agency goals to help choose the direction of such change. Using psychiatry as a force of innovation raises serious ethical questions when community consent is absent.

Specifically, mismatched service technology threatens five cultural systems (see Higginbotham, 1979b for a broader accounting of these threats). First, indigenous conceptions of dysfunction and disease are replaced by psychiatric nosologies and standards of normality. Second, certain social values, life styles, and child rearing customs are judged pathological. From the psychiatric perspective, changes are demanded at the social systems level. Third, medical institutions represent unique sub-cultures, hierarchically structuring roles and relationships of their members (Kleinman, 1980). These sub-cultures undermine an intricate pattern of interpersonal relationships between the patient and significant others who seek to care for his/her needs. Fourth, fostering family and community dependency on institutional resources erodes the informal network's ability to competently cope with stressful occasions and "illness" episodes. Fifth, medical technology, under the control of the urban power elite, strengthens their positions vis-a-vis the rural peasant majority. It bolsters government efforts to impose new administrative frameworks on heretofore autonomous village units. Lastly, government sanctions against traditional medicine may actually decrease assistance for those in need. Native specialists are curative, useful in mediating social change, stress, and massively relied upon by rural and urban citizens alike. Official disapproval and suppression of folk institutions would create a psychological care vacuum since modern mental health systems maintain only token resources and still suffer the stigma of community rejection.

In short, without cultural sensitivity, institutions created according to Western strictures of organization and purpose are discontinuous with Asian patterns of psychological healing. Unless services are integrated with basic sociocultural elements, they impose social change. Change without the participation of those affected is unethical. Imposition of influential yet incongruent institutions may hasten sociocultural disintegration. This is counter to cultural adaptation, a necessary, ongoing process in the face of modernization pressure and national development.

REQUIREMENTS OF A NEW MODEL

Given the problematic status of mental health delivery in parts of Asia and the brave but fragmented attempted to "indigenize" Western therapeutics, there remains a pressing need for a unified, culture-specific approach to guide the design of helping services. This new approach must be capable of coping with the current dilemmas outlined above while offering a testable vision of how cultural sensitivity is achievable. The concept "culture accommodation" aptly satisfies these two demands. Constructing a working model of culture accommodation begins by delineating the tasks which accommodation must perform. These tasks, viewed as outcome variables or "consequences" of accommodation, are manifested at three levels:

Level 1: Structural Qualities

(1) *Low Resource Intensive*: Programs created are low budget, non-demanding of professional manpower, operative without elaborate infra-structure, and need minimal administrative functions or institutional facilities.

(2) *Enhanced Accessibility*: (i) Helping service is sited in natural gathering place easily reached on foot or by bike; (ii) System entry procedures most attractive to users are followed, especially operating hours, intake questions, cost, time delays, architecture, child care for waiting mothers, etc.

(3) *Maximum Administrative Openness*: Program is open to local community review and control of policy formulation, hiring, finances and so forth, generating a sense of community responsibility and "ownership" of services.

Level 2: Social Ecology Qualities

(1) *Enhanced Acceptability*: Helping service is non-stigmatizing, non-alienating and engenders positive attitudes among community members.

(2) *Health Network Inclusive*: The program is intimately linked with informal referral pathways used by help-seekers once "illness" management moves beyond the immediate family nexus thus promoting "psychological sense of community".

(3) *Increased Community Competency and Self-Management*: Program reinforces existing community skills and coping strategies; already available helpers are supported in case management only when necessary; the overarching aim is to secure community independence from reliance upon formal intervention.

(4) *Continuity with Prevailing Social Norms, Beliefs, and Power Relationships*: Program practices respect pluralistic life styles and philosophies – no attempt is made to disrupt or modify the unique explanations of disorder, learning styles, standards of community adjustment, beliefs regarding efficacious curing techniques, etc.

Level 3: Healing/Helping Qualities

(1) *Reducing Community Stressers*: Helping service has far-reaching effects when it supports community social action efforts to remove community identified sources of distress, including unemployment, discrimination, unresponsive government bureaucracies, etc.

(2) *Heightened Prognostic Expectancies*: Service users manifest a strong expectation of treatment success stimulated by the qualities of staff members helping them and the therapeutic procedures undertaken.

(3) *User Satisfaction*: Clients and family members positively evaluate treatment efficacy; users don't unexpectedly drop out, are willing to re-use program and recommend it to kinsmen, friends and neighbours.

What antecedent conditions help determine these outcome variables? Figure 1 represents a three-phase model of culture accommodation, showing the linkage between antecedent and consequent conditions. As seen in Figure 1, two antecedent phases are necessary: first, culture assessment of the local community constructing an ethnographic description of relevant dimensions; second, *accommodation implementation* or the translation of assessment findings into the design of helping systems. Literature in the disciplines of medical anthropology, transcultural psychiatry and minority mental health converge to suggest important culture assessment dimensions.

FOUNDATIONS OF CULTURAL ASSESSMENT

The study of culture and psychopathology, ethnomedicine, and informal support networks provide departure points for determining attributes of a

Antecedent Conditions

Phase One:
Culture Assessment

Semantic Illness Network

1. Analysis of Culturally Defined Problem:
   a) Explanatory Model:
      classification;
      labelling;
      etiology;
   b) Attitude.
2. Norms of Personal Adjustment
3. Expected Ways and Means of Curing:

   social support networks;
   healers;
   tactics of social influence.
4. Expected Community Relationship with Agency:

   community control;
   structure and social climate;
   folk healer integration;
   personnel characteristics and manners.

Phase Two:
Accommodation Implementation

Translate culture assessment data into helping program in terms of:

1. Siting/architecture
2. Goals/objectives
3. Policies/procedures
4. Organizational social "climate"/ manning level
5. Personnel
6. Therapeutics
7. Administrative style
8. Community relationship

Consequent Conditions

Outcome & Validating Criteria

1. Structural Qualities:

   Low resource intensive;
   enhanced accessibility;
   maximum administrative openness.
2. Social Ecology Qualities:

   enhanced acceptability;
   health network inclusive;
   increased community competency and self-management;
   "psychological sense of community".

   continuity with prevailing social norms, beliefs, power relationships.
3. Healing/Helping Qualities:

   reducing community stressers;
   heightened prognostic expectancies;
   user satisfaction.

Fig. 1. Culture Accommodation Model

culture/community group which must be understood prior to implementing an accommodation program. The literature offers three contributions: (1) culture-specific (emic) definitions of abnormality and causal explanations; (b) sociocultural causes of disorder, including models relating sociocultural stress, disintegration, immigration, and rapid social change to rates for psychological problems; and (c) sociocultural responses to disorder including family involvement and formally prescribed procedures for healing and psychotherapy.

These three domains can be transformed into a set of assessment questions and administered through interviews with community recipients. Briefly, the design of a cultural accommodation treatment program follows an assessment of: cultural perceptions of problem behaviour; philosophy and norms of individual adjustment; social support networks; folk healing practices; and expected community relationship with the agency.

Department of Psychology,
University of Waikata,
Private Bag,
Hamilton, New Zealand

REFERENCES

Benyoussef, A.
1977 Monitoring and Servicing National Health: Health Service Delivery in Developing Countries. International Social Science Journal 29: 396–418.

Carstairs, G. M.
1973 Psychiatric Problems of Developing Countries. British Journal of Psychiatry 123: 271–277.

Higginbotham, H. N.
1976 A Conceptual Model for the Delivery of Psychological Services in Non-Western Settings. In: R. Brislin (ed.), Topics in Culture Learning (Vol. 4). Honolulu: East-West Center.

Higginbotham, H. N.
1979a Culture and the Delivery of Psychological Services in Developing Nations. Transcultural Psychiatric Research Review 16: 7–27.

Higginbotham, H. N.
1979b Culture and Mental Health Services. In: A. J. Marsella, R. Tharp, and T. Ciborowski (eds.), Perspectives in Cross-Cultural Psychology. New York: Academic Press.

Higginbotham, H. N.
1979c Delivery of Mental Health Services in Three Developing Asian Nations: Feasibility and Cultural Sensitivity of 'Modern Psychiatry. Doctoral dissertation, University of Hawaii.

Kleinman, A.
1980 Patients and Healers in the Context of Culture. Los Angeles: University of California Press.

Marsella, A. J. and Higginbotham, H. N.
1979 Applications of Traditional Asian Medicine to Psychiatric Services in Developing Nations. Paper presented at the International Conference of Traditional Asian Medicine, Canberra, Australia.

World Health Organization
1975 Organization of Mental Health Services in Developing Countries. Sixteenth report of the WHO Expert Committee on Mental Health. Geneva: WHO Technical Report Series, No. 564.

Father ROBERT J. RONALD, S. J.

"IF YOU PINCH ME, I'LL HURT" – DISABILITY ADJUSTMENT: MINE AND THINE

As a disabled person, I face two kinds of problems every day: how to cope with my disabilities and their limitations and how to cope with the reactions of other people to me. In a way the latter is harder because I can often control my own reactions, but there is little I can do to control the reactions of others. I wish to address both issues: first, to point out some significant elements of adjustment to disability and how non-disabled persons can help in this adjustment; and secondly, to identify some concerns about the reactions of others to disability.

PERSONAL ADJUSTMENT TO DISABILITY

For me to become rehabilitated, I need proper medical treatment, assistive devices, training, placement, etc. To stay rehabilitated I need society's acceptance of my integration and its removal of barriers. On top of these external things I have to add my own person willingness to take advantage of them. The response of a disabled person to disability is a major factor in rehabilitation's success or failure.

In my experience, there can be no long-term healthy response to disability without honesty, which means admitting that the disability exists. Here are some of the facts I have to admit:

– My disabilities and handicaps cause frustrating limitations.
– They make me different from others.
– They make my life more difficult.
– I cannot go into public without being stared at.
– I must be pushed wherever I go.
– I live with the memories of lost abilities.
– I must watch others do things I used to enjoy.
– For the rest of my life I must look up from my wheelchair at even short people towering over me.

When these were the only facts I thought of, as when I first became disabled, I was tempted to say "To hell with life! Life without walking isn't worth living." But I discovered there are other facts equally true:

– I can still relate to people.
– I can still do or learn to do many things.
– To say my life with disability will never be the same is true, but to say I will never be happy again is false, unless I make it true by quitting or complaining.
– Human worth is not measured by how many pounds I can lift or how fast I can run.

Richard C. Nann, Dorcas Susan Butt, and Lourdes Ladrido-Ignacio (eds.), Mental Health, Cultural Values and Social Development, 287–294.

- Life is what I choose to make of it. I cannot always control the outcome of my actions or avoid unpleasant happenings, but I can control the way I act.
- Happiness is something I have to create for myself out of my responses to the environment.
- Adjustment does not mean I must like my limitations and restrictions. It only means I am not afraid to admit them or to live with them or even to laugh about them.
- Adjustment means I opt for the fullest possible life and will do my best to make sure that my disabilities get in the way as little as possible.

SUGGESTIONS FOR DISABLED PERSONS

From my own experience and from what I have seen of others, I offer the following advice for those trying to adjust:

- Be yourself. Assert yourself. Have confidence in yourself. Don't measure yourself by the standards of others. Growth comes from setting one's own goals and from comparing oneself against one's own blueprint. God did not make you the way you are just so you could become someone else.
- If you put all your energy into mourning your losses or into desiring only what you don't have, you'll be unhappy most of the time. If you are flexible enough to make the most of whatever is at hand, you can find happiness anywhere.
- Don't let yourself stay bogged down in sadness, frustration or anger when your disability upsets you. If you do, you'll have no energy or spirit left for coping. The first step toward rehabilitation is looking up and away from yourself. You must begin to recognize and use your remaining powers and abilities.
- Find someone more upset or unhappy than yourself and try to encourage that person. This is one of the best ways of encouraging yourself.
- Disabilities are not funny, but life is. If you can laugh at yourself and at the situations your disability causes, you can pick yourself up and keep going. Laughter is one of life's lubricants.

I cannot stress strongly enough the need for us disabled people to have confidence in ourselves and take pride in our human dignity. And this positive image of ourselves must be projected to others. People will not respect us if we don't respect ourselves and reveal our competence. We must act like we really are what we want to be before people will believe we are what we are.

I believe that strong religious belief and practice is an important source of self-confidence and courage. Faith in God and in spiritual values is what gives my faith in myself its foundation and security, for I know that I am not alone and that all which is most essentially good and important in me has not been touched or devalued by my disabilities. I have a dignity and destiny that disability cannot destroy or impair.

SUGGESTIONS FOR NON-DISABLED PERSONS

To all those who would like to help us disabled persons adjust better I have the following advice:

- Please don't deny our disabilities or dismiss them lightly or try to persuade us they don't matter, because they do. They are a permanent presence and influence in our lives.
- Please don't deny us the opportunity to feel and express our grief and anger at the losses we suffer when we become disabled, because these losses are serious and real.
- Please don't take as personal insults or rejection the anger we might express in your presence in frustration at our restrictions.
- If however, we become too absorbed in or hindered by our grief and anger, and you wish to shake us out of our lethargy, depression or fear don't tell us to "Wake up and live" until you can also offer us some concrete hope worth waking up for.

Let me explain why: It is a basic human experience that no one is motivated to make an effort for something, especially for something that cannot be immediately realized, unless three conditions are met:

(1) The goal is really considered worth striving for.
(2) There is a real expectation that the goal can actually be reached.
(3) In the meantime the day to day efforts in the direction of the goal are rewarding, or at least there is some positive feedback.

Therefore, if you want me to embark on the long road to rehabilitation, you will have to somehow show me some concrete goal for my life that I will find valuable and worthwhile and which I believe I can actually attain even with my disability, and then, as my friend, you must let me know regularly that I am making progress.

People say we disabled persons are prone to inferiority and depression, that we would rather keep in the background and stay with our own kind. This is sometimes true. If we manifest fear, frustration, anger, hostility, or distrust it is usually the result of bitter experience.

People avoid us, stare at us, laugh at us, pity us, overprotect us. Everywhere we meet barriers.

If we have grown up with our disabilities and our parent or other grown-ups have shielded us from outsiders, protected us from all risks, set no challenging goals for us, given us no responsibilities at home, or worse, made us feel we were burdens or worthless, then of course we grow up immature or feeling inferior. Frustration, anger, hostility, depression, futility are natural by-products of rejection, repression, and relegation to inferior status.

- If you non-disabled people really want to help us disabled persons come out of ourselves, then give us positive feedback.
- We will the more readily learn to value ourselves and put ourselves forward the more we experience you valuing us, accepting us as friends and associates,

encouraging us, providing us opportunities for participation and self-expression and for growing and giving and loving.

– Disabled people are beautiful people, when they are seen as people. Treat us like what we are and we will become what we should be.

Another observation I would like to leave with those who deal with disabled persons is this: Don't put too much emphasis on the external trappings of success. We are all familiar with the spotlights turned on outstanding disabled persons who have made notable achievements in spite of overwhelming obstacles. They do deserve this recognition and praise. But for every giant, there are hundreds of ordinary disabled persons who have not had the advantages of super-parents, super-friends, super-talents, super-funds, super-equipment or super-opportunities and have not accomplished or distinguished themselves as much.

I submit that any disabled person who is not afraid to look life squarely in the eye and face its difficulties with patience and human dignity is just as giant even if his/her contribution to society is very limited.

THE REACTIONS OF NON-DISABLED PERSONS TO DISABILITY

I wish to turn my attention now to that other problem we disabled persons face, namely the reactions of others to us. None of these remarks, of course, are applicable to you good people because of your experience and understanding, but the world at large is full of strangers who tremble with apprehension, shake with curiosity, shiver with grief or stumble over themselves (and us) in their haste either to get away from us as fast as they can or to smother us with sympathy.

I hope that no one will be offended if I approach this serious subject in a humorous way. You have all heard, of course, of bird watchers, folks who tramp the woods to observe birds in their natural habitats. We disabled persons are like birds, fair game for all the world to watch. What I want to do is turn the tables on those who watch me by watching them.

1. *Birds Who Invariably Radiate Distress*: This is a common species. Whenever I begin to think that maybe things are alright after all, one of these specimens swoops down oozing sadness at the sight of my misfortune. Females of this species are sometimes known to pat you on the head and murmur, "You poor dear. Does it hurt?" Being wept over is not very comforting, seeing how it is such a powerful reminder of pitiable limitations, but I have found that trying to comfort these would-be sympathizers is a great way to forget my own problems. Seriously, while not wanting to deny anyone the right to express sincere emotions, even at my own expense, if you really want to help me, consider what you might do or what we might do together to eliminate some of my limitations. Now, if I am the one who is weepy and discouraged, then you might try weeping with me – empathy and all that – or at least respect the fact that I probably

have a good reason, even if only a subjective one, for my sadness. So after showing you understand, suggest some measures that may help solve my problem or turn me to a more positive frame of mind.

2. *Birds Who Insist on Rejoicing and Denial*: This happy-go-lucky species doesn't know what sadness is. "Everything is going to be alright! You better believe it!" With a slap on your back and a hearty cheerio, he flies out of sight believing that if you acclaim everything is OK long and loud enough, the difficulties will automatically disappear. Such cheerful banter may be a pleasant distraction, but it denies reality rather than copes with it. No one hopes for a cure to reverse the effects of polio more than I but, I for one, am not going to sit around waiting for that to happen. If you want to help me, don't deny or belittle the hard work that lies ahead of me, but express your encouragement and confidence that I can make the best of it.

3. *Birds Who Intently Regard Deviation*: I am so used now to people staring at me, I expect it and if no one looks, I wonder what is wrong. Young birds poke their mothers on the wing and exclaim, "Look at that!" Some older ones have elaborately developed ways of looking while pretending to do something else. I'm not bothered much by staring anymore. After all, it isn't the starer's fault I look strange. But consider for a moment the devastating effect staring can have on a sensitive youngster just trying to face the outside world or on a newly disabled individual who has not yet accepted the disability. Being looked at like an animal in the zoo re-opens wounds of inferiority and self-pity.

4. *Birds Who Interrogate With Relentless Demands*: The song of this species is, "Who, What, Why, How". You know, it's really tiring to be asked the same question over and over again day after day. I have a friend who relieves the monotony with myths: he has the envious record of answering the same question about his disability, thirty-seven different ways. Myself, I usually don't mind answering questions so long as inquirers are sincerely interested. But what really burns me up is when someone's sole interest is in my sickness or my wheelchair as though they hadn't noticed or thought about the person in the wheelchair. Please don't be afraid to ask questions, but check to see whether the disabled person minds or not. And by all means let it be obvious that you respect the individual and are interested in his/her success and welfare just like you are in the non-disabled.

5. *Birds Who Make Inaccurate Remarks and Demands*: These advisors are self appointed experts who try to tell us all about our disabilities. Especially if they were once in a wheelchair for a week or their grandfather had a stroke, they know all about disability. They tell you what medicine to take and what exercises to do regardless of what your disability is, for to them all disabilities are the same. They become rather upset if you don't accept their advice or try

to tell them your doctor doesn't agree. The worst of this kind is the one whose uncle was paralyzed but can now walk because of his strong will-power or because he prayed to God for a cure. If you're still in your wheelchair the next time this bird appears, well, it's your own fault – you just haven't tried or prayed hard enough! (Birds like this treat us disabled persons like ignorant children, create false hopes, confuse the insecure and thoroughly exasperate those whose rehabilitation is already proceeding quite well.) Please don't be afraid to give advice or speak out if you are aware of something important that I should know, but be sure of your facts and realize there are thousands of different reasons why a person may be in a wheelchair. Show some respect for me, for my intelligence and for my right to make my own decision.

6. *Birds Who Insist on Restraining the Disabled*: This kind of smothering would-be defender of the weak has an overpowering urge to save us trouble, protect us from harm and nourish our strength. The problem is they insist on doing everything in accordance with what they imagine we need. We are handled as fragile invalids, only allowed to desire or enjoy what they think best. A good time with the boys, working hard, facing risks, really enjoying yourself are against their rules. A wheelchair in their clutches is a dull person. I'll never forget the lady who actually got mad at me because I was joking about my disability. "Here you are crippled and miserable for the rest of life. How dare you make light of something so serious!" Undoubtedly, had she been disabled she would have felt miserable and she wasn't about to let me feel any differently. Then I've been shouted at in the mistaken notion that being in a wheelchair also affected my ears. Grownups have spoken to me with the vocabulary they reserve for small children. I've been told that, "naturally I wouldn't enjoy watching a ballgame." A hostess once tried to send me to bed early since being an invalid I should retire early like the children. Look, I do have limitations and special needs, but please, if you want to help, let me tell you what they are before you act.

Another type of restriction we meet is rejection by people who, never sick themselves, believe the world belongs only to them. There is no room in their consideration for the weak nor any patience for the different. So far as they are concerned the crippled and deformed should mind their own business and keep out of other people's way. At best, these proud birds tolerate the disabled with cold politeness. At worst, they tenaciously obstruct wheelchair integration. It is an uphill battle for us disabled persons to prove our worth in their eyes. A shortcut might be to pray they'll break a leg and join our ranks for three months.

Incidentally, some disabled persons object to being called "crippled"; others oppose "disabled"; still others hate "handicapped". It is not the words that hurt, but the meanings people give to the words. As for me, you can use any word you want, but know this: I and all disabled persons will be offended and angry, if by any of these words you imply we are an inferior class of person or unwholesome or pitiable or incompetent or somehow unfit for the ordinary company of men. Perhaps we shouldn't be so sensitive – we wouldn't be if people wouldn't back up their words with prejudicial conduct. Please, all of you understanding and accepting people out there, help break down these social barriers by making your own positive attitudes contagious.

7. *Birds Who Improperly Ransom the Distressed*: This species of eager-beaver scouts is always on the lookout for good deeds. They snatch the knife out of your hand and cut your meat. Or they rush up to your wheelchair crying, "Can I help?" and before you answer they're pushing you down the corridor at breakneck speed and they haven't even asked where you're going yet. And they usually don't know how to push a wheelchair. I always wear good strong shoes not because I can stand up – I can't – but that is my only protection against banging into furniture, walls and other people's legs. I've been dumped out of my chair more than once by people who just would not listen when I told them directions. Please don't be afraid to offer me help if you see I need it. But, ask first if the assistance is wanted and be sure to ask how you should do it if you haven't had experience. And another thing, please do it inconspicuously. It is embarrassing to me if someone gleefully crashes my wheelchair through a crowd shouting "Out of the way" or demands a busy salesgirl at a crowded counter to immediately wait on "This cripple here" out of turn. Please remember it can be uncomfortable sometimes for a grownup to be seen needing assistance in public. Ordinarily the best way for you to help me is the way that draws the least attention.

8. *Birds Inexperienced in Relating to the Disabled*: These are well-intentioned fellows who just haven't learned yet what to say or do in the presence of someone disabled. Common reactions are running away in the opposite direction or pretending the wheelchair isn't there by looking away or talking only to the person pushing me, or even asking that person how I am as though I can't talk for myself. Sometimes they break the silence with a rapid monologue, talking wildly about any subject that comes to mind except, of course, myself or the disability. Occasionally someone dares to meet the issue head on, like blurting out, "Gee, it must be fun to ride around in a wheelchair all day", or "My grandfather was in a wheelchair too before he died". Many a time I've been the captive audience of someone who thinks I only want to hear about his own ill health and a stitch by stitch account of his last six operations.

Do you want to know how to act with me? Just be yourself. Do not be afraid to notice my disability. After all I've already noticed you aren't disabled. Talk directly, openly, honestly. If I'm depressed, show you understand. Don't feel guilty if you can't cheer me up. In fact, I don't think you have an obligation to make me smile no matter what. But if I can laugh at myself and the world, laugh too. If I'm the quiet type, don't feel obligated to keep the conversation going, even if you have nothing to day. In short, relate to me the same as you would to any other person with a similar personality.

In dealing with others, we disabled persons aren't without blame either. We sometimes are grumpy or in the dumps, sometimes on cloud nine, sometimes lazy, demanding help we don't need, sometimes stubborn or hostile, sometimes bitter, sometimes angry. No wonder people are confused how to deal with us. In this respect, we disabled are all too normal. I don't ask you to ignore our faults; we should be held accountable for our actions like everyone else. But at least show as much tolerance for our shortcomings as you show for those of your other friends and co-workers.

9. And now, the final species, which I am happy to relate is on the increase, namely the millions of *Birds Who are Impartial Reactors to Diversity and Beautiful Insusers of Respect and Dignity*: This is what all of you are when you accept us as we are, put up with our foibles, encourage us, give us helping hands just when we need them, listen to us, share with us your companionship and your dreams.

Mental health is being able to look reality in the eye without denial, touch it without rejection and shape it without distortion. Not all your efforts succeed, but things are sure a lot easier with friendship and acceptance. Disability is not the only significant part of my reality, you too are there. My reality is either richer or poorer when you are a part of it. Let's join hands and remake the world.

Operation des Handicapped,
Taipei, Taiwan

T. H. TSE

ATTITUDES AND INTEGRATION

One of the main objectives this year, the International Year of Disabled Persons, is to help the integration of disabled people into society. To this end, we are faced with two barriers. One is a physical barrier, due to the physical limitations of disabled people. The second is a psychological barrier, i.e. the hindrances caused people's attitudes towards the disabled, as well as the disabled's attitudes.

At first sight, the physical barrier cannot be helped, whereas the psychological barrier could be reduced easily. Quite the contrary. Because of the vast improvements in modern living conditions and the advances in modern technology such as micro-electronics, the physical limitations have actually been diminishing. On the other hand, people's attitudes on the disabled seem to have remained at the traditional level. It is the purpose of my presence here to point out how some of these attitudes affect the integration process, and to make suggestions as to how they might be overcome.

Before we look at the attitudes, however, let us make one position clear.

When we talk about integration, there is a question often raised, especially by able-bodied decision makers. The question is, would be disabled people be better off if they live together in a special home, attend special schools and work in sheltered workshops? They would not have to suffer the same frustrations or intimidating experiences that they have to face in an able-bodied society.

Experience in integration programs shows that disabled people do have difficulties and frustrations at times, just as their able-bodied counterparts. But, given the choice, most integrated disabled people do not want to go back to a sheltered society. I think this justifies the need for integration more than any theoretical argument. So let us now turn to the attitudes of various people who help to shape our integration process.

We are living in a work-oriented community. In order to be fully integrated, the disabled person must be able to obtain employment and make himself financially independent. So what are the attitudes of employers? Employers tend to look at the disabled collectively as people having sub-normal intelligence, people who can only do handicraft or unskilled factory work. Under this view, therefore, employers would consider them unsuitable for the keen competition in a highly industrialized market. To solve this problem, it would be best to publicize the employers who have already recruited disabled people. This would give a chance for the employers to express their first-hand experience of disabled people's abilities. It would also enable the rehabilitation service to show their appreciation of these employers.

Another area of concern of employers is that of absenteeism of disabled

Richard C. Nann, Dorcas Susan Butt, and Lourdes Ladrido-Ignacio (eds.), Mental Health, Cultural Values and Social Development, 295–298.

people. This is often expressed by employers who have never recruited any disabled people. Would disabled people be less physically fit and, hence, more likely to be absent from the job? To answer this question, we must see firstly that physical disability is not in contradictory terms with physical fitness. Secondly, it is found that absenteeism is more connected with the loss of morale rather than of physical fitness. In fact, employers who have actually recruited disabled people find that they are more loyal to the company than the average workers. This is because disabled people realize that their job mobility, or the chance of switching to another job, is considerably less than others.

To answer another worry of employers, accident rates of disabled people have been found to be less than the overall average, probably because disabled people are careful not to cause a second disabling incident in their life. So employers must have a word with their insurance company to alleviate their fear.

Despite the statistics, however, some insurance policies do have a clause stating that the people covered must not suffer from any physical deformity or mental illness. They make use of this clause to overcharge the disabled clients. Such practices should either be regulated by the government or made known to the public so that employers could turn to other insurance companies that have a more reasonable premium rate.

Managers also complain about the onset cost of special facilities for the disabled, such as computer braille terminals and special toilet cubicles. Actually some of these are general facilities recommended by the building codes anyway. Others may be the needs of individual employees. We suggest that the government should give tax relief or special subsidy to such provisions in order to encourage more disabled people to be recruited.

Another important area that we must look at is the attitudes of rehabilitation professionals. It has been some years since we tried to avoid giving discriminating labels to disabled people. So words like "cases" have been deleted from the professionals' dictionaries and replaced by words like "clientele" or "consumers". I had been happy to be referred to as a client, until recently when I was asked to produce a short paper on the International Year of Disabled Persons. When the paper was translated into another language, the word "clients" became "beneficiaries", or someone receiving an aid or a handout, because this was what they thought the clients were after. So we see that although changing the label could help a little, it is rather superficial and the concepts in people's minds might not be affected at all.

Furthermore, when a person is struck by a disability, he has no idea what the rest of his life will be like, and most of his self-conceptions are given to him by the rehabilitation workers. Besides being taught how to take care of himself, he is given vocational training from a very limited number of choices. If the client is blind, he is taught as a telephone operator. If he is otherwise physically disabled, he is taught woodwork or electronics.

These choices are the excellent work of innovative professionals early in our rehabilitation history. To copy them might seem likely to lead to success. But this is no reason to believe that these are the only choices for the clients. There are clients who are young and ambitious and who want to try something new. Such people should not be brushed aside as unrealistic. They should be given the chance and the assistance from the rehabilitation workers.

After training, the disabled client will have to go out and attend job interviews. He will be bombarded with questions similar to those we have just discussed. The client, who is a novice in the job, has neither the competence nor the confidence to answer these questions.

What we need is a very understanding rehabilitation worker, say the placement officer, who has the experience and expertise to deal with these questions. He meets the potential employer before the job interview, so that the confidence of the client would not be challenged. This is more easily said than done. Very often, unless it is a well-established placement, the placement officer himself is not very convinced about the client's potential for filling the job. What happens then could be that the client is rejected before the job interview even starts.

So the attitudes of the professionals are very important. They not only shape the whole rehabilitation process, but help to impose attitudes on the minds of disabled people, their families and potential employers. It is recommended that we should conduct ongoing training sessions and seminar workshops for rehabilitation workers at all levels, especially those who have been in the trade for so long that they have been affected by current practices and prejudice.

Let us now look at the disabled people themselves. It is estimated that about 10 percent of the world's population is disabled. This alone is sufficient reason for making provisions for the disabled. But people's reaction to this estimate is: "Where are the disabled people? I don't see any." There are two main reasons for this.

First, there are already disabled people who have fully integrated into the community. They may be working as professionals or in the factory. They may be married and raising their own family. But many of them no longer want to identify themselves with disabled people, but rather as an accountant, a teacher or a father.

It is these people to whom we must make a particular appeal. They have undergone the entire rehabilitation process, have seen the shortcomings, and have managed to overcome the barriers. They are the ideal people to help in the planning or policy-making of services to other disabled people. They see problems that ablebodied decision makers don't. They must make themselves seen and heard.

To quote an example, many architects think that the installation of elevators is the end of the story on physical access to buildings. Blinking lights and bells outside elevators are simply luxurious accessories. But this is not the case for the deaf and the blind, especially if the bells could help to differentiate an elevator going up from one going down. Even the physically handicapped would appreciate the blinking lights because they give them an early notice to the appropriate elevator. Such simple conveniences are not easily conceivable unless one has a first hand experience of a disability.

A second reason why disabled people are not seen is due to the attitudes of the man in the street. In some cultures, young children are taught not to stare at disabled people nor to talk about them. This, however, is not true in other parts of the world. People are left free to make gratuitous remarks and gestures. This is particularly disconcerting to the people who are about to recover from the disabling incident and, hence, most vulnerable. As a result, they want to stay invisible and withdraw from the community. So the attitudes and behaviour of the man in the street is also a big concern.

People do not normally have a chance to meet enough disabled people to understand them. Their impressions are gained through the stereotypes portrayed by the media, or handed down from the older generations. It has been found, unfortunately, that whenever disabled people appear on television series, fiction or children's story books, they are usually portrayed as a victim or a villain. This tendency is in fact rising because nowadays criminal behaviour in fiction is frequently attributed to mental disorder of one form or another. We hope that the mass media could instead do more investigative reporting on the life of disabled people and present the other side of the story.

When voluntary agencies ask for contributions, their description of the disabled people also affects the attitudes of everyday people. Disabled people are portrayed as very dependent. They need sympathy and hence donations. Actually, a more positive attitude would be to ask for understanding and assistance, so that the disabled people could live an independent life.

To summarize, the smooth integration into society for disabled people must be a joint effort of rehabilitation professionals, employers, the media and disabled people themselves. The attitudes of all these people could alter the entire integration process. So we hope that their minds are set on the right track from the very beginning to the very end.

University of Hong Kong

LOUIS REYES

MY EXPERIENCES WITH SERVICE PROVIDERS AND EMPLOYERS

When we arrived this afternoon, I was surprised to learn that I was one of those scheduled to be a panel member. I would like, therefore, to deviate a little from the established format of presentation and give a brief description of the problems I faced in coping with my disability. I would then welcome questions from the conference gathering.

I was disabled by a gunshot accident. I was sent to Hawaii for physical therapy and rehabilitation and returned home after one year in hospital. After being at home for approximately three months, I asked myself, "What shall I do; what kind of life will I have?" I decided that I did not want to stay home nor spend my life in a nursing home. I was then determined to make a life for myself.

My experiences with service providers and with a vocational rehabilitation in particular, were difficult. In my first attempt, I was denied service but, because of my persistence, I was finally accepted. But, before too long, my case was dropped. However, I was determined to complete my education with or without DVR. I applied for a government scholarship and was able to accomplish the goal that I set for myself. It was ironic that this was a service provider for the disabled, yet, I was denied this service. Of course, this happened a long time ago.

As far as employment is concerned, one of the employment agencies initially gave me a hard time for two years. It was very apparent that my disability was the primary factor in denying me employment, since it was not based on my qualifications and training for the job. When I was finally employed, I had to put in much extra effort to prove that I was as capable as any other individual.

So you see, disabled individuals at times may encounter difficult problems even with service providers, and certainly with many employers.

University of Guam

Richard C. Nann, Dorcas Susan Butt, and Lourdes Ladrido-Ignacio (eds.), Mental Health, Cultural Values and Social Development, 299.

MIGUEL P. BALBIN

COPING WITH MY DISABILITY

There is an old Filipino folksong which all school children in this country have learned by heart. Its simple lyrics go like this:

Planting rice is never fun,
Bent from morn 'til the set of sun.

Being disabled is never fun but, unlike planting rice when the planter is relieved of his aching back at the setting of the sun each day during planting season, being disabled means being handicapped to do some things normal people do, and that is for eternity, unless a miraculous cure or process is evolved. Being disabled is never fun, not only for us who are personally afflicted, but also for the members of our family who live with our disabilities.

Someone has said that when God closes a door, he opens a window. I like to believe that this is so because I looked through that window and saw that the world outside was beautiful. Had I retreated into my own shell shutting the world outside from my view, things would have been different. I became resigned to the fact that rehabilitation by surgery could no longer work for me having been disabled from walking at the very tender age of two years, just after I had learned to walk.

My mother was a teacher so I went to school with her, just as my older brother and sisters did. In the beginning, I could hop and skip without a crutch but, as I grew in height, my afflicted limb could no longer touch the ground. My parents hired an Igorot helper to carry me to school for a time.

School was interesting and after I finished my elementary grades, I went to high school and, finally, college. I had a special interest in music so I took voice lessons for a little while. As I was pursuing a course in college, I thought about what I would do to earn a living, taking my disability into consideration. One of my instructors mentioned to me at one time that I had a good speaking voice so I thought of training in radio broadcasting and with my appreciation for good music, I thought I would make a fine disc jockey.

Maybe it was a blessing for me that our family moved to Davao City in 1951 where the pace of life is much slower than in Manila. There, when you hail a passenger jeepney, it would come to a full stop and take you right to your doorstep. Of course, I saw to it that no one was in its front seat, which I find more comfortable and more convenient. Davao City was a growing community and I feel I also grew with it. Because it was a melting pot of different ethnic tribes coming from all parts of the country, it seemed easy for me to integrate into the mainstream of community life.

An American gentleman, Alfred J. Wills, hired me as newscaster and disc

Richard C. Nann, Dorcas Susan Butt, and Lourdes Ladrido-Ignacio (eds.), Mental Health, Cultural Values and Social Development, 301–302.

jockey and sooner than I realized, I started getting fan mail from school girls. It's a good feeling to be appreciated and one strives to do even better. In the quiet evenings, I spiced light classical music with poetry readings and more fan mail came pouring from young professionals and housewives.

Since I had a college degree at 18 years old, I thought of applying fo a teaching job at the University of Mindanao and they also took me in. I taught English poetry and drama and also Filipino language in the teacher training department. It was in this job that I met the girl who thought that beneath my crippled physical self was the real person whom she could love. Since then, I have never given her cause to regret her initial impressions of me. It might seem too early – as we are both 47 – but my wife and I plan to retire soon as our youngest child is out of college and ready to start on her own. Our youngest is now 15 years old and a first-year college student at the Ateneo, trying and determined to follow my lead in communication arts.

How did all these things happen, and you might even add, so fast and so soon?

While I complained that being disabled is never fun, I did not say that I can never be happy and enjoy life. I would like to present to this distinguished gathering my own personal experience, observations and views on how I coped with my disability.

First, I almost always live in hope. I seldom completely accept my physical limitations for there is always a hope that I shall conquer and overcome my physical drawbacks.

Second, I have always considered by personal obligation to take part in the everyday life of my family and the community I live in. Therefore, I strived harder and looked for better opportunities to be just one among the people, to succeed, or even to excel. But should it be, I am not afraid to fail after doing the best I know how just like anyone else in my community.

Third, it has been my dream to lead a dignified life so that in the end I gain fulfillment by working to improve the lives of others – others who may be disabled like me and others who may be physically able but have not been afforded the opportunities that I have.

With these as my experiences, observations and views, I must be very quick to add with strong conviction that without the right people backing me up, the right time and the right place, I may not be as happy as very certainly as I am tonight. When is the right time? Where is the right place and how?

As I close my presentation, may I invoke the UN General Assembly, through its Resolution 34/154 which should infuse the international symposium of experts to take place this month of July – the reason why concerned people are in Argentina, at the Development Academy of the Philippines in Tagatay, and elsewhere in the world. As UN Secretary General, Kurt Waldheim, stressed in the International Year of Disabled Persons – "Disabled persons have the right to participate fully in the life and development of the society to which they belong. It is our duty to enable them to exercise that right. Now what are we going to do?"

University of Mindanao, Philippines

Dr. JOHN A. NESBITT, Ed.D.

RECREATION, ATTITUDES AND HANDIPEOPLE

A RATIONALE FOR SPECIAL RECREATION FOR DISABLED PERSONS

Recreation participation is vital to the normal growth and development of children and youth and to the functioning of adults and seniors. Recreation is an activity of experience in which a participant engages voluntarily during leisure or free time, which is inherently satisfying. Recreation's satisfactions are usually described as amusement, diversion, enjoyment, fulfillment, pleasure, relaxation or self-expression. An essential characteristic is the attitude of the participant in that he or she anticipates satisfaction from the recreation experience. Recreation activity is as diverse as human activity ranging from art to hobbies to sports to travel.

Recreation often imparts aesthetic, creative, emotional, intellectual, physical, and social benefits to the individual. Recreation opportunity provided by service agencies encompasses planning to achieve social goals such as citizenship, personal growth, physical and mental health, and social training.

Recreation service is organized help, aid or assistance which provides individuals with the opportunity to have the experience known as recreation. Generally, local recreation service is characterized by the provision of financing, personnel and leadership, equipment, facilities, supplies, and the organization of activities. Recreation personnel include superintendents or directors of recreation and/or parks; recreation centre or recreation program directors and supervisors; recreation leaders; recreation or camp counsellors; play or playground leaders; volunteers, etc.

Recreation for persons in institutions who are ill, injured or disabled is often called therapeutic recreation service or recreation therapy. Recreation for handicapped and special recreation are terms that are used to describe recreation provided on an adapted basis in the community.

Recreation service for handicapped children, youth, adults and seniors is vital, for the following reasons:

(1) *The Human and Civil Right to Recreation*: All people regardless of sex, age, nationality, etc., or handicap are entitled to participate in the recreation lifestyle of their community, seeking to achieve their highest potential in and through recreation.

(2) *Normalization in Recreation is Necessary*: Normalization in recreation, as well as other basic dimensions of life, is necessary for normal growth and development of children and youth. For adults, normalization in recreation provides reward, relaxation and renewal.

Richard C. Nann, Dorcas Susan Butt, and Lourdes Ladrido-Ignacio (eds.), Mental Health, Cultural Values and Social Development, 303–306.

(3) *Contribution of Recreation to Rehabilitation in Treatment and Community Functioning*: Day-to-day experience, as well as a growing body of professional knowledge, substantiates the fact that professional recreation services contribute to the achievement of medical, social, educational and vocational rehabilitation goals and the pursuit of a healthful recreation lifestyle contributes to independent community living.

INEQUITABLE OPPORTUNITY AND PREJUDICE

It is generally recognized that disabled persons are excluded from recreation opportunity because of prejudice and barriers (architectural, service and transportation). In the United States, I estimate that the exclusion rate of disabled persons is approximately 90%. The following generalization about attitudes toward disability have been made:

- The different in society are less desirable.
- The self-image of the sheltered person is undermined.
- Non-disabled decide who may join – at school, at work, at recreation.
- Negative characteristics create negative attitudes.
- One's self-image is dependent on acceptance by others.
- The public's unconscious attitude toward the disabled is disabled.
- Some professionals perceive low competence among the disabled.
- Enjoyable, voluntary contact with the disabled increases favourable attitudes.
- Higher frequency of contact with the disabled increases positive attitudes.
- Closer contact with disabled persons increases acceptance.

Some "attitude sets" or "syndromes" that create attitude blocks may be described as follows:

The Futility Syndrome: "What can I do to help? The situation is impossible. There are no laws. No money. There are only barriers."

The Leprosy Syndrome: "If I touch them, I may get it. These conditions, like cerebral palsy, are contagious."

The Deuteronomic Syndrome: "They must have done something wrong. God means for them to be punished. If they repent, they will get well." This attitude is classical Deuteronomic Code right out of the Old Testament, which says in essence, "Do good and ye will be blessed; sin, and God will punish you." There are many people whose "gut-level" thinking and feeling follow this line, and for these people, attitudes make them negative facilitators.

The Punishment Syndrome: "They are not in jail to be coddled and play games; they're there to be punished."

The Hypocrisy Syndrome: "We serve the handicapped; that doesn't mean that we have to employ them." This syndrome is characteristic of some individuals and agencies in education, special education, recreation and parks, therapeutic recreation, welfare and social work, rehabilitation, etc. Count the number of handicapped employed in your agency, university, hospital.

The Charity Syndrome: "I gave to Cerebral Palsy but that doesn't mean that I want my daughter to marry one."

The Civic-Pride Syndrome: "Why sure I am concerned about the handicapped. Our local chapter of the Royal Order of Roosters gives a Christmas party at the rehabilitation centre every year." This syndrome is especially pernicious because well-intended people delude themselves into thinking about how they can solve the horrendous problems of disease, disability, poverty, inequality, ignorance, and violence. There is no room for Pollyanna in the fight against prejudice.

The Me-Me-Me Syndrome: The handicapped person speaks: "I am here at this meeting with my problem. I want it solved this minute. I refuse to do the staff work, the surveying or joining with other handicapped persons in order to give really sound advice and guidance to civic-minded citizens or professionals." The role of consumer spokesperson is no less demanding than any other professional role.

The "I-Want-To-Be-Left-Alone" (like Greta Garbo) Syndrome: Some disabled people who simply do not face up to their civic and social responsibility to assist the public agencies, etc.

The Defense Syndrome: "I don't see what your recreation-for-handicapped people are squawking about; we are meeting our social and professional obligation by running a once-a-month social night for the mentally retarded and 25 kids show up pretty regular." Yes, 25 out of a population of maybe 2,500 that need creation service.

The All-Those-Others Syndrome: "I simply can't divert money, personnel, and resources away from the 500,000 able-bodied that I serve to the 500 severely handicapped that I don't serve. I have all those others to worry about and I can't be concerned with a handful of handicapped."

The Lack-of-Training Syndrome: "I can't have these people in my program. I don't have the trained staff to handle epileptic fits, convulsions, slobbering, soiled clothing, poor speech."

The Smooth-Waters Syndrome: "I can't have those people in my centre because the other participants, the regular people, their parents, the staff, the food suppliers, the janitors, the WCTU – they would all just quit my program. I can't make waves or the whole thing will just come down on me. We don't want that, do we?"

SOME THOUGHTS ON RECREATION AND HANDIPEOPLE

Use of terms such as "handicapped, disabled, disabled persons" all serve to reinforce the negative perception of people who are disabled that the public holds almost "naturally". Further, while we all recognize the real and profound pain and suffering that disease and injustice cause, it is the positive side of rehabilitation that we wish to emphasize. Rehabilitation is a philosophy, a goal and a method in working with people who are disabled. We in rehabilitation believe that through recreation every disabled person should achieve his or her highest potential medically, socially (in terms of psychological and social adjustment), educationally, vocationally and recreationally. It is, in fact, the "handiness" of people who are disabled that makes it possible for them to achieve success in living, in education, in work, and in recreation. Thus, I propose that we refer to people who are disabled as "handipeople, handiyouth, handichildren", and so on, in order to emphasize their capabilities and the positive side of their achievements.

PUBLIC ATTITUDES TOWARD HANDIPEOPLE

A strategy for creating positive public attitudes toward handipeople:

I. Preparation.
II. Initial Exposure.
III. Direct Involvement.
IV. Observe Involvement.
V. Recreation Activities that may be Used.

Director, Special Recreation Project,
U.S. Office of Special Education

RICHARD HUNTER

ATTITUDES TOWARD DISABLED PERSONS FROM THE POINT OF VIEW OF A SERVICE PROVIDER

I feel a bit uncomfortable about sailing under false colours – I am not a service provider. The National Mental Health Association in the United States of America is not a provider but is instead a consumer advocate. If one thinks of a provider sitting across the desk from the client, the MHA is sitting on the same side of the desk as the client, ready to help the client secure whatever services are needed. From that spot we have a chance to observe providers and how they work.

There are three kinds of providers that I would like to mention.

(1) The first represents the most cynical view of providers. This is the provider who views his or her client primarily as a source of income.

> The number of clients multiplied by the dollars charged per client represents the level of income. Fortunately there are not many of this sort and I am sure there are none who travelled so far to come to this place.

(2) The second is the provider who finds his or her symbiotia fulfillment in the client.

> The provider is trained but this training is nothing without a client.
>
> The client becomes the object required by the provider to achieve fulfillment.
>
> If the client gets better, he or she can be replaced by another. This condition often shows up in an institutional setting such as clinics.
>
> A limit is set on the size of the case load and on the nature of the disorder to be seen. When the limit of those who can be comfortably cared for has been reached, intake is closed. What happens to those not admitted is of only passing concern. The providers from the several professions are each engaged in what they have been trained to do having a suitable number of acceptable clients available to assure filfillment of their function. This category viewed in the extreme can also be somewhat cynical.
>
> The difference is that this is at least patient- or client-oriented even if on the provider's terms.

(3) The third kind of provider is client oriented and on terms related to the client's special needs. The handicapped person is viewed not as an object to be altered but as a unique human being with a condition that puts

Richard C. Nann, Dorcas Susan Butt, and Lourdes Ladrido-Ignacio (eds.), Mental Health, Cultural Values and Social Development, 307–308.

him at a disadvantage in the culture in which he lives. The therapist has tools that he or she can make available as the provider and client set out together to cope with a shared concern. If the therapist does not have the tools, then he or she will be a resource in the search for the tools needed. The basic aim in the relationship is to enable the client to maintain independence while building competence to cope in the culture. This is accomplished through the following means. (a) If possible, by correcting the condition which puts the disabled at a disadvantage; (b) This might be surgery, physical medicine, psychotherapy; and for some handicapped people, this approach is going to be successful and brings prompt resolution of the problem. (c) By providing support and encouragement if the condition cannot be removed. This may be simple counselling or deeper grief work. The client is prepared to be able to take positive steps on his or her own behalf. (d) By assisting in the development and operation of a sub-culture in which clients can feel safe and supported while struggling with adaptation to the dominant culture. Self-help groups provide a haven of protection. They are not to be seen as leper colonies where people are isolated, but as a safe base of operations. The same applies to group homes. (e) By working with the handicapped to modify the dominant culture to make it more acceptable. The work of the physically handicapped to assist on the removal of architectural barriers is an excellent example of successful efforts to modify the dominant culture. Modification of the U.S. Government Employment Application forms to remove the question concerning prior mental illness is another example. (f) By carefully avoiding the role model which casts the providers as "superior" and the client as "inferior". The provider is able to learn from the client. The provider is honest enough to acknowledge his own handicaps so that while in this instance he may have needed skills and experience to give positive help, that does not make him superior but only in a better position to provide help. While the client acknowledges the need for help, he retains his dignity and self respect while he and the provider enter into a joint effort.

Acting Director,
U.S. Mental Health Association

KENNETH BAYES (U.K.)

THE EFFECT OF THE ENVIRONMENT ON ATTITUDES TOWARDS HANDICAPPED PEOPLE

I believe that the theme of this seminar is one of the most important issues in helping handicapped people today. However much we succeed in providing services and programs, and the professional staff to run them (in all of which we are pitifully short), they cannot succeed fully without a new attitude towards the handicapped by people in general and without a new attitude by the hanid-capped towards themselves.

This was not true in the past when the pattern of services was different. When the attitude was "out of sight, out of mind" and handicapped people were isolated from everybody else, either in the back room of the house or in a large institution, it made no difference what the man in the street felt. In those days the only important thing was the attitude of the professionals and custodians within the institution. I know many of the big institutions still exist, especially in the West and in developed countries, but what we are talking about in this seminar is services and attitudes which lead to and permit integration and rehabilitation.

I have been asked to speak to you as an architect involved in the design of buildings for handicapped people, and to describe ways in which the physical environment affects attitudes towards the handicapped.

The first thing I want to point out is that the kind of buildings that one provides depends on the kind of services and programs one wants to create. Each is dependent on the other. If one wants to improve public attitudes, the services must be provided within the community, because the public must see handicapped people about and get to know them. In this context, if properly handled, familiarity does *not* breed contempt, but acceptability. The relationships which will free the person imprisoned in his handicap are with family, friends, neighbours and community. We must remember that integration within the community helps not only the handicapped person but is salutary also for the non-handicapped.

How can the physical environment help people towards this acceptance? The answer is to design buildings which allow the handicapped people to live, work and play in as normal an environment as possible so that they can be accepted as "one of us". As far as living conditions are concerned this means as many of the handicapped people as possible living at home as part of a family. In terms of services it means domiciliary help rather than special buildings. It necessitates the handicapped being included in family activities and outings. It assumes the same contact with neigbours and friends as are enjoyed by the rest of the family.

Only if family circumstances demand it will the handicapped person live away from home in a group home or hostel. If this is necessary there should be a

Richard C. Nann, Dorcas Susan Butt, and Lourdes Ladrido-Ignacio (eds.), Mental Health, Cultural Values and Social Development, 309–311.

variety of facilities available to cater to the individual's ability to be independent. These may range from a shared house or flat with visiting support staff, to a group home or hostel with live-in staff. The facilities must appear as normal and homelike as possible, must fit into the community and be unobtrusive. This means that it must be small in its occupancy and domestic in its architecture, similar to the surrounding buildings. It should be among other houses and not grouped, as so often happens, with institutional buildings. Even its address is important – give it a number like the other houses and do not proclaim its otherness by a plaque which says "Lady Somebody's Home for the Handicapped".

The institution, as we have already suggested, is not a facility which improves public attitudes. It encourages unacceptable and peculiar behaviour among those who live there for any length of time and emphasizes to the outside world everything that is different, dangerous, abhorrent and frightening about handicapped people far beyond the actual reality. It is architecture's most lamentable contribution to the handicapped.

If we are aiming to improve attitudes to handicapped people, it is important to start at an early age. There is no reason why handicapped children should not be fully integrated into pre-school play groups and nursery schools. Children at that age are happily still immune from prejudice (unless indoctrinated by adults) and their play can assimilate all sorts and variety of children. During school age, integration in the regular school should be achieved where possible even if this demands specialist teachers, special resource rooms or special classes. Only when this is found to be quite inappropriate should be handicapped child go to a special school.

Work should follow the same pattern as school. If possible, employment should be found among non-handicapped peers in the general workshop or market place. Only when this is clearly impossible should work be found in the sheltered workshop. For the retarded person, a period in the advanced training centre can of course be a prelude to the open workshop.

All *leisure* activities which the abilities of the handicapped person permit him to pursue should be available to him.

All that I have said so far applies to all handicapped people, whether they are mentally retarded, mentally ill, blind, deaf, elderly infirm, or physically disabled in other ways. For all of these people, the kind of physical environment in which they live matters and can help others to accept them.

With the *physically* disabled, especially the non-ambulant, there is the additional problem of mobility. This is obviously an essential ingredient of the formula for integration and acceptability. There is now a lot of useful information on how to make buildings accessible. But let us remember that accessibility is a means to an end. The purpose of accessibility is to achieve maximum normalization for the handicapped person.

So to sum up, one can use that rather overused phrase, the normalization principle, to express the way in which the environment can best help to improve attitudes towards the handicapped. This principle, as you know, has been defined as "making available to the handicapped patterns and conditions of everyday life which are as close as possible to the norms and patterns of the mainstream of society". The *acceptance* of this principle, which relates to any country or culture is, I believe, the key to changing attitudes. Its actual *application* depends a great deal on providing the right physical environment, whether for living, schooling, working or playing. Within the time available, I have suggested only daily basic principles for the right environment for handicapped people. In the workshop I hope you will help in developing, expanding and adding to these ideas.

Architect Consultant,
Design Research Unit International

NENITA Y. DAVADILLA

HOW I AS A PARENT HAVE COPED WITH A DISABLED CHILD IN THE FAMILY

This is one occasion on which, not even by choice, could I reject this invitation to be with you here today. Personally, I had made a commitment on behalf of disabled persons through my daughter to invest myself in any small measure for the welfare of the mentally retarded and other disabled persons in our country.

To the planners and organizers of this Pre-Congress Seminar, allow me to extend to you my appreciation for giving me this opportunity to realize my commitment.

To trace back the events that relate to coping with the daily stress of having a disabled child is not easy. However, if this sharing will prove to be helpful in modifying some of our stereotyped and unhealthy attitudes toward disabled persons today, I will take the risk of sharing my own experiences in coping, from the very first day my child was handicapped.

From the beginning when I learned that the baby I had carried for nine months was disabled, I felt the most painful thing that a mother could in life.

If one has a baby that does not fit with one's expectation, it is indeed painful and traumatic. This is even harder to accept when the child who happens to be disabled was not intentionally conceived. This is true with our daughter Ninette.

Ninette was only two days old when I visited her in the hospital. This visit was prompted because I became impatient waiting for her to be delivered into my room for breast feeding. As I was longing to touch her and to put my arms around her and I could hardly wait to see her, I found myself in front of the nursery.

As soon as I reached the glass window, I lost no time in asking for her from the charge nurse. Slowly, the nurse held her up in order for me to have a good glimpse of her face. Ninette began to move her arms and turned her head from side to side. Unexpectedly, she opened her eyes. The first encounter with Ninette had a deadening effect on my whole being. I felt shocked and stunned in silence for a moment. "Oh, no!" I whispered to myself. I thought there was something strange about her, but more strongly, I felt my love for her. However her squint eyes left a lasting impression on my memory as I ushered myself back into my room. Everything about Ninette during this first meeting appeared to be like a flashing thought and, indeed, within a very short time, all about her unusual appearance had totally escaped my memory. Unknowingly, I avoided the idea of discussing my observation with anyone, not even with my husband. We somehow managed to take all that there was about Ninette as normal.

Two weeks had passed and it was time to bring her home. The pediatrician had to see Ninette for a routine check-up in his office. Everything appeared okay until the time I was preparing to take her from the examining table and the

Richard C. Nann, Dorcas Susan Butt, and Lourdes Ladrido-Ignacio (eds.), Mental Health, Cultural Values and Social Development, 313–320.

doctor said: "I would like to see your baby once a month without fail. Your baby has some features of a mongoloid. But let us observe her further. Besides, you may want to consult a geneticist for her."

His words awakened me to full awareness. I knew that I was all ears to every word the doctor had said but it all sounded as though there was nothing unusual. We left the doctor's office and the idea about Ninette's abnormal condition was kept repressed. Instead, the great desire and joy to bring her home prevailed, with a sister and three brothers all waiting and eager to see a new baby after years without one.

After five months, my husband and I decided to take counsel from a geneticist. On our way to the clinic, we were hoping that this consultation would offer us some kind of support and relief from our feelings of uncertainty. As Ninette's name was called, we entered the doctor's office, where she looked at me straight in my face, gave a quick stare at Ninette and said: "You should not have given birth anymore!" Her greetings caught me in surprise and disbelief! "Oh, my God!" was the only phrase I muttered to myself. Never in my life have I felt so frustrated and disgusted. I was in a rage. At the same time, I felt pain inside me, and a big choking lump in my throat. I could almost feel the blood rushing up into my head. It was like a big slap on my face. Within me, there was an initial impulse to hit back but I found myself too weak to say anything. I wanted to leave right away, but I decided to stay if only to allow her to finish whatever examination she had to do in fairness to Ninette. It was very difficult to succumb to such an unsolicited, anxiety-provoking climate, but, I had no choice.

All the while I was feeling miserable, I religiously watched the doctor as she held Ninette's hands, at the same time pressing each of her palms on a stamping pad, then moving them one at a time to a clean piece of paper to print. Then she continued to work with a ruler on the prints. After about five minutes, she looked up at us and announced: "She is a mongoloid."

I looked at my husband who was standing beside me and he was looking at me in painful silence. We calmly accepted the label, but deep inside me I asked the question, "Why has it to be she?" I felt too numb to say a word. A little later, the geneticist hinted that we could submit for chromosomal examination, but it would cost us money. Besides, she further explained: "Considering your age (I was 41) I am almost positive that your child's condition is brought about by a genetic aberration."

At this point, we realized that our quest for the much-needed enlightenment, understanding and emotional support for our concerns was to no avail. It was very frustrating to realize that a specialist of her kind could fail us, especially when we needed her most. Not having enough courage and energy to talk, we hurriedly made an exit, paid the bill and left.

On our way home, we dropped by the pediatrician's office for Ninette's regular check-up. The doctor patiently explained to us that everything about Ninette was all right, except that she would be different from the rest of her siblings. Her physical, mental, emotional and social development may be impaired, he added emphatically. We left the pediatrician's office feeling a little bit better.

Around 10:30 a.m. of the same day, another doctor shared with me the story of two disabled children of another family. In time, these children had to be kept in a locked room and finally in an institution because of uncontrollable and destructive behaviours. Somehow, the doctor had insinuated that we should prepare a trust fund for Ninette and should she become unmanageable in the future, she would be placed in an institution where she would be assured of good care.

While listening to the doctor's story, I found myself shaking my head in protest at the fate of the two children under discussion. Within me, I thought, Ninette will be a different child. She will never be placed behind locked doors. I will see to it that she will live with the family where she belongs. She will be taught and be guided how to live with us her family and with other people within her capacities and limitations. Yes, I promised myself and Ninette that I would show and prove to the whole world that, regardless of her condition and her label, she could become another human being capable of a modest life that would be worthy of respect from others. I took this commitment and challenge as I never had before in my life.

Finally, when we reached home, I was almost exhausted. I lay on my bed and closed my eyes to relax. Then my thoughts began to linger over the happenings at the geneticist's clinic, the pediatrician's and the sharing of the other doctor earlier in the morning. Within a short time, I was submerged in painful depression. There seemed to be no way to hold back so I let go the painful feelings. I went into crying spells. All too soon, I came to realize that being a psychiatric nurse could not spare me from painful feelings in response to a stressful situation such as this. Through this experience, I was convinced that this is only one of the many risks one has to take in being human. Yes, let us face the situation frankly: having a disabled child is one of the most painful realities to accept. This is especially true when you realize that the burden is all yours and your family's alone.

The interactions I had with the three specialists mentioned earlier had not in any way helped to give me directions on what to do after telling that my child, Ninette, was a mongoloid. As a matter of fact I would say that the two of them had even succeeded in adding insult to the injury that was already there. Of course, I did not expect miracles from them. But, I did expect that some kind of help, psychological or otherwise, could have been initially extended to us. That might have made it a lot easier for us to accept Ninette's disability. Moreover, I wished that some kind of services could have been suggested for intervention as Ninette passes through the early developmental periods. Following these traumatic encounters with the specialists, I decided that no one could better help Ninette and I overcome her disability than me, her mother, and her family.

The long hours seemed to drag and I could not seem to stop crying in pain.

Unexpectedly, my eleven year old son walked into the room and saw me sobbing in pain. Without hesitating, he approached me at the bedside and asked: "Mother, why are you crying? Why? What happened to Ninette? Is she sick?" I could hardly answer his queries. It was hard even to say a word. Nevertheless, I decided to take this opportunity to explain to my children about Ninette's very unique personality. I thought that there could be no better time to involve them, so I asked for all of them and started to explain:

"Nerissa, Rene, Ruel, Raul, I wanted to talk to you. I wanted to tell you that Ninette was born in her natural form as you can see her. But she is and will be different from each of you in many ways. She has a pair of tiny but squint eyes and so she is called a mongoloid child. And she will continue to be that way all her life. Also, for most of you, at the age of 10 to 12 months, you were learning to walk, but for Ninette, she may not be able to do it then. At the time when you learned to talk, Ninette may not be able to speak and at five or six, you may have learned to read and write, but for Ninette that might be a difficult task to do. However, one thing is very important for us to remember – Ninette needs support from all of us. In order to help her overcome the difficulties she might encounter in growing up, we should be ready to help her.

"Some families around the world have also children with conditions similar to Ninette, but often they send them away. For Ninette, we will do the opposite. We should be happy to tell our friends and relatives that she is one of our family.

"Before anything else, Ninette needs our love and acceptance of her handicap and of her as a person. This means that we must accept her being different in her physical looks, her limited intellectual abilities and maybe her occasional unacceptable or distinctive behaviour. For only when we are able to do this will Ninette be able to grow and be happy with us. I believe that if we treat Ninette with love and respect in front of other people, they will tend to follow. However, if we treat her with cruelty and indifference, other people will likely do the same. Ninette will definitely take her cue from all of us around her. If we look at her as an upsetting state of life not worth living, so will she. Or, if we are bitter against an unjust fate, she will feel the same. And if we expect her to measure her ability to accomplish or succeed against that of ordinary children, we may not only increase our sorrow, but also put an addition burden on her.

"Finally, Ninette's attitude toward herself, her relations with us and other people and her ability to respond to her environment can be shaped. And here is where we are the key persons to help her."

After a while, I felt the need to talk to someone. Crying my heart out did not seem to be enough. My husband had left for work and I felt so alone. I telephoned a close friend of mine and found myself pouring out all my painful feelings and confusion to her. It was hard, but afterwards I felt so relieved. Also, my friend who happened to be a child psychiatric nurse offered to undertake therapy for Ninette. It was reassuring to carry out a positive, planned program for Ninette and the whole family. Aware of the fact that constructive action is always the best way to relieve emotional strain, my husband and I agreed to submit Ninette for therapy.

Thus, as young as five months old, Ninette started to undergo therapy with the child psychiatric nurse at the Lamp Centre for three consecutive years. I saw to it that she attended her therapy sessions as scheduled, three times a week without fail. At the same time, working closely with the nurse therapist was a must for me to be able to carry out planned program of activities at home to be consistent with the goals of her therapy.

Ninette grew with time and eventually the landmarks of her motor development gradually appeared. The supportive emotional climate and the stimulating environment afforded her at home, as well as in the clinic, have had a tremendous impact on her consistent growth physically, emotionally, socially and mentally.

At the age of three and a half, Ninette entered the Preschool Program at the Lamp Centre, which I established two years ago. Feeling inadequate to handle the training she badly needed at home, I left my job at the hospital and enrolled in the graduate program as education major in Special Education at the State University. In one summer and four semesters, I finished the program. Thus, the Therapeutic Learning Program for Handicapped Children was born, with Ninette as the first child to enroll among three other children.

Raising Ninette from 0 to 3 years old was easy, but as she learned to move about the house it became more difficult. She began to throw around everything she picked up. There was a time when I almost lost patience, when I felt so fed up with her seemingly aimless, destructive behaviour, but I did not give up. One day, at the dining table, Ninette seated herself in her usual place. I spooned some rice into her plate and, without any warning, she pushed it away. The next thing we knew, everything in front of her was thrown on the floor and broken. She went into a tantrum, so I moved her down to the floor for safety. My initial reaction then was to spank her, but I controlled myself. I tried to understand what could have provoked her tantrum. I asked for another set of plate and silverware for her. Surprisingly, when she noticed this, she wiped her tears away and quickly climbed back into her chair. Then, I moved the rice bowl close to her so she could reach for it and, seeing this, she looked up at me and smiled. Happily, she scooped some rice and continued to feed herself.

It was only later that I realized she no longer liked the idea of my serving her food in her plate. She wanted to do it by herself, but could not communicate it. So she became frustrated and angry, which could explain her destructive behaviour. From that day on, I learned to accept her need for independence in the area of self-help skills. This particular experience made me aware of her need to have a room where she could be allowed to explore the environment in her own way. Thus, gradually, a room was arranged that provided for Ninette a kind of laboratory equipped with simple but varied home-made learning tools and equipment to facilitate the development of gross/fine motor skills, language skills, self-help skills, socialization skills, as well as cognitive skills. Since Ninette loves to dance and sing, an old radio and record player were added to her equipment, which she herself has been allowed to operate with some guidance. Lately, she showed great interest in reciting nursery rhymes and songs, so I allowed her to use my old portable tape recorder. Last week, I began to teach her to tape her poems and songs. Then, I allowed her to listen to her voice, which has, incidentally, stimulated her to recite them over and over again. This was a great help in her language development, too. Varied books are made available to her for picture-reading. Watching "Sesame Street" is a regular habit and from it she has learned to read all letters of the alphabet, numbers from 1 to 12, and much more.

Once a week I take her for a stroll around the nearby grocery or department stores. How she enjoys riding the escalator, but hates the elevator. At least once a month I give her a treat in a restaurant for either fried chicken, her favourite dish, noodles, or ice cream. Gradually, her aimless and seemingly destructive behaviour stopped, and instead, more adaptive behaviours began to appear.

However, though I wholeheartedly devoted myself to this program, I was careful not to neglect the needs of my other children and other family obligations. As a matter of fact, each of us in the family have our own share of helping Ninette develop her abilities, through games or play. In addition, but within time and energy limitations, I see to it that my other children and I maintain outside interest and activities of our choice to continue growing as persons. This arrangement, in some ways, enables us to extend ourselves more unselfishly to her.

At home, my role as a mother of a disabled child and four non-disabled children becomes complicated when there are occasional conflicts between them, as in the following situations.

One afternoon, Ninette picked up a hairbrush on top of the dining table. Without apparent provocation, she hit it against the edge of the table and it broke. Nerissa, her elder sister, upon learning about the incident, came out of her room in anger, screaming at Ninette: "There you are again. All that you do in this house is to destroy things. Look at what you did to my hairbrush." As expected, Ninette cried and went into a tantrum.

At this point, I remained as an observer. I could not say anything but, in my mind, I was working on something. After a few minutes, both children in the situation returned to normal. Purposely, I allowed Nerissa to release her anger without intervening, as is always true in many other situations so long as she does not inflict physical harm. A little later, I invited Nerissa into my room for a talk. I tried very hard to gain my composure, to be able to convey my message without distortion. As I look at her face, she appeared to be waiting for a reprimand, so I said:

"Nerissa, I wonder if you remember what I explained to you and your brothers about Ninette's condition? She is a person whose mental functioning may not be appropriate to her age, and her judgement may be impaired, so much so, that she is not capable of making accurate judgement of what is right or wrong. Also, she may have limited ability to understand the meaning of things in the world around her. Therefore, it is possible that she may respond to things in a destructive way, as in the way she handled your hairbrush this afternoon. But, to her, it could be her way of discovering about things in her environment. I suppose yourr hairbrush attracted her. She picked it up, but she simply didn't know what to do with it. She struck it against the table and it broke, perhaps without even intending to break it.

"On second thought, I think that if your hairbrush had been kept in a safe place, perhaps Ninette could not have broken it.

"Nerissa, I hope you don't mind, but we must remind ourselves that Ninette needs help from everyone of us. This is one situation where she needs your understanding of her limitations. Maybe her actions could be taken to mean a cry for help. No one else outside of this home could possibly give her the caring and understanding she needs so badly."

I paused for a few minutes waiting for her to talk, and then she said in a low voice: "Mother, I'm sorry. (I noticed her teary eyes.) Sometimes, I forget that Ninette cannot yet understand the many things she does. Many times I hate myself for doing the things I do, like this afternoon. But, why is it like that? Sometimes I can't control myself."

Another afternoon, Ninette came into the room where Nerissa was fixing a little gift for a friend's birthday. Beside her was a pink ribbon, lying peacefully and waiting to be picked up when, all too quickly without any warning, Ninette snapped it from the table. Of course, upon realizing it, Nerissa ran after her almost shouting desperately: "Ninette, please! Don't crumple my ribbon! Give it back to me! Give it back to me, please!" But Ninette held on tightly as she ran around the room in a circle, almost tickled with laughter and enjoying every minute of the chase. Finally, Nerissa caught up with her and grappled hard with her to get back the ribbon, but it was ruined.

At this point, Nerissa, who was boiling with anger and frustration, had to let go her emotion. She grabbed Ninette's hand and spanked her palm three times, at the same time admonishing her. Ninette cried in confusion. All the fun and excitement had turned into unexpected punishment.

After witnessing this, I remained calm and quiet where I stood. I gave Nerissa an emphatic look to convey to her that I understood how she felt. At the same time, I wanted to communicate to her the question in my mind: "Can you really blame Ninette for what she did?" Inside me, I felt a mixed emotion of pity and at the same time, disappointment in how she had handled Ninette. I had convinced myself that, considering the previous incident, Nerissa could have very well understood Ninette's limitations and that should have been enough explanation for her. But, I knew that her anger and frustration were real and had to be released. Still, my main concern was how I could help her see the ways to prevent similar incidents in the future.

I had an appointment at four o'clock that afternoon. I left without saying a word to her about the incident, but I said that I will be back in 30 minutes. On my way home, later, I felt a little better. As I entered the house, I noticed a note for me, folded nicely on top of my notebook. I opened it and it read:

Dear Nanay (Mother),

I am sorry for what I did to Ninette this afternoon. I know, I was wrong. Again, I was not able to control myself. I felt bad and angry.

Nanay, I'm sorry! I'll try not to do it again.

Love,
Riza.

Aware of the stereotyped reactions and attitudes of people in general toward the disabled, I felt I had to protect Ninette from any unnecessary traumatic experience in her relations with other people. I thought that if I talked about Ninette and her condition with friends and relatives before she was exposed to them, this would probably lessen the need for them to whisper to each other (which I do not like Ninette to see) or stare at her with surprise or indifference. At first, it was difficult to do, but through repeated experience I got used to it. As I anticipated, now, the moment they see Ninette with me, they greet her with a smile or by calling her name, which creates an atmosphere of acceptance and warmth. And Ninette enjoys all these encounters with others.

Ninette is now 5 years old. I am happy to say that she is a "bundle of joy" to the family who allowed her to grow to what she now is – a sweet, lovable and beautiful person. I am proud to be her mother, and I would say this a million times over and over again. I have come to realize too that in the process of parenting a disabled child, I have discovered abilities and creativity that I was not aware that I had. These I owe to Ninette.

In closing, I wish that each and everyone of you participants and guests in this Pre-Congress Seminar, being specialists in your own right, are part of that breed of professionals who are capable and willing to play the role as agents of change, with parents as partners, in developing new desirable attitudes towards disabled persons. More power to you!

RN, MSN, M.Ed. Special Education

CHESTER M. PIERCE, M.D. (U.S.A.)

RESPONSE TO THE SEMINAR ON THE DISABLED

Words are a handicap in attempting to convey my thanks and appreciation at being able to participate in this conference. With all the participants, I extend my compliments to our hosts and salute them for their generous hospitality and matchless arrangements. Their abundant efficiency and dedication will be remembered. In addition to these riches, we have been rewarded by the unforgettable magnificence of the scenic splendour at the venue. With all these blessings it is not surprising that the scholarship and enthusiasm of the conference members was able to yield a productivity and fellowship that have been superb.

Such was the depth and breadth of the seminar that a summarization is impossible. Thus, I will try only to submit a portion of what I distilled at the conference. From this distillate, filtered through my personal and professional background, will come some modest suggestions in the service of our aim to improve attitudes about the handicapped and disabled. Like everyone else, I wrestled with insoluble definitional problems such as the meaning and usefulness of the word handicapped and disabled. I vacillated between focussing on the physically and mentally handicapped and I wandered between the covertly and overtly disabled. Often, I was unsure of whether we should be pursuing a discussion of tactics or strategy.

However, I concluded that, at the minimum, both the structure and substance of the seminar demanded that I examine an equation. On one side was the moving material presented so honestly by the panelists who were themselves disabled or a parent of a disabled individual. On the other side of the equation were the multi-disciplinary and multi-national insights provided by professional providers of service. Yet all this was superstructure to the sobering insistence our keynoter provided when we were told that we all are close to disabled people and even more, that we all are more or less disabled, at any given time. But mostly we were reminded that all of us are potentially more fully disabled.

Personal Response:

Therefore, I will begin my observations on the personal side of the equation, then proceed to some comments from the professional side. Moreover, I will give a few brief suggestions.

My overwhelming personal response was to compare the plight of the disabled and handicapped to that of being a Black American. In both instances, general society acts as an oppressor and victimizer. In both instances, the fundamental negotiation that must be made is to accept the reality of the awfulness of one's situation. This helps to sustain one against the hostile, harsh and unforgiving actuality as it is encountered daily. The victim never knows whether he is being

Richard C. Nann, Dorcas Susan Butt, and Lourdes Ladrido-Ignacio (eds.), Mental Health, Cultural Values and Social Development, 321–325.

tolerated or accepted. The victim cannot be certain that he or she is being regarded in terms of what is visible or in terms of more intrinsic, non-stereotyped aspects of his or her own person.

As I listened to the panelists, it seemed that, like Black Americans, they are burdened by something which they can never change. Others almost always will respond to them as if they are inferior and without civil or human rights. Almost always too, no matter how much or how little they achieve, they must work much harder and much longer and against more barriers for less reward. Victims can expect that they will be forced into dependency in all interactions. They will be condescended to, patronized, and either totally ignored or surveyed with more negative and punitive intensity.

In both instances, the oppressed will have interactions initiated toward them in an insolent, careless, offensive manner. These offensive mechanisms are delivered in the form of subtle, stunning, cumulative microaggressions. A single one would seem harmless and inocuous and could be shrugged off. Yet, we were told that a person in a wheelchair can anticipate people coming to move him without pausing to ask him if he wished to be moved or where he wished to go. When these anticipated interactions go on ruthlessly, each day, countless times, the victim must ask difficult and often unanswerable questions. He or she must ask if it is possible for the victimizer and the victim to be mentally healthy at the same time. Thousands of times in one's life one must ask if one should attempt to break out of an oppressive, offensive interaction or should one accommodate and adjust to the social injustice and inequity.

It is at this juncture that the victim must manage rage and anger. It is here he or she must confront the chief enemy. This enemy is the feeling of helplessness. This helplessness is compounded by the societal insistence that one must be deferential, patient and, above all, grateful for whatever little bit of respect and dignity any victimizer chooses to expend.

In a very real manner, the ingredients for the desired respect the victim wishes is related to feeling worthwhile. That is, one dwells on how much time, energy and effort are given to him by others. The unhappy and quantitatively predictable answer is that any oppressed person has his time, space, energy and freedom of mobility restricted, controlled, ignored, abused and misused by all oppressors. The more one's time, space, energy and mobility are beyond one's command, the more oppressed one must be and the more concerned one must be about being overwhelmed by helplessness.

This formulation of the psychology of the disabled and handicapped offers clinicians sites for engagement. For now we can move to the other side of the equation. How can the general society, as well as the specialist professional, interact with the handicapped/disabled? However the interaction proceeds, all who are human-hearted will demand that the method is under the aegis of respect, dignity and regard for individual sanctity of time, space, energy and mobility.

PROFESSIONAL RESPONSE

Each of our own professional persuasions will affect our reaction to the seminar. In my instance, I distilled the seminar content in terms of my experience as an investigator of how individuals adapt to extreme environments. Such environments include human ajdustment in space or under the sea or on polar deserts.

Let me say at the outset that, in my view, there can be no comparison between the courage and adaptive skill that it takes to be severely handicapped versus that which it takes to be an astronaut or a polar explorer. The person in space or at the South Pole is a volunteer. He or she elected to go to the situation. Society provides virtually limitless resources for highly trained, highly selected companions for him- or herself. Usually, there is a known time limit, which the individual knows must be traversed. One knows too, that should one have trouble, immense efforts would be launched to effect rescue. Further, upon return to the society handsome rewards may be waiting.

Of course, in the case of the disabled, there are slender resources, no mode of escape and no reward. In fact there is never-ending debt (emotionally and, perhaps, financially), and incessant worry and grief about why one was chosen for such a wretched lot.

My next point is that both the disabled and the spaceman are stressed. Technically, stress is what one perceives of one's situation. It is known that stresseful events, such as breaking an arm or losing a spouse, are easier to overcome than stressful circumstances. A stressful circumstance is something that is ongoing, such as bickering with a family member or getting through each day when one is in abject poverty. So, here too, the comparison is far more favourable for the polar scientist than the disabled. For, in one instance, one is stressed as an event or period of time. In the other instance, one is stressed as a circumstance or for an indefinite period of time.

For those who roam extreme environments, the chief enemy is hopelessness. In order to combat hopelessness, one can delineate components of stress that characterize life in extreme environments. I will list these component parts for they offer sites for prevention, intervention or postvention for inhabitants of extreme environments. From what I have said, you can conclude that I place the disabled in the category of human begins who must adjust to extreme environmental conditions.

The more of each of these component parts of stress that one has, the more one is under stress. Further, the more stress one is under, the more courage one must have to adapt and the more vulnerable one is to being overwhelmed by feelings of hopelessness.

The component parts are: (1) forced socialization; (2) spatial isolation; (3) depression; (4) boredom; (5) monotony; (6) anxiety; (7) panic; (8) information fractionalization; (9) biological dysrhythmia; (10) sociological disrhythmia; (11) time elasticity; (12) noise/silence extremes; (13) inability to escape.

Time does not permit me to elaborate how I heard all these components mentioned in our seminar. However, as an example of an application, let me mention that a ghetto child who is crippled and lives on the fifth floor of a walk-up tenement may perforce have drastically reduced possibilities for personal contacts. He or she is unavailable to the open, general social network, hence is obliged and forced to socialize with a narrow band of individuals. Theory would predict his or her stress could be reduced if ways were found to increase the variety and depth of social contacts.

In general, to ameliorate stress, one finds ways to increase social support, autonomy and decision-making capacity. During the conference, I heard many instances of these suggestions from both sides of the equation. I would add that the model from extreme environments also offers many areas for research and social action. It is in this vein that I would turn now to some suggestions.

SUGGESTIONS

After such a stimulating seminar, it is our duty to marshall our efforts to make some improvements. Rather than lofty, unobtainable goals, I will try to institute modest changes where I can do so. For instance, I can use the lessons learned here to improve the teaching I do by including more sensitization and information about the handicapped and disabled. I can continue as a private citizen to support and endorse the sort of reforms we have heard recited.

Then, in the relevant national organizations with which I am connected, I can advocate on behalf of the disabled. For this I may call upon you to help me. For the more groundswell that can be achieved, the more likely there will be positive reform.

In American psychiatry thirty years ago, one could be certified as a specialist without ever seeing a child patient. It was later decided by relevant authoritative bodies that, henceforth, every psychiatrist must have some experience with children. This fiat helped change medical education, service and research as well as the organization of the specialty of psychiatry in the U.S.A. For it meant teaching departments had to serve an under-aged population. It meant more knowledge had to be found and shared. It led to the guarantee of minimal standards and exposure in undergraduate education. It helped lead to different attitudes and expectations about psychiatry from the general public.

Simply put, I would like for all of us to seek in our relevant national organizations and disciplines, to be sure that they have considered such sort of "legislative" efforts. In most cases, the idea may not be contested. Yet, in many instances, mass problems such as financing, curriculum time, and deployment of manpower may complicate the immediate enactment of such "legislations". I will pledge to try to get a fiat discussed by the relevant bodies in the U.S.A. In fact, I will attempt, too, to get such a discussion initiated in other English-speaking countries which have credentialling and certifying bodies.

If these several bodies have interest and/or need, I may need direct assistance, information and support from many of you. Similarly, if any of you choose to undertake initiatives where I could be of any assistance I request you to call upon me.

Finally, I would say that I distilled one more aspect that I would like to present to you. Over and over I heard the plea for emphasizing strengths rather than weaknesses in the disabled. This leads me to reinforce that perhaps the best and most important clinical research direction is to learn more about how people *do* survive and how they employ different strengths when they live each day, each hour with an unsung but highly admirable, if generally unrecognized, heroism.

Thank you for instructing me so abundantly in these past few days. I hope that participants of the World Congress in a decade will be amazed at how crude, unimaginative and simple our approach was this weekend. By that measure, we will have made monumental progress.

U.S.A.

JULITA C. BENEDICTO (Philippines)

SUMMARY REMARKS

During the observance of the Third National Disability and Rehabilitation Week, many activities were organized, with many people participating. Old and new methods for improving the conditions of the handicapped were presented through forums, programs, projects, and activities. Aside from the lead programs of the National Commission Concerning Disabled Persons (NCCDP) and the International Year of Disabled Persons (IYDP) Secretariat, numerous rehabilitation agencies, public and private launched projects. These activities, when put together, formed a kind of a festival, and I am sure that the different modes of celebration – music, competitions, exhibits, awards, conferences, fairs, and actual projects – will have a beneficial and lasting effect.

This year's theme, the "Disabled As True Partners in Nation-Building", supports the IYDP theme, "Full Participation and Equality". What we tried to emphasize was that improving the plight of the handicapped would allow them to be active citizens, working rather than worked for, serving (as equals) rather than served, participating rather than just passive receivers of benefits. The fact is that the handicapped themselves have shown no need for charity – they only need opportunities which unfortunately for them, are not plentiful because of the many factors that we in the movement have been trying to eliminate – such as prejudice and consequent unemployment. If, after this week, things do not turn out as expected, we can only conclude that we have a lot more to do.

We have also discovered that, in some areas, people have been responsive, creating potential for greater breakthrough. One thing is certain – many people from different walks of life are sincerely interested in assisting the handicapped to be independent, productive and self-reliant. We hope that our efforts, like Longfellow's arrow, will find their way into more people's hearts because good ideas will always flower into activities and benefit more and more people.

Ladies and gentlemen, mental health, because it strikes at the root of health, occupies a most important place in our lives. Mental health makes for a pleasurable existence, and what else have we all been working for but to create a worthwhile social symbiosis amongst us all? In tackling this problem, therefore, this Pre-Congress Seminar underscores that, as a part of the disability prevention and rehabilitation strategies, projects assigned to make everybody as mentally healthy as possible should be a prime concern. Therefore, from the stage of prevention through to crisis and rehabilitation we should, as you have emphasized here, pool our resources.

It is fitting that this Seminar has considered a wide scope of participation involving representations from the family, the service providers, the business community, the disabled persons, the educational and cultural field, the media,

Richard C. Nann, Dorcas Susan Butt, and Lourdes Ladrido-Ignacio (eds.), Mental Health, Cultural Values and Social Development, 327–328.

the environmental accessibility field, the recreation-leisure field, the legislative field, and the church. Few problems have taken a deeper hold on our lives than disability, since it chooses no special place and persons, and involves each and everyone everywhere. Yet, no problem has met with so much prejudice, disinterest and passive concern than disability, a fact which has been an error of many generations and has been given world-wide attention only recently through congresses, international conventions, and observances like the International Year of Disabled Persons.

On July 27th, the Congress will discuss the subject of disability – its prevention and rehabilitation – more elaborately. I hope that, while you discuss it against the backdrop of the Congress theme, you will also keep in mind the theme of the International Year of Disabled Persons, "Full Participation and Equality". For rehabilitation alone is not the end of our efforts, it is rather that the rehabilitated individual be our partner in building society. There are about 450 million disabled all over the world. A great many of them are independent and self-reliant. The rest need our assistance.

Philippines

Min. JESUS C. AZURIN

1981 World Congress CLOSING RMARKS

I am deeply honoured by this privilege of addressing the distinguished delegates of the World Congress on Mental Health. The international character of this Congress signifies the prevalent global concern on diverse issues that have important bearing on mental health and mental illness. As such, we are happy that the Philippines had been selected as the venue for this Congress.

For a developing society, the improvement of health of the population is not only an end but is also an essential means to attain its social and economic goals. Thus it is imperative that the health effort should be directed by clearly perceived aims and geared toward the attainment of national objectives. Health needs will be based therefore on an overview of the state of health of the country at specific time periods. The health status of the Republic of the Philippines is reflected in the following health indicators –

The population of the country will be 50.4 million by the year 1982; will increase to 70 million by the year 2000. The population growth will be reduced from 2.28% to 2.1% by 1985.

One of the health indicators is the life span which has increased from 50 years in 1972 to 63 years today.

The crude death rate continues to decline from 15/1000 to an expected 6/1000 in the year 2000.

Infant deaths will continue to decrease. By 1982 infant deaths will decrease from 54.1 to 50.0 deaths per 1000 live births.

Communicable diseases will still be a problem by the year 2000 but emphasis shall shift from communicable to non-communicable diseases by year 1985 due to an intensive communicable disease control program.

Cardiovascular degenerative diseases and other stress-induced diseases will increase as health problems between the years 1981 – 2000.

Water supply and waste disposal will continue to be a problem due to an increased population.

Pollution will worsen due to industrialization.

These indicators show that the country has today a level of health status that is favourably comparable to that of developing countries.

Mental ill-health to date remains a topic that is not so well understood, where there are still prevailing dark areas of ignorance. In any country, I believe mental illness is still an unsolved problem. The mental patient continues to be rejected and feared even by his own relatives and friends. This Congress then represents a significant step in our common efforts to continuously understand the disease and to search for innovative approaches and strategies for improving health and the quality of life of our people.

Richard C. Nann, Dorcas Susan Butt, and Lourdes Ladrido-Ignacio (eds.), Mental Health, Cultural Values and Social Development, 329–330.

While we are aware that mental health problems are recognized around the world as a part of public health, still, mental health programs especially in underdeveloped and developing countries have not received priority attention because communicable and infectious diseases, nutrition and family planning continue to require urgent attention.

Mental health programs comprise a part of the health care delivery system of our Ministry. A variety of services has been instituted, the majority of which are located in urban and sub-urban centres. These include a wide range of traditional psychiatric services in mental hospitals, psychiatric units in general and regional hospitals, out-patient psychiatric services in general hospitals and mental hygiene clinics.

Another component of our mental health program is the training of our field health workers as they integrate mental health activities at the primary care level.

While the Ministry of Health is the lead agency in all aspects of health, it cannot work effectively in isolation. The involvement of other ministries and of the private sector are vital to ensure a viable and multi-sectoral approach in the management of relevant health and mental health concerns. Hence, it becomes imperative that a national co-ordinating group in mental health be established. This group shall be responsible for assessing mental health needs, priorities for action, and plans for implementation. Hopefully, in this country a national co-ordinating group will be organized within this year.

The Philippine Mental Health Association, your host for this Congress, has been the Ministry's consistent partner in providing mental health services to our people. Together, we are fully committed to the Filipino people for a strong mental health program.

I should like to convey to each and every delegate our deep appreciation for taking time from their busy schedules in their own countries to come to the Philippines to discuss and share their expertise on the various critical issues confronting our world today. I hope that there will be a continuing exchange of information between participating countries even after this Congress, so that we may achieve our common goals for mental health.

Let me take this opportunity to commend and congratulate the Philippine Mental Health Association and the World Federation for Mental Health for the very successful conduct of this affair.

Thank you.

Ministry of Health,
The Philippines

EUGENE B. BRODY, M.D., President 1981–1983

WFMH: AN AGENDA FOR THE 1980'S

Now into its fourth decade this Federation has had its ups and downs in growth rate and effectiveness during the past 33 years. However, our goals and ideals have been remarkably consistent. It is to these, and to ways of implementing them in the 1980's, that I now address myself.

As we consider an agenda for the '80s, we look back to the ideals of our predecessors. These were initially the members of the United States National Committee for Mental Hygiene which organized the first International Congress of Mental Health – a courageous and pioneering act in itself. This Congress drew 4,000 people – volunteers, professionals, clinicians, behavioural scientists, planners and administrators – to Washington, D.C. in 1930. They were the first to embrace an ideal of global mental health and they organized the International Committee for Mental Hygiene, representing 29 countries. In 1930, it was their hope that an international ideal of mental health might draw the disparate peoples of the world together in pursuit of peace and a better life.

Today, half a century and several wars later, aware of continuing poverty and political oppression, we are less sanguine about "mental health", narrowly defined, as a rallying slogan. We remain committed, however, to the ideal of collaboration between individual citizens of good will, and between non-governmental organizations across political, social and cultural boundaries. We remain convinced because our interest, our investment, in the long-run is with individual human beings, human feelings and human lives. Social organizations, institutions and governments have powerful advocates and constituencies. Persons, however – the self-aware individuals who actually experience the anguish of loneliness, illness, injury and loss of liberty – have few advocates and we count ourselves among them.

ADVOCACY ROLE

In its narrowest perspective, our commitment is to the lives and well-being of the socially deprived, disenfranchised, chronic, mental hospital patients and their families. Our traditional role is to be their advocate and constituency, and our agenda for the '80s must always take them into account.

The Federation's broader goal and ideal reaches beyond the individual to confront the problems of communities and social organizations. This goal reminds us that despite the efforts of mental health volunteers and professionals to deal with people already sick, the flood of social system casualties continues to overwhelm existing services. There is no way in which we can excuse a lack of concern with social systems by saying that our responsibilities are more narrowly

Richard C. Nann, Dorcas Susan Butt, and Lourdes Ladrido-Ignacio (eds.), Mental Health, Cultural Values and Social Development, 331–335.

defined. This Manila Congress has underscored the importance of promoting social and familial conditions that make for optimal growth and development, an optimal quality of life, and the continued possibility of persons to realize their latent potentials.

WORLD NETWORK EMERGES

In an effort to translate these ideals into action, a second International Mental Health Congress in Paris in 1937 moved in this direction by strengthening a worldwide network of concerned citizens and by disseminating information which might be used as the basis for local action. Plans for a third world congress, however, were interrupted by World War II.

It was not until 1946 that a preparatory commission for the third congress, scheduled for London in 1948, laid the groundwork for a new organization which was to become the World Federation for Mental Health. Its members envisioned a Federation which would not confine its activities to periodic congresses, but would be a continuing force for mental health throughout the world. The commission included people from many countries with a wide range of backgrounds. Its work was based, in part, on a suggestion which had already been made by UNESCO: that a thoroughly interprofessional and completely international body representing voluntary and non-governmental services in the mental health field was needed to co-operate with UN agencies. These last included WHO which, still in the planning stage, did not become a formal entity until 1949.

A major operating modality of WFMH, thus, became its relationship with the United Nations and its relevant health and welfare agencies, specifically WHO, the International Labour Organization, the Economic and Social Council, UNICEF and UNESCO. WFMH began auspiciously, as the International Preparatory Commission's (IPC) recommendation was among those at the World Health Assembly in which the WHO mental health section was brought into being. This relationship between WFMH and the UN has continued and we are still the unique non-governmental organization with consulting status in mental health to the United Nations. Ways of enhancing the effectiveness of this relationship, especially in regard to WHO, have been on our agenda for some time, and remain high on our list.

WFMH PROBLEMS NOT YET SOLVED

In 1946 the members of the IPC also produced a document called Mental Health and World Citizenship. The name alone implies a basic relationship between the existence of individual human rights expressed through social organizations, and mental health – not so much the absence of illness as well-being and optimal function. It reminds us of a fundamental issue repeatedly faced but never totally resolved by our Federation. That is, how to maintain our vital stand in favour of individual rights and human dignity while at the same time retaining a focus on particular projects, necessarily discrete, which can be completed and in their cumulative impact further the cause of human rights and the quality of individual life.

A number of such issues have been on previous agendas, especially in the years between 1948 and 1966 under the executive directorship of the distinguished British psychiatrist, Jack Rees, through whom WFMH achieved much of its international stature. These have included problems of racial prejudice and discrimination; of migration, especially the involuntary migration of those uprooted by war and political oppression; of community development, especially as it is influenced by urbanization and technical change; and of the life cycle, especially in terms of early mother-infant interaction, child-rearing and old age.

TWO MAIN PROBLEMS

As I consider the basic mental health issues of this decade, aside from those fundamental ones dealing with defined mental patients, two general groups of problems come to mind.

Minority Status

A minority is a group of people distant from the sources of societal power. They have no voice in the great decisions which affect their own destinies. Minorities are most typically defined on the basis of race, ethnic or religious status. However, they may be migrants, newcomers into old communities. Or they may be defined on other bases. Age is one of these. The elderly comprise a minority which is just becoming self-aware and militant. Gender is one. Women are still disadvantaged members of patriarchal societies in a great many countries of the world. The physically handicapped are a minority which, in the United States, has just begun to wield political power. The chronic mentally ill are a minority which still depends on others to speak for them. In many regions endemic poverty has shaped successive generations into a permanent minority or underclass. Many in numbers, they remain undereducated, underemployed and excluded from the cultural mainstream of those who control their society. A newly identified minority includes victims of violence, particularly politically inspired by violence. This has already been the topic of joint work between WFMH, Princeton University's Woodrow Wilson School of Foreign Affairs and the US National Institute of Mental Health.

A salient feature of being a member of a minority is that one is placed at a disadvantage through no fault of one's own. Discrimination, prejudice, and exclusion from opportunity are suffered because one happens to belong to a socially visible category of people. These inflicted wounds have in common the fact that they are dehumanizing. When a person is treated in a particular way because of a category to which he or she happens to belong, this constitutes a denial of one's unique past history and the individuality shaped by it, and of the reflective self-awareness crucial to being human. Those who suffer dehumanizing treatment have a special claim upon a Federation committed to the welfare of persons. For this reason, if for no other, the mental health problems associated with minority status will be significant in our agenda for the '80s.

Community Opportunities

The second set of problems associated with a range of mental health impairments overlaps with those of minority status. They are clustered around failures in how communities serve individual human needs. Central are needs for opportunity. I refer particularly to opportunities for those early developmental and educational experiences, and later for jobs and information on the basis of which a person can make choices about his/her own life.

Among the community problems which concern us are lack of leadership, poor communications between people, inadequately developed health and educational institutions, and severe socioeconomic stress which may threaten family stability. WHO is recognizing this as a matrix in which illness and inability to function are frequently encountered. It has, therefore, moved its focus to the area which it calls psychosocial functioning. This involves both attention to social settings, and a new emphasis on primary care carried out by people, who while not trained to the most sophisticated medical levels, are very familiar with the communities in which they work. Social and community development emphasize opportunities for self-determination. These can range from co-operative work endeavours, to adult education programs, to family planning services which give women the knowledge allowing them to make choices about their own fertility.

In June 1981, at the meeting of the Sociedad Interamericana de Psicologia in Santo Domingo, WFMH along with the Pan-American Health Organization of WHO co-sponsored a half-day workshop on "Personal fertility regulation: co-operative research in the Americas". Exploration of avenues for relevant mental health development will continue as part of our agenda. In these and similar efforts we expect the support of various divisions of WHO which have included among their chief priorities the development of primary case services utilizing non-medical personnel.

Without listing other agendae for the '80s, I remind you that these two clusters of problems require the most effective collaboration between members of voluntary and professional mental health associations, and governments. This is the topic of a workshop planned for London in the late spring of 1982.

Finally, I cannot over-emphasize the symbolic and emblematic importance of a worldwide federation of mental health associations – especially one which includes both volunteers and professionals. As the only truly global mental health coalition, one which does not represent only a profession or only a specific group of voluntary agencies, and one which deliberately excludes governments from membership, we have a rare and unique responsibility. Yet, we work with governments if they want our help, as well as with and through the United Nations. Yes, we are concerned with specific issues, and specific populations at-risk, and, thus, we do engage in practical moves and projects. Our very existence and nature, however, have inherent within them a humane obligation to be sensitive to the thinking, feeling, self-aware persons who actually experience health and illness, pain and pleasure.

Our view of social contexts is not that of powerful governments, and institutions concerned with the management of people. It, instead, symbolizes advocacy of the citizen trying to earn a living and raise a family, and participate in the decisions necessary to manage him or herself. These decisions are influenced by the socially inherited rules of culture, the man-made rules of government, and one's place in the socioeconomic hierarchy. From the viewpoint of mental health they may be either conforming, or in the direction of creative change. This is equally true for the patient within the constraints of the mental hospital. It is self-deceiving for us to be concerned with the liberties and opportunities of one and not the other.

WFMH WORK DEFINED

With these considerations in mind, then, I remind you again of the symbolic meaning and significance of our actions as a worldwide federation devoted to the cause and ideal of mental health. We are highly visible and constantly examined as to our goals, where we stand, whose interests we really represent in respect to the integrity and opportunity of individuals and their families. This is true for our public pronouncements, publications, decisions about where to meet, who will be our officers, which projects and groups we choose to support.

I believe that it is only by the most sensitive adherence to our goals and ideals, and the most sensitive awareness of the public meaning of what we do, that we will be able to effectively further the ideal of mental health in this decade of the 1980's. With these considerations in mind, the primary theme for our 1983 World Congress to be held in Washington, D.C., U.S.A. will be "Personal and social responsibility in the search for mental health". The subsidiary theme will be "Collaboration between volunteers, professionals and governments in the formation of mental health policy and the delivery of services". We will be looking for new patterns of collaboration, new alliances, new ideas and ways of doing things. I invite your participation in this collective task.

Department of Psychiatry,
Institute of Psychiatry and Human Behavior,
University of Maryland School of Medicine
645 West Redwood Street,
Baltimore, Maryland,
U.S.A. 21201

INDEX OF NAMES

INDEX OF SUBJECTS